Obstetrics and Gynaecology

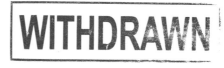

Obstetrics and Gynaecology

Lawrence Impey

BA, MRCOG
Consultant in Obstetrics
and Fetal Medicine,
The John Radcliffe Hospital,
Headington, Oxford

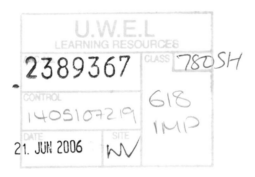
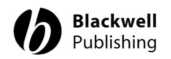
Blackwell
Publishing

© 1999 by Blackwell Science Ltd
© 2004 by Blackwell Publishing Ltd
Blackwell Publishing, Inc., 350 Main Street, Malden,
Massachusetts 02148-5020, USA
Blackwell Publishing Ltd, 9600 Garsington Road, Oxford OX4
2DQ, UK
Blackwell Publishing Asia Pty Ltd, 550 Swanston Street,
Carlton, Victoria 3053, Australia

First published 1999
Reprinted 2000, 2001, 2002, 2003
Second edition 2004
Reprinted 2005

ISBN 10: 1-4051-0721-9
ISBN 13: 978-1-4051-0721-1

A catalogue record for this title is available from the British
Library

Library of Congress Cataloging-in-Publication Data
Impey, Lawrence.
    Obstetrics and gynaecology / Lawrence Impey.– 2nd ed.
    p. ; cm.
Includes bibliographical references and index.
    ISBN 1-4051-0721-9
    1. Gynecology–Outlines, syllabi, etc.
2. Obstetrics–Outlines, syllabi, etc.   [DNLM:
1. Pregnancy–Outlines.   2. Genital Diseases,
Female–Outlines.   3. Pregnancy Complications–Outlines.
WQ 18.2 I340 2003]   I. Title.
    RG101.I47 2003
    618′.02′02-dc22

                                              2003026247

Set in 9½/11.5 pt Minion by
SNP Best-set Typesetter Ltd., Hong Kong
Printed and bound in Italy by G. Canale & C. SpA, Turin

Production Editor: Rebecca Huxley
Commissioning Editor: Fiona Goodgame
Managing Editor: Geraldine Jeffers
Production Controller: Mirjana Misina

For further information on Blackwell Publishing, visit our
website:
http://www.blackwellpublishing.com

Contents

Preface to the Second Edition

Second editions always seem to be longer than the first, probably because it is easier to put more in than take things out. I have tried not to do this. Because the layout and conciseness seemed to work well, the structure of this book has been changed little. However, things change fast in medicine and I have brought the book right up to date, and made it more 'evidence-based', including Cochrane references wherever possible. The reading lists have also been expanded. Feedback has come from many sources, particularly medical students, and has been very helpful. More is always welcome.

Lawrence Impey
2004

Preface to the First Edition

This book is written for the UK medical student, in line with changes in medical education and the advent of the core curriculum. The level of information is enough to allow a high mark in the final obstetrics and gynaecology examinations. But its strong emphasis on management should also be useful for practising doctors and those about to take postgraduate examinations.

As a student and then a lecturer I was always surprised at the deficiencies of many textbooks: how they failed to emphasize what was common or important, how little emphasis they placed on 'what to do' in a real situation, and how little they allowed understanding of the subject. Problem-based learning is in part a backlash against this. Yet there remains a need for a comprehensive yet straightforward textbook. In this, the space given to each topic reflects it importance. Subjects are cross-referenced (page cross-references are indicated by superior square brackets). The information is up to date, evidence-based where possible, and referenced, at least for important, new or contentious issues. At the end of each chapter, summaries of all the major topics should aid revision and prevent the need for a separate revision text. At the end of the book, separate management sections describe what to do in all the common clinical situations, from the management of slow progress in labour to the management of the subfertile couple.

Lawrence Impey
1999

Acknowledgements

I am grateful to the many friends and colleagues in the UK and Ireland who have made criticisms in their areas of expertise and have helped with the preparation of this book. These are Mr Mike Bowen, Dr Bill Boyd, Dr Bridgette Byrne, Dr Paul Dewart, Dr Valerie Donnelly, Dr Anne Edwards, Dr Michael Foley, Miss Michelle Fynes, Mr Mike Gillmer, Dr Jonathan Hobson, Mr James Hopkisson, Miss Pauline Hurley, Mr Simon Jackson, Dr Catherine James, Dr Declan Keane, Mr Stephen Kennedy, Dr Peter Lenehan, Dr Graham Lloyd-Jones, Dr Graz Luzzi, Dr Dermott MacDonald, Dr Pamela MacKinnon, Dr Peter McParland, Mr Enda McVeigh, Miss Kathryn MacQuillan, Dr Jane Mellanby, Dr Breda O'Kelly, Miss Meghana Pandit, Dr John Picard, Miss Charlotte Porter, Professor Chris Redman, Miss Margaret Rees, Dr Robin Russell, Miss Susan Sellers, Dr Sarah Sheikh, Dr Orla Sheil, Mr Alexander Smarason, Professor Philip Steer and Dr Mary Wingfield. I am indebted to Blackwell Science, particularly Ms Rebecca Huxley, Dr Andrew Robinson and Dr Michael Stein for their faith, help and encouragement, and to the medical students of The Royal College of surgeons in Ireland and of Oxford University for their criticisms. And I am particularly grateful to Ms Jane Fallows for her illustrations. Most of all, however, I thank Susan and Cicely Impey for their support and patience during the writing of this book.

Acknowledgements for the second edition

In addition to those who helped with the first edition, I am very grateful to Dr Patricia Boyd, Miss Kirsten Duckitt, Ms Jane Fallows, Miss Catherine Greenwood, Ms Rebecca Huxley, Miss Cicely Impey, Mr Simon Jackson, Professor Sean Kehoe, Mr Stephen Kennedy, Dr Gillian Lockwood, Dr Graz Luzzi, Dr Nicky Manning, Mr Enda McVeigh, Ms Sally Newman, Miss Meghana Pandit, Professor Chris Redman, Miss Margaret Rees, Miss Susan Sellers, Miss Geraldine Tasker and Mr Danny Tucker for their help and advice.

L.I.

List of Abbreviations

ACE	angiotensin-converting enzyme
ACTH	adrenocorticotrophic hormone
ADH	antidiuretic hormone
AFP	alpha fetoprotein
AIDS	acquired immune deficiency syndrome
AP	antero-posterior
APH	antepartum haemorrhage
ARDS	adult respiratory distress syndrome
ARM	artificial rupture of membranes
BCG	Bacille bilié de Calmette-Guérin
BP	blood pressure
BNA	borderline nuclear abnormalities
BSO	bilateral salpingo-oöphorectomy
BV	bacterial vaginosis
CA	carcinoma/cancer antigen
CGIN	cervical glandular intraepithelial neoplasia
CIN	cervical intraepithelial neoplasia
CMV	cytomegalovirus
CNS	central nervous system
CNST	Clinical Negligence Scheme for Trusts
CO_2	carbon dioxide
COC	combined oral contraceptive
CPR	cardiopulmonary resuscitation
CRP	C-reactive protein
CSF	cerebrospinal fluid
CT	computed tomography/graph
CTG	cardiotocography/graph
CVA	cerebrovascular accident
CVP	central venous pressure
CVS	chorionic villus sampling
CXR	chest X-ray
D&C	dilatation and curettage
DCDA	dichorionic diamniotic
DI	detrusor instability/donor insemination
DIC	disseminated intravascular coagulation
DNA	deoxyribonucleic acid

DoH	Department of Health
DVT	deep vein thrombosis
DXA	dual-energy X-ray absorptiometry
DZ	dizygotic
ECG	electrocardiogram/graph
ECV	external cephalic version
EDD	expected day of delivery
ELISA	enzyme-linked immunosorbent assay
ERPC	evacuation of retained products of conception
EUA	examination under anaesthetic
FBC	full blood count
FBS	fetal blood sampling
FFP	fresh frozen plasma
FHR	fetal heart rate
FIGO	International Federation of Gynaecology and Obstetrics
FISH	fluorescence *in situ* hybridization
FSH	follicle-stimulating hormone
G&S	'group and save'
GFR	glomerular filtration rate
GI	gastrointestinal
GIFT	gamete intrafallopian transfer
GnRH	gonadotrophin-releasing hormone
GSI	genuine stress incontinence
Hb	haemoglobin
HCG	human chorionic gonadotrophin
β-HCG	human chorionic gonadotrophin beta-subunit
HELLP	haemolysis, elevated liver enzymes and low platelet count
HFEA	Human Fertilization and Embryology Authority
HIV	human immunodeficiency virus
HPV	human papilloma virus

HRT	hormone replacement therapy		OA	occipito-anterior
HSV	herpes simplex virus		OP	occipito-posterior
HVS	high vaginal swab		OT	occipito-transverse
IA	intermittent auscultation		PAPPA	pregnancy-associated plasma protein A
IBS	irritable bowel syndrome		PCA	patient-controlled analgesia
ICSI	intracytoplasmic sperm injection		PCB	postcoital bleeding
i.m.	intramuscularly		PCO	polycystic ovary
IMB	intermenstrual bleeding		PCOS	polycystic ovary syndrome
IUD	intrauterine device		PCR	polymerase chain reaction
IUGR	intrauterine growth restriction		PE	pulmonary embolus
IUI	intrauterine insemination		PGD	preimplantation genetic diagnosis
IUS	intrauterine system		PGE_2	prostaglandin E_2
i.v.	intravenous		$PGF_{2\alpha}$	prostaglandin $F_{2\alpha}$
IVF	*in vitro* fertilization		PI	Pearl index
IVP	intravenous pyelogram		PID	pelvic inflammatory disease
			PLDH	pegylated liposomal doxorubicin hydrochloride
KCl	potassium chlorine		PM	postmortem
KOH	potassium hydroxide		PMB	postmenopausal bleeding
			PMS	premenstrual syndrome
LFT	liver function test		PPH	postpartum haemorrhage
LH	luteinizing hormone/laparoscopic hysterectomy		PRL	prolactin
LLETZ	large loop excision of transformation zone		PSV	peak systolic velocity
LMP	last menstrual period		PV	per vaginum
LMWH	low-molecular-weight heparin			
LN	lymph node		RCOG	Royal College of Obstetricians and Gynaecologists
LSCS	lower segment Caesarean section		Rh	rhesus
LUNA	laser uterosacral nerve ablation			
			SBR	serum bilirubin
MC&S	Microscopy, culture and sensitivity		SERM	selective oestrogen receptor modulator
MCA	middle cerebral artery		SFD	small for dates
MCDA	monochorionic diamniotic		SHBG	sex hormone-binding globulin
MCHC	mean cell haemoglobin concentration		SIDS	sudden infant death syndrome
MCMA	monochorionic monoamniotic		SLE	systemic lupus erythematosus
MCV	mean cell volume		SSRI	selective serotonin reuptake inhibitor
MESA	microsurgical epididymal sperm aspiration		SROM	spontaneous rupture of membranes
MRI	magnetic resonance imaging		STI	sexually transmitted infection
MSU	mid-stream urine			
MZ	monozygotic		TAH	total abdominal hysterectomy
			TB	tuberculosis
NAAT	nucleic acid amplification test		TEDS	thromboembolic disease stocking
NHS	National Health Service		TENS	transcutaneous electrical nerve stimulation
NICE	National Institute for Clinical Excellence		TESA	testicular sperm aspiration
NSAID	non-steroidal anti-inflammatory drug		TFT	thyroid function test
NTD	neural tube defect		TOP	termination of pregnancy
NVP	nausea and vomiting of pregnancy		TSH	thyroid-stimulating hormone
			TV	trichomoniasis

TVS	transvaginal sonography	VDRL	Venereal Disease Research Laboratories
TVT	tension-free vaginal tape	VE	vaginal examination
		VH	vaginal hysterectomy
UA	umbilical artery	VIN	vulvar intraepithelial neoplasia
U&E	urea and electrolytes	VMA	vanillylmandelic acid
USS	ultrasound scan		
UTI	urinary tract infection	WBC	white blood cell count

List of Journal Abbreviations

Acta Psychiatr Scand	Acta Psychiatrica Scandinavica
AmJOG	American Journal of Obstetrics and Gynecology
Ann Intern Med	Annals of Internal Medicine
Ann Neurol	Annals of Neurology
BMJ	BMJ (Clinical Research Ed.)
BJOG	BJOG: an International Journal of Obstetrics and Gynaecology [2000+]; British Journal of Obsterics and Gynaecology [1975–1999]
Clin Obstet Gynecol	Clinical Obstetrics and Gynecology
Cochrane	Cochrane Database System Review (Online: Update Software)
Drug Saf	Drug Safety: an International Journal of Medical Toxicology and Drug Experience
Eur J Obstet Gynecol Reprod Biol	European Journal of Obstetrics, Gynecology, and Reproductive Biology
Fertil Steril	Fertility and Sterility
Gynecol Endocrinol	Gynecological Endocrinology
Hum Reprod	Human Reproduction (Oxford, England)
Infect Dis Obstet Gynecol	Infectious Diseases in Obstetrics and Gynecology
Int J Gynaecol Obstet	International Journal of Gynaecology and Obstetrics
JAMA	JAMA: the Journal of the American Medical Association
J Matern Fetal Neonatal Med	The Journal of Maternal–Fetal & Neonatal Medicine
J Matern Fetal Med	The Journal of Maternal–Fetal Medicine
J Med Genet	Journal of Medical Genetics
J Natl Cancer Inst	Journal of the National Cancer Institute
Minerva Ginecol	Minerva Ginecologica
NEJM	The New England Journal of Medicine
Neurourol Urodyn	Neurourology and Urodynamics
Obstet Gynecol	Obstetrics and Gynecology
Obstet Gynecol Clin North Am	Obstetrics and Gynecology Clinics of North America
Prenat Diagn	Prenatal Diagnosis
Ultrasound Obstet Gynecol	Ultrasound in Obstetrics & Gynecology

Gynaecology Section

1 The History and Examination in Gynaecology

The remit of the doctor is to improve quality of life, not just to treat life-threatening disease: if a symptom is causing distress, treatment should be considered. The type and extent of treatment is determined largely by the patient: the doctor gives information and advice, so the patient can give her *informed* consent. The patient's history should be used not only to help make a diagnosis but also to discover how much her symptom(s) is/are affecting her. Or she may simply be concerned as to the cause of her symptoms (e.g. malignancy) and reassurance is enough.

The gynaecological history

Personal details

Ask her name, age and occupation.

Presenting complaint(s)

How long has the problem been present and how much does it affect her? If it is pain, what alleviates and what exacerbates it, where is it and what is its nature? Allow the patient to elaborate as there may be more than one problem, initially without asking direct questions, perhaps asking her to rate her problems in order of severity. Has she ever consulted a doctor about this problem before and, if so, what has been done? If there are multiple presenting complaints, these should be put in order of severity/effect on her life.

Specific gynaecological questions

These are asked next, starting with ones that are relevant to this presenting complaint. For example, if it is a menstrual problem, the most appropriate next questions concern menstruation; if it is a urinary problem, one should ask all the appropriate urinary tract questions next.

Menstrual questions. How often does she menstruate and how long does menstruation last? (4/28 means bleeding lasts for 4 days and occurs every 28 days.) Is it regular or irregular? Is it heavy? (Number of pads/tampons used or the presence of clots can be useful.) Is it or the days leading up to it painful? Is there ever intermenstrual bleeding (IMB) [→ p.10]? Is there ever postcoital bleeding (PCB) [→ p.16]? Is there ever a vaginal discharge and, if so, what is it like? Does she experience premenstrual tension? When was her last menstrual period (LMP)? If postmenopausal, has there been postmenopausal bleeding (PMB)?

Menstrual questions
How often and for how long?
Heavy or painful?
Regularity?
Intermenstrual bleeding (IMB) or postcoital bleeding (PCB)?
When was her last menstrual period (LMP)?

Sexual/contraceptive questions. Is she sexually active? If so, is it painful? If so, is it on penetration (superficial dyspareunia) or deep inside (deep dyspareunia). What contraceptive (if appropriate) does she use and what has she used in the past?

Cervical smear questions. When was her last cervical smear? (This should be done every 3 years.) Has she ever had an abnormal smear? If so, what was done [→ p.29]?

Urinary/prolapse questions. Does she experience frequency, nocturia, urgency or enuresis? Does she ever leak urine? If so, how severe is it and with what is it associated (e.g. coughing or urgency)? Is there ever dysuria or haematuria? Does she ever get a dragging sensation or feel a mass in or at the vagina?

Other history

Past obstetric history: This should be brief. Start with 'Have you ever been pregnant'? If the answer is 'No', go on to past medical history. If 'Yes', ask details about previous pregnancies in chronological order. Of deliveries, ask when, what weight, how was the infant born and how the infant is now. Ask about any major complications in the pregnancy or labour.

Past medical history: First ask about any previous, particularly gynaecological, operations, however distant. Then directly ask about venous thrombosis, diabetes, lung and heart disease, hypertension, jaundice, etc. as in any medical history. If you elicit no significant history, ask 'Have you ever been in hospital'?

Systems review: Ask the usual cardiovascular, respiratory, abdominal and neurological questions.

Drugs: Does she take any regular medication?

Family history: Is there a family history of breast or ovarian carcinoma, of diabetes, venous thromboembolism, heart disease or hypertension?

Personal/social history: Does she smoke? Does she drink alcohol? If either, how much? Is she in a married or stable relationship and, if not, is there support at home? Where does she live and what sort of accommodation is it?

Allergies: Ask specifically about penicillin and latex.

Presenting the history

Start by summing up the important points, including relevant gynaecological questions:
This is . . ., who is a . . . year-old . . . (parity), *with a . . .* (time) *history of . . ., who . . .* (most significant findings in history).

Example: This is Mrs X, who is a 38-year-old nulliparous woman, with a 3-month history of postcoital bleeding (PCB), who has a normal menstrual cycle and last had a cervical smear 7 years ago.

N.B. By mentioning the last smear, you have shown understanding that PCB may be a symptom of cervical carcinoma.

Now go through the history in some detail.

Then sum up again, in one sentence.

Gynaecological history: specific essential questions

Presenting complaint, its history
Menstrual questions: last menstrual period (LMP), cycle, flow, intermenstrual bleeding (IMB), postcoital bleeding (PCB)
Urinary/prolapse questions
Sexual/contraceptive questions
Cervical smear history
Past obstetric history

Other questions

Now ask 'Is there anything else you think I ought to know'? This gives her the opportunity to help you if you have not discovered all the important facts.

Summarizing the history

1 Could the symptoms be a manifestation of underlying disease that needs to be treated? (For example, erratic menstrual bleeding may be a sign of malignancy.)
2 Are the symptoms themselves causing physical damage? (For example, erratic menstrual bleeding may lead to severe anaemia.)
3 Are the symptoms themselves causing distress? (For example, erratic menstrual bleeding may disrupt a woman's life such that she may feel unable to leave the home.) Or is she unconcerned?

The gynaecological examination

General examination

This is to:
1 Seek the effects (e.g. secondary spread of malignancy) or more rarely the causes (e.g. thyroid abnormalities cause menstrual disturbances) of gynaecological problems.
2 Assess general health and incidental disease, particularly if an anaesthetic may be needed.

General appearance and weight, temperature, blood pressure and pulse, and possible anaemia, jaundice or lymphadenopathy should be noted. More detailed examination of the rest of the body is often perfunctory in the young, fit patient, but is important in the older or more sick patient, or in those about to have an anaesthetic.

Breast and axillary examination

This is performed as a screening test for breast cancer (Fig. 1.1). The patient sits back, the breasts are inspected for irregularities and all four breast quadrants are palpated as the patient lies supine with her hands behind her head. The axilla, a principal area for lymph drainage, is then palpated with the patient's arm resting on the examiner's shoulder.

Abdominal examination

The patient lies comfortably on her back with her head on a pillow, discreetly exposed from the xiphisternum to the symphysis pubis. The bladder should be empty.

Inspect
Look for scars, particularly just above the symphysis pubis and in the umbilicus. Look at the distribution of body hair, for irregularities, striae and hernias.

Palpate
Ask about tenderness first, then palpate gently around the abdomen looking for masses or tenderness. Then palpate specifically for masses from above the umbilicus down to the symphysis pubis (Fig. 1.2). If any masses are present, do they arise from the pelvis (i.e. can you get below them)?

Percuss
Go around the abdomen. The bowel is resonant; fluid-filled and solid cavities (e.g. masses, full bladder) are dull (Fig. 1.3). Look for shifting dullness (free fluid).

Auscultate
Listen to the bowel sounds.

Gynaecological examination
General
Breast
Abdomen
Pelvic palpation: digital
Cervical/vaginal inspection: speculum

Vaginal examination

Ensure privacy, explain simply what you intend and ask for the patient's permission. A chaperone must be present, whether you are male or female. Use lubricating jelly. A speculum should be warmed. Internal examination is often uncomfortable, but severe tenderness is abnormal.

Inspect
The vulva and the vaginal orifice are inspected first.

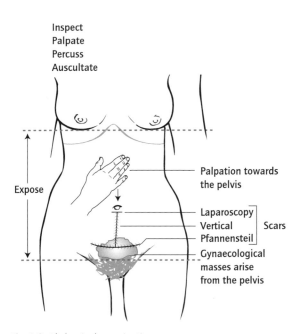

Fig. 1.2 Abdominal examination.

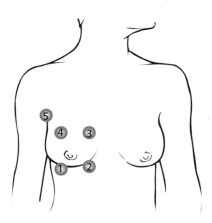

Fig. 1.1 Examination of the breast.

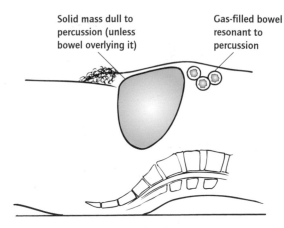

Fig. 1.3 Percussion of the abdomen.

Are there any coloured areas, ulcers or lumps on the vulva? Is a prolapse evident at the introitus? Three types of examination have different purposes.

Digital bimanual examination

This assesses the pelvic organs. The patient lies flat, with her legs apart. The left hand is placed on the abdomen above the symphysis pubis and is pushed down into the pelvis, so that the organs are palpated between it and two fingers are gently inserted into the vagina (Fig. 1.4a,b).

The uterus is normally the size and shape of a small pear. Size, consistency, regularity, mobility, anteversion or retroversion and tenderness are assessed.

The cervix is normally the first part of the uterus to be felt vaginally and the os is felt as an opening like a toy car tyre. Is the cervix hard or irregular?

The adnexa (lateral to the uterus on either side, containing tube and ovary): tenderness and size and consistency of any mass are assessed. Is it separate from the uterus?

The pouch of Douglas (behind the cervix): the uterosacral ligaments should be palpable. Are these even, irregular or tender, or is there a mass?

Cusco's speculum examination

This allows inspection of the cervix and vaginal walls. The patient lies as for the digital examination. With the blades closed and parallel to the labia and the opening mechanism pointing to the patient's right, gently insert the speculum (Fig. 1.5a). Then rotate it 90° and insert it as far as it will go without causing discomfort (Fig. 1.5b).

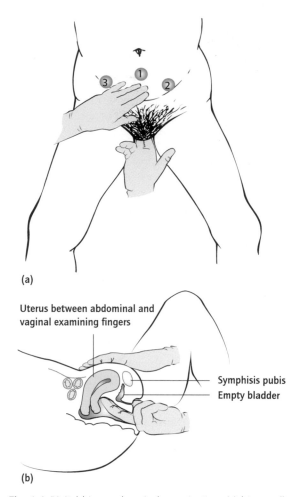

Fig. 1.4 Digital bimanual vaginal examination: (a) bimanually palpate areas 1, 2, 3 in order; (b) digital bimanual palpation of the pelvis.

Open it slowly under direct vision and the cervix will come into view (Fig. 1.5c). Look for ulceration, spontaneous bleeding or irregularities. A cervical smear can be taken. Now slightly withdraw the speculum under direct vision and partly close it without catching the cervix. Slowly withdraw it just open, allowing inspection of the vaginal walls to the introitus, and then close the speculum and remove it.

Sims' speculum

This allows better inspection of the vaginal walls and, specifically, the prolapse. The patient should be positioned in the left lateral position with the legs partly

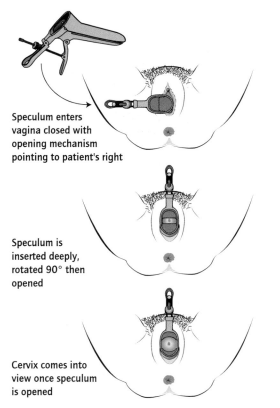

Speculum enters vagina closed with opening mechanism pointing to patient's right

Speculum is inserted deeply, rotated 90° then opened

Cervix comes into view once speculum is opened

Fig. 1.5 Cusco's speculum examination of the cervix and vaginal walls. (a) Speculum enters vagina closed with opening mechanism pointing to patient's right. (b) Speculum inserted deep, rotated 90°, then opened. (c) Cervix comes into view once speculum is opened.

curled up. Insert the curved speculum into the vagina from behind, with one end pressing against the posterior wall to allow inspection of the anterior wall. Then reverse the speculum, pressing back the anterior wall so that the posterior wall can be seen (Fig. 1.6). If the patient is asked to bear down, the prolapse of either wall can be assessed.

Rectal examination

This is occasionally appropriate if there is posterior wall

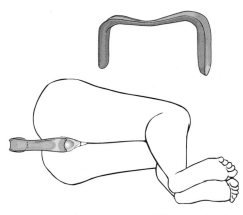

Fig. 1.6 Sims' speculum examination of the vaginal walls.

prolapse, to distinguish between an enterocele and a rectocele, and in assessing malignant cervical disease.

Presenting the examination

Present the examination findings, including relevant positive or negative findings:
Mrs X is . . . (describe general appearance sensitively), *her blood pressure, temperature and pulse are . . . and abdominal and pelvic examination reveals . . .. There is . . .* (mention important positive and negative findings).

Example: Mrs X looks thin and clinically anaemic, her blood pressure is 120/60, temperature is normal and pulse is 90; abdominal examination reveals a mass arising from the pelvis up to the level of the umbilicus, with no obvious ascites. There is no lymphadenopathy or breast abnormality.
N.B. By mentioning ascites, lymphadenopathy and the breasts, you demonstrated your understanding of the possible aetiology and effects of a pelvic mass.

Management plan. Now decide on a course of action. Plan what investigations (if any) are needed and what course of action (if any) is most appropriate.

Gynaecological History at a Glance

Personal details	Name, age, occupation	
Presenting complaint	Details, time-scale, any previous treatment. Prioritize	
Gynaecological questions	(Start with most relevant to complaint)	
	Menstrual:	Last menstrual period (LMP), cycle, heaviness, intermenstrual bleeding (IMB), postcoital bleeding (PCB)
	Sex/contraceptive:	Sexually active, dyspareunia, contraception?
	Cervical smear:	Last smear, ever abnormal?
	Urinary/prolapse	Frequency, incontinence, lump at introitus
Other history	Past obstetric history:	Ever pregnant? If so, details
	Past medical history:	Operations, major illnesses. Ever in hospital?
	Systems review, drugs, personal (smoking, alcohol), social, family history (particularly breast/ovarian/heart disease), allergies	
Summarize	Presenting complaint and relevant history findings	

Gynaecological Examination at a Glance

General	Appearance, anaemia, lymph nodes, blood pressure, pulse
Breasts/axillae	Inspect, palpate
Abdomen	Inspect, palpate (particularly suprapubically), percuss, auscultate
Vaginal	Inspect vulva; digital examination; Cusco's speculum, Sims' speculum if prolapse
Summarize	Positive and important negative findings; consider management

2 The Menstrual Cycle and its Disorders

Physiology of puberty

Puberty is the onset of sexual maturity. It is marked by the development of secondary sex characteristics. The *menarche*, or onset of menstruation, is normally the last manifestation of puberty in the female, and in the West occurs on average at 13 years of age. Normal puberty is controlled centrally. The hypothalamic–pituitary axis can be considered as 'waking' and then 'waking up' the ovaries. After the age of 8 years, hypothalamic gonadotrophin-releasing hormone (GnRH)-pulses increase in amplitude and frequency, such that pituitary follicle-stimulating hormone (FSH) and then luteinizing hormone (LH) release increases. These stimulate oestrogen release from the ovary (Figs 2.1, 2.2).

Oestrogen is responsible for the development of secondary sexual characteristics: the *thelarche*, or beginning of breast development, occurs first at 9–11 years; the *adrenarche*, or growth of pubic hair (also dependent on adrenal activity), starts at 11–12 years; the final stage is the *menarche* (Fig. 2.2). Menstruation may be irregular at first; as oestrogen secretion rises, it will become regular. Pregnancy is now possible. These changes are accompanied by the growth spurt, due to increased growth hormone release. By the age of 16 years, most growth has finished and the epiphyses fuse. The average age of the menarche is reducing.

Physiology of the menstrual cycle

The hormonal changes of the menstrual cycle cause ovulation and induce changes in the endometrium that prepare it for implantation should fertilization occur.

Days 1–4: menstruation
At the start of the menstrual cycle (designated as the start of menstruation) the endometrium is shed as its hormonal support is withdrawn. Myometrial contraction, which can be painful, is accompanied by vasoconstriction to reduce blood loss.

Days 5–13: proliferative phase
Pulses of GnRH from the hypothalamus stimulate LH

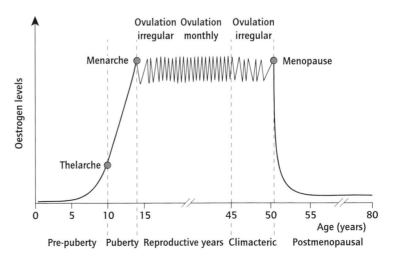

Fig. 2.1 Oestrogen levels in a lifetime.

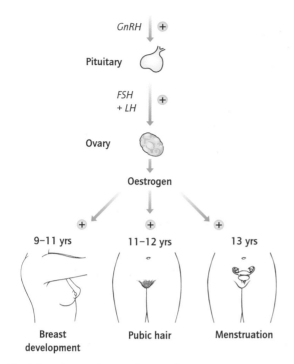

Fig. 2.2 Endocrine changes during puberty.

Normal menstruation
Menarche < 16 years
Menopause > 40 years
Menstruation < 8 days in length
Blood loss < 80 mL
Cycle length 21–35 days
No intermenstrual bleeding (IMB)

Abnormal menstruation and definitions of terms

Excessive menstruation (frequency or volume):
Heavy but regular:	Menorrhagia
Irregular and often frequent:	Polymenorrhoea
Between menses:	Intermenstrual bleeding (IMB)
N.B. These often coexist	

Too little bleeding [→ p.14]:
Never starts (>16 years):	Primary amenorrhoea
Ceases (>6 months):	Secondary amenorrhoea
Infrequent (>every 35 days):	Oligomenorrhoea

Other variants and abnormalities:
Traumatic:	Postcoital bleeding (PCB)
After cessation of menses (> 1 year):	Postmenopausal bleeding (PMB)
Occurs too early (< 8 years):	Precocious puberty [→ p.17]
Painful:	Dysmenorrhoea
Preceded by cyclical symptoms:	Premenstrual syndrome (PMS)

and FSH release. These induce follicular growth and these follicles produce oestradiol. This suppresses FSH secretion in a 'negative feedback', such that (normally) only one follicle and ovum matures. As oestradiol levels continue to rise and reach their maximum, however, a 'positive-feedback' effect on the hypothalamus and pituitary causes LH levels to rise sharply: ovulation follows. The oestradiol also causes the endometrium to re-form and become 'proliferative': it thickens as the stromal cells proliferate and the glands elongate.

Days 14–28: luteal/secretory phase
The follicle from which the egg was released becomes the corpus luteum. This again produces oestradiol, but relatively more progesterone, levels of which peak around day 21. This induces 'secretory' changes in the endometrium, whereby the stromal cells enlarge, the glands swell and the blood supply increases. Towards the end of the luteal phase, the corpus luteum starts to fail if the egg is not fertilized, causing progesterone and oestrogen levels to fall. As its hormonal support is withdrawn, the endometrium breaks down, menstruation follows and the cycle restarts (Fig. 2.3). Continuous administration of exogenous progestogens maintains a secretory endometrium, preventing breakdown and menstruation.

Excessive menstruation: volume (menorrhagia)

Menorrhagia occurs (objectively) when menstrual loss regularly exceeds 80 mL or (subjectively) when the loss is unacceptable to the woman, although in only 40% of the latter group is the loss more than 80 mL. Irregular menstruation and intermenstrual bleeding (IMB) often occur in conjunction with menorrhagia and some of the causes as well as management options are similar. However, irregular periods are more likely to be anovulatory and, particularly in older women, are more commonly associated with malignancy.

Epidemiology

This very common: each year 1 in 20 women between

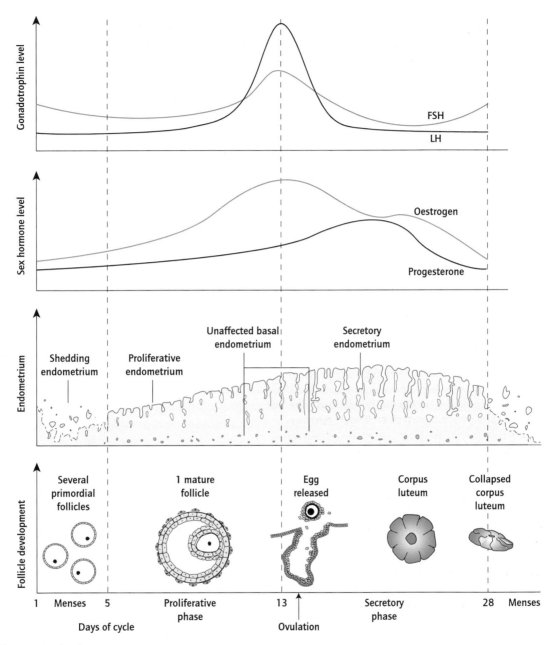

Fig. 2.3 The menstrual cycle.

the ages of 30 and 49 years will seek medical help for menorrhagia.

Causes
Unexplained
This is when no anatomical or systemic cause is found and this accounts for 60% of women. The term dysfunctional uterine bleeding is seldom used nowadays. Mechanisms vary. Most women with regular cycles are ovulatory and menorrhagia may result from subtle abnormalities of the endometrial fibrinolytic system or uterine prostaglandin levels.

Systemic problems

Thyroid disease, haemostatic disorders, such as von Willebrand's disease, and anticoagulant therapy are rare causes of menorrhagia. No other endocrine tests are required when bleeding is regular.

Local anatomical disorder (see Chapter 7)

Causes include fibroids, uterine and cervical polyps, adenomyosis and endometriosis. Chronic pelvic infection, ovarian tumours, and endometrial and cervical malignancy (Fig. 2.4) are rare and all likely to cause irregular bleeding.

Clinical features

History: This should assess both the amount and timing of the bleeding. A menstrual calendar is helpful. 'Flooding' and the passage of large clots indicate excessive loss. Other symptoms may be helpful: severe dysmenorrhoea before the menses suggests an anatomical cause. Any method of contraception should be ascertained.

Examination: Anaemia is common. Pelvic signs are often absent. Irregular enlargement of the uterus suggests fibroids; tenderness suggests adenomyosis. An ovarian mass may be felt; tenderness and immobile pelvic organs are common with endometriosis and infection.

Investigations

To assess the effect of blood loss and fitness, the patient's haemoglobin is checked.

To exclude systemic causes, coagulation and thyroid function are checked.

To exclude local organic causes, a *transvaginal ultrasound* of the pelvis is performed. This will assess endometrial thickness, exclude a uterine fibroid or ovarian mass and detect larger intrauterine polyps. If the endometrial thickness is more than 10 mm or a polyp is suspected, an *endometrial biopsy* (at out-patient hysteroscopy or with a Pipelle) (Fig. 2.5) should be performed to exclude endometrial malignancy or premalignancy [→ p.24]. *Hysteroscopy* allows, in addition to biopsy, an inspection of the uterine cavity, and therefore detection of polyps and submucous fibroids that could be resected. A dilatation and curettage (D&C) is not a treatment for menorrhagia, is less effective at detecting malignancy, and is largely obsolete.

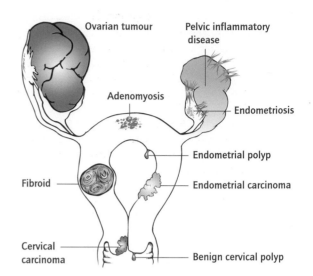

Fig. 2.4 Anatomical causes of too much menstrual bleeding.

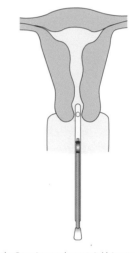

Fig. 2.5 Pipelle de Cornier endometrial biopsy going through the cervix.

Treatment

Once malignancy and systemic disorders are excluded, management is of symptoms, not clinical entities: the patient with very heavy periods and a normal uterus needs treatment more than one with small asymptomatic fibroids.

Medical treatment

Antifibrinolytics (tranexamic acid) are taken during menstruation only. By reducing fibrinolytic activity they can reduce blood loss by about 50%. There are few side effects (*Cochrane* 2000: CD000249). *Non-steroidal anti-inflammatory drugs* (NSAIDs; e.g. mefanamic acid) inhibit prostaglandin synthesis, reducing blood loss in most women by about 30% (*Cochrane* 2000: CD000400). They are also useful for dysmenorrhoea. Side effects are similar to those of aspirin. *The combined oral contraceptive* usually induces lighter menstruation, but is less effective if pelvic pathology is present. Its role is limited because its complications [→ p.81] are more common in older patients and it is these patients who have the most menstrual problems.

Intrauterine system (IUS): This progestogen-impregnated intrauterine device (IUD) (Fig. 2.6) is a 'coil' [→ p.84] that reduces menstrual flow by > 90% with considerably fewer side effects than systemic progestogens. It is a highly effective alternative to both medical and surgical treatment of menorrhagia (*Fertil Steril* 2003; **79**: 963). It is a contraceptive and most useful in the management of the older woman. It should be distinguished from inert IUDs which may increase menstrual loss.

Gonadotrophin-releasing hormone [→ p.58] agonists produce amenorrhoea.

Progestogens [→ p.80] in high doses will cause amenorrhoea, but bleeding will follow withdrawal.

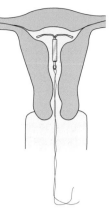

Fig. 2.6 Progestogen impregnated intrauterine device (IUD) (intrauterine system, IUS) *in situ* in the uterus.

still required. Gonadotrophin-releasing hormone agonists are often used to reduce the size of fibroids first. *Hysterectomy* should be the last resort in the treatment of abnormal uterine bleeding. Nevertheless, 20% of all women in the United Kingdom will have a hysterectomy, mostly for bleeding problems. The operation can be vaginal, abdominal or laparoscopic.

First-line treatments for menorrhagia
Antifibrinolytics (tranexamic acid)
Non-steroidal anti-inflammatory drugs (NSAIDs)
Combined oral contraceptive
Consider intrauterine system (IUS)

When to do an endometrial biopsy (Pipelle or hysteroscopy)
If endometrial thickness > 10 mm in premenopausal; >4 mm in postmenopausal
If ultrasound suggests a polyp
Before insertion of intrauterine system (IUS) if cycle not regular
Prior to endometrial ablation/diathermy
If abnormal uterine bleeding has resulted in acute admission

Surgical treatment

Hysteroscopic

Polyp removal: If localized abnormalities such as polyps are seen they can be resected.

Endometrial resection, *ablation* or *diathermy* all involve removal or destruction of endometrium. Amenorrhoea or lighter periods usually follow. Long-term patient satisfaction with endometrial destructive techniques is less than with hysterectomy, although surgical complications and hospital stay are less (*Cochrane* 2000: CD000329). Such techniques are most effective in older women with pure menorrhagia.

Radical

Myomectomy is the removal of fibroids from the myometrium. It can be open or laparoscopic [→ p.103] and is used if fibroids are causing symptoms but fertility is

Excessive menstruation: frequency (polymenorrhoea and intermenstrual bleeding)

Epidemiology

This often coexists with excessive blood loss and is more common at extremes of reproductive age.

Causes

Anovulatory cycles are common in younger women and near the climacteric.

Local anatomical disorder: Non-malignant causes include fibroids, uterine and cervical polyps, adenomyosis, endometriosis and chronic pelvic infection. However, with older women, particularly if there has been a recent change, the chances of malignancy, ovarian and cervical, and most particularly endometrial (Fig. 2.7), are slightly increased.

Clinical features

Women should be assessed as for menorrhagia. Speculum examination may reveal a cervical polyp.

Investigations

To assess the effect of blood loss and fitness, the patient's haemoglobin is checked.

Investigations should exclude malignancy, except in young women where malignancy is rare, and exclude local treatable pathology. A cervical smear is taken. An *ultrasound* examination of the cavity is performed for women over the age of 35 years with irregular or intermenstrual bleeding, and for those younger if medical treatment has failed, and will also detect a uterine fibroid or ovarian mass. *Endometrial biopsy,* preferably at hysteroscopy, is then used if the endometrium is thickened, a polyp is suspected or if ablative surgery or the IUS are to be used. *Diagnostic laparoscopy* is useful if endometriosis or chronic pelvic infection are suspected.

Treatment

Medical treatment

This is appropriate where no anatomical cause is detected: cycles are considered anovulatory. *The combined oral contraceptive* usually induces regular and lighter menstruation. Its role is limited because its complications are more common in older patients and it is these who have most menstrual problems. *Progestogens* in high doses these will cause amenorrhoea, but bleeding will follow withdrawal. They induce secretory changes in the endometrium and so, when given on a cyclical basis, can mimic normal menstruation. *Hormone replacement therapy* (HRT) may regulate erratic dysfunctional uterine bleeding during the climacteric. Use of the IUS [→ p.13] should be considered. *Other treatments* that are second-line treatments for menorrhagia may also be used on a short-term basis.

Surgical treatment

A cervical polyp can be avulsed and sent for histological examination. Surgery is as for women with menorrhagia, except that ablative techniques tend to be less helpful.

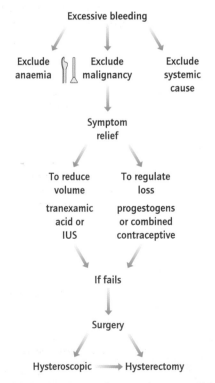

Excessive bleeding

Exclude anaemia — Exclude malignancy — Exclude systemic cause

Symptom relief

To reduce volume — To regulate loss

tranexamic acid or IUS — progestogens or combined contraceptive

If fails

Surgery

Hysteroscopic → Hysterectomy

Fig. 2.7 The common causes of too much menstrual bleeding vary with age.

Amenorrhoea and oligomenorrhoea

Definitions

Amenorrhoea is the absence of menstruation. *Primary amenorrhoea* is when menstruation has not started by the age of 16 years. It may be a manifestation of *delayed puberty,* which is when secondary sex characteristics are not present by the age of 14 years. Amenorrhoea may also occur in girls with otherwise normal secondary sexual characteristics, when a problem of menstrual outflow is likely. *Secondary amenorrhoea* is when previously normal menstruation ceases for 6 or more months (Fig. 2.8). *Oligomenorrhoea* is when menstruation occurs less frequently than every 35 days.

Classification of causes

Physiological amenorrhoea occurs during pregnancy, after the menopause and, usually, during lactation. Constitutional delay is common and often familial.

Pathological causes may lie in the hypothalamus, the pituitary, the thyroid, the adrenals, the ovary or the uterus and 'outflow tract'. Drugs such as progestogens, GnRH analogues and sometimes, major tranquillizers cause amenorrhoea.

Where pathological, primary amenorrhoea is due either to rare congenital abnormalities or acquired disorders that arise before the normal time of puberty. Where pathological, secondary amenorrhoea or oligomenorrhoea is due to acquired disorders that arise later. The most common causes of secondary amenorrhoea or oligomenorrhoea are the premature menopause [→ p.88], polycystic ovary syndrome [→ p.70] and hyperprolactinaemia [→ p.72].

Hypothalamus

Hypothalamic hypogonadism [→ p.71] is common and is usually due to psychological factors, anorexia nervosa or athleticism. Gonadotrophin-releasing hormone and therefore FSH, LH and oestradiol are reduced. Treatment is supportive; anorexia nervosa is life threatening and requires psychiatric treatment.

Pituitary

Hyperprolactinaemia is usually caused by pituitary hyperplasia or benign adenomas. Treatment is with bromocriptine, cabergoline or, occasionally, surgery. Rare pituitary causes include other pituitary tumours and Sheehan's syndrome [→ p.72], in which severe postpartum haemorrhage causes pituitary necrosis.

Adrenal or thyroid gland

Over-activity or under-activity of the thyroid can cause amenorrhoea. Congenital adrenal hyperplasia or virilizing tumours are rare.

Ovary

Acquired disorders: The commonest is *polycystic ovary syndrome.* This can cause primary or secondary amenorrhoea, although oligomenorrhoea is more common. It is extremely important as it is common, is also associated with subfertility and has long-term health consequences (*BJOG* 2000; **107**: 1327). The *premature menopause* occurs in 1 in 100 women. Rare *virilizing tumours* can arise in the ovary.

Congenital causes: The commonest is *Turner's syndrome,* in which one X chromosome is absent, producing the 45 XO genotype. These women have short stature and poor secondary sexual characteristics, but normal intelli-

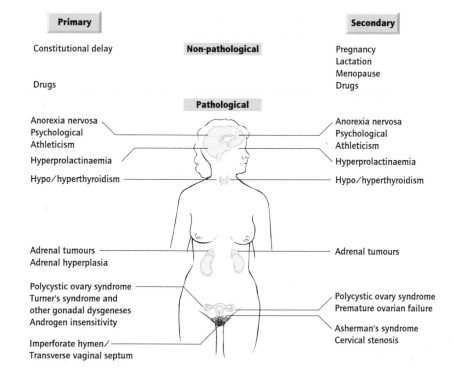

| Primary | Non-pathological | Secondary |

Constitutional delay

Drugs

Pregnancy
Lactation
Menopause
Drugs

Pathological

Anorexia nervosa
Psychological
Athleticism

Hyperprolactinaemia

Hypo/hyperthyroidism

Anorexia nervosa
Psychological
Athleticism

Hyperprolactinaemia

Hypo/hyperthyroidism

Adrenal tumours
Adrenal hyperplasia

Adrenal tumours

Polycystic ovary syndrome
Turner's syndrome and
other gonadal dysgeneses
Androgen insensitivity

Polycystic ovary syndrome
Premature ovarian failure

Asherman's syndrome
Cervical stenosis

Imperforate hymen/
Transverse vaginal septum

Fig. 2.8 Causes of amenorrhoea.

gence. In other forms of *gonadal dysgenesis* the ovary is imperfectly formed due to mosaic abnormalities of the X chromosomes. Gonadal agenesis, the resistant ovary syndrome and androgen insensitivity [→ p.17] are extremely rare.

Outflow tract problems: menstrual flow is obstructed or absent

Congenital problems cause primary amenorrhoea with normal secondary sexual characteristics. The *imperforate hymen* and the *transverse vaginal septum* obstruct menstrual flow, which therefore accumulates over the months in the vagina (haematocolpos) or uterus (haematometra), which may be palpable abdominally. Treatment is surgical. Rarer causes include absence of the vagina with or without a functioning uterus.

Acquired problems usually cause secondary amenorrhoea. *Cervical stenosis* prevents release of blood from the uterus, causing a haematometra [→ p.23]. *Asherman's syndrome* is a rare consequence of accidental excessive curettage at D&C; *endometrial resection* or *ablation* [→ p.103] produces this effect intentionally.

Management

The important conditions of premature menopause [→ p.88], polycystic ovary syndrome [→ p.70] and hyperprolactinaemia [→ p.72] are discussed elsewhere.

Postcoital bleeding (PCB)

Definition

Vaginal bleeding following intercourse that is not menstrual loss. Except for first intercourse, this is always abnormal and cervical carcinoma must be excluded.

Causes

When the cervix is not covered in healthy squamous epithelium it is more likely to bleed after mild trauma. Cervical ectropions [→ p.27], benign polyps [→ p.27] and invasive cervical cancer [→ p.30] account for most cases. The bleeding occasionally comes from the vaginal wall, usually if it is atrophic.

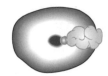

Fig. 2.9 Cervical carcinoma.

Causes of postcoital bleeding
Cervical carcinoma (Fig. 2.9)
Cervical eversion or ectropion
Cervical polyps
Cervicitis, vaginitis

Management

The cervix is carefully inspected and a smear is taken. If a polyp is evident, it is avulsed and sent for histology: this is normally possible without anaesthesia. If the smear is normal, an ectropion can be frozen with cryotherapy. If not, colposcopy [→ p.30] is undertaken to exclude a malignant cause.

Dysmenorrhoea

This is painful menstruation. It is associated with high prostaglandin levels in the endometrium and is due to contraction and ischaemia of uterine muscle.

Causes and their management

Primary dysmenorrhoea is when no organic cause is found. It usually coincides with the start of menstruation and is very common (50% of women, 10% severe), particularly in adolescents. Pain usually responds to NSAIDs, glyceryl trinitrate patches or ovulation suppression (e.g. the combined oral contraceptive) (*Cochrane* 2001: CD002120). Reassurance in the young adolescent is important. Pelvic pathology is more likely if medical treatment fails.

Secondary dysmenorrhoea is when pain is due to pelvic pathology. Pain often precedes and is relieved by the onset of menstruation. Deep dyspareunia and menorrhagia or irregular menstruation are common. Pelvic ultrasound and laparoscopy are useful. The most significant causes are fibroids, adenomyosis, endometriosis, pelvic inflammatory disease and ovarian tumours, which should be treated appropriately.

Precocious puberty

This is when menstruation occurs before the age of 10 years *or* other secondary sexual characteristics are evident before the age of 8 years. It is very rare. The growth spurt occurs early, but final height is reduced due to early fusion of the epiphyses. Investigation is essential, as it may be a manifestation of other disorders. Treatment is essential to arrest sexual development and allow normal growth.

Causes and their management

In 80% of cases, no pathological cause is found. Gonadotrophin-releasing hormone agonists [→ p.58] are used to inhibit sex hormone secretion, causing regression of secondary sex characteristics and cessation of menstruation.
Central causes: increased GnRH secretion: Meningitis, encephalitis, central nervous system tumours, hydrocephaly and hypothyroidism may prevent normal prepubertal inhibition of hypothalamic GnRH release.
Ovarian/adrenal causes: increased oestrogen secretion: Hormone-producing tumours of the ovary or adrenal glands will also cause premature sexual maturation. Regression occurs after removal. The McCune–Albright syndrome consists of bone and ovarian cysts, *café au lait* spots and precocious puberty. Treatment is with progestogens.

Ambiguous development and intersex

There are many causes and degrees of ambiguous genitalia. Psychological support is important and gender assignation should be consistent.

Increased androgen function in a genetic female

Congenital adrenal hyperplasia is recessively inherited. Cortisol production is defective, usually as a result of 21-hydroxylase deficiency: adrenocorticotrophic hormone (ACTH) excess causes increased androgen production. The condition normally presents at birth with ambiguous genitalia; glucocorticoid deficiency may cause Addisonian crises. Occasionally it presents at puberty with an enlarged clitoris and amenorrhoea. Treatment involves cortisol and mineralocorticoid replacement: lack of these can be fatal. Androgen-secreting tumours and other causes of Cushing's syndrome are rare.

Reduced androgen function in a genetic male

Androgen insensitivity occurs when a male has cell receptor insensitivity to androgens, which are converted peripherally to oestrogens. The individual appears to be female: the diagnosis is only discovered when 'she' presents with amenorrhoea. The uterus is absent and rudimentary testes are present. These are removed because of possible malignant change and oestrogen replacement therapy is started.

Premenstrual syndrome (PMS)

This encompasses psychological, behavioural and physical symptoms that are experienced on a regular basis and in relation to menstruation.

Epidemiology

Eighty-five per cent of women experience some cyclical symptoms; in about 5% they are severely disabling (Fig. 2.10).

Aetiology

This is unknown, but is dependent on normal ovarian

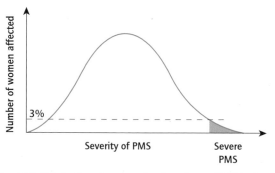

Fig. 2.10 Distribution of premenstrual syndrome (PMS) in the population.

function and the hormone progesterone. Exogenous progestogens are known to cause PMS-like symptoms. Differing neurochemical responses to ovarian function (certain neurotransmitter levels may be altered during the luteal phase in severely affected women) may account for the differing severities of the syndrome.

Clinical features

History: These vary and it is the cyclical nature rather than the symptoms themselves that enable diagnosis. Behavioural changes include 'tension', irritability, aggression, depression and loss of control. In addition, a sensation of bloatedness, minor gastrointestinal upset and breast pain can occur.

Examination: This is necessary to exclude 'organic' disease. Psychological evaluation may be helpful as depression and neurosis can present as PMS. There are no biochemical markers for PMS.

Management

Any treatment must be evaluated against the high (≤94%) placebo response. Support and reassurance are often helpful.

Drug treatments

Selective serotonin reuptake inhibitors (SSRIs) are effective (*Cochrane* 2002: CD001396). Some patients experience relief with the combined contraceptive pill, but not with progestogens alone. High-dose oestrogen is helpful, but progestogens are needed to prevent endometrial ma-lignancy. Gonadotrophin-releasing hormone agonists abolish ovarian activity, but can only be used for 9 months and are used if confirmation of the diagnosis is needed or to predict the response to oöphorectomy, an extreme solution that should be the last resort.

Alternative treatments

The use of these is widespread, but most are of unproven or limited benefit. These include oil of evening primrose, vitamin B_6, borage seed oil and other dietary supplements such as calcium, magnesium and vitamin E.

Further reading

Duckitt K. Menorrhagia. *Clinical Evidence* 2002; **7**: 1716–32.

Lethaby A, Cooke I, Rees M. Progesterone/progestogen releasing intrauterine systems versus either placebo or any other medication for heavy menstrual bleeding. *Cochrane Database of Systematic Reviews (Online: Update Software)* 2000: CD002126.

Lethaby A, Hickey M. Endometrial destruction techniques for heavy menstrual bleeding. *Cochrane Database of Systematic Reviews (Online: Update Software)* 2002: CD001501.

Slap GB. Menstrual disorders in adolescence. *Best Practice & Research Clinical Obstetrics & Gynaecology* 2003; **17**: 75–92.

Vleck JP, Safranek SM, What medications are effective for treating symptoms of premenstrual syndrome (PMS)? *The Journal of Family Practice* 2002; **51**: 894.

Excessive Menstrual Bleeding at a Glance

Types	Menorrhagia, irregular menstruation, intermenstrual bleeding (IMB)
Epidemiology	Common, more frequent with age
Aetiology	Menorrhagia: usually ovulatory cycles Irregular bleeding: often anovulatory Local anatomical problem: e.g. endometrial or cervical carcinoma (usually irregular or intermenstrual bleeding, also postcoital bleeding), fibroids, endometrial/cervical polyps; also endometriosis, pelvic inflammatory disease, ovarian tumours Systemic problem: e.g. disorders of thyroid or coagulation
Investigations	Full blood count (FBC), thyroid function tests (TFTs), clotting, pelvic ultrasound, ± endometrial biopsy and hysteroscopy if thickened endometrium
Treatment	Treat systemic disease appropriately. Then symptom relief Medical: To reduce volume: tranexamic acid, mefanamic acid, intrauterine system (IUS) To regulate timing: combined contraceptive or progestogens Surgical: Hysteroscopic surgery: resection or ablation, hysterectomy occasionally, myomectomy/embolization if fibroids

The Uterus and its Abnormalities

Anatomy and physiology of the uterus

Anatomy and function

The uterus nourishes, protects and, ultimately, expels the fetus. Inferiorly it is continuous with the cervix, which acts as its neck and communication with the vagina. The superior part is the fundus; on either side of this the uterus communicates with the fallopian tubes at the cornu. It is supported predominantly at the inferior end, at the cervix, by the uterosacral and cardinal ligaments. In 80% of women it tilts up towards the abdominal wall—anteversion. In 20% of women it is retroverted, tilting back into the pelvis. The wall is made of smooth muscle (the tissue of origin of the benign tumours *fibroids*) that encloses the uterine cavity. This is lined by glandular epithelium—the endometrium (the tissue of origin of *endometrial carcinoma*). The outside coat of the uterus, or serosa, is the peritoneum posteriorly. This also covers the uterus anteriorly down to the bladder, which is on the anterior surface of the lower uterus, the cervix and the vagina. (The proximity of the bladder to the lower uterus and vagina explains the ease with which it can be damaged at surgery or in childbirth.) Laterally this peritoneum is continuous with the broad ligaments that run between the uterus and pelvic side wall. These have little function as supports, but are continuous with the fallopian tubes and round ligaments superiorly, and inferiorly contain the uterine blood supply, ureters and parametrium (Fig. 3.1).

Blood and lymph

The uterine blood supply (Fig. 3.1) is from the uterine arteries, which cross over the ureters lateral to the cervix and pass inferiorly and superiorly supplying the myometrium and endometrium. At the cornu there is an arterial anastomosis with the ovarian blood supply. Inferiorly, there is an anastomosis with the vessels of the upper vagina. Lymph drainage of the uterus (Fig. 3.1) is mostly via the internal and external iliac arteries.

The endometrium

The endometrium is supplied by the spiral and basal arterioles. The former are important in menstruation and in nourishment of the growing fetus. The endometrium is responsive to oestrogen and progesterone. In the first 14 days of the menstrual cycle, it proliferates: the glands elongate and it thickens largely under the influence of oestrogens (proliferative phase). After ovulation, under

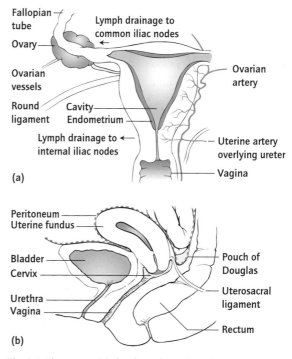

Fig. 3.1 The uterus. (a) Blood supply and lymph drainage. (b) Relations of the pelvic organs.

the influence of progesterone, the glands swell and the blood supply increases (luteal or secretory phase) (see Fig. 2.3). Towards the end of this phase, progesterone levels drop and the secretory endometrium disintegrates as its blood supply can no longer support it: menstruation occurs. Poor hormonal control commonly causes erratic bleeding patterns.

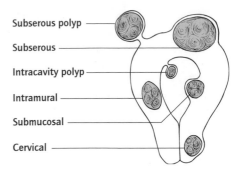

Fig. 3.2 Sites of fibroids showing intramural, subserosal and submucosal.

Fibroids

Definition and epidemiology

Also known as leiomyomata, these are benign tumours of the myometrium. They are present in about 25% of all women and are more common approaching the menopause, in Afro-Caribbean women and those with a family history. They are less common in parous women and those who have taken the combined oral contraceptive.

Pathology and sites of fibroids

The sizes vary from a few millimetres to massive tumours filling the abdomen. The fibroid may be intramural, subserosal or submucosal (Fig. 3.2). Submucosal fibroids occasionally form intracavity polyps. Smooth muscle and fibrous elements are present, and in transverse section, the fibroid has a 'whorled' appearance.

Aetiology

Fibroid growth is oestrogen- and probably progesterone-dependent. Growth increases in pregnancy and with combined contraceptives and regresses after the menopause.

Clinical features

History: Fifty per cent are asymptomatic and discovered only at pelvic or abdominal examination. Symptoms are related more to the site than the size.
● Menstrual problems: menorrhagia occurs in 30%, although the timing of menses is usually unchanged. Intermenstrual loss may occur if the fibroid is submucosal or polypoid. Fibroids are common in the perimenopausal woman and may be incidental:

menstrual problems may also be the result of hormonal irregularities or malignancy.
● Pain: fibroids can cause dysmenorrhoea. They seldom cause pain, unless torsion, red degeneration or, rarely, sarcomatous change occur.
● Other symptoms: large fibroids pressing on the bladder can cause frequency and occasionally urinary retention, those pressing on the ureters can cause hydronephrosis; other pressure effects may also be felt. Fertility can be impaired if the tubal ostia are blocked or submucous fibroids prevent implantation.
Examination: A solid mass may be palpable on pelvic or even abdominal examination. It will arise from the pelvis and be continuous with the uterus. Multiple small fibroids cause irregular 'knobbly' enlargement of the uterus.

Symptoms of fibroids
None (50%)
Menorrhagia (30%)
Erratic/intermenstrual bleeding (IMB)
Pressure effects
Subfertility (rare)

Natural history/complications of fibroids

Enlargement can be very slow. Fibroids stop growing and often calcify after the menopause, although the oestrogen in hormone replacement therapy (HRT) may stimulate further growth. In mid-pregnancy they enlarge. Pedunculated fibroids occasionally undergo torsion, causing pain.
'Degenerations' are normally the result of an inadequate

blood supply: 'red degeneration' is characterized by pain and uterine tenderness; haemorrhage and necrosis occur. In 'hyaline degeneration' and 'cystic degeneration' the fibroid is soft and partly liquefied.

Malignancy: Between 0.1 and 0.5% of fibroids are leiomyosarcomata [→ p.25]. This may be the result of malignant change or *de novo* malignant transformation of normal smooth muscle.

Complications of fibroids	
Torsion of pedunculated fibroid	
Degenerations:	Red (partic. in pregnancy)
	Hyaline/cystic
	Calcification (postmenopausal and asymptomatic)
Malignancy:	Leiomyosarcoma

Fibroids and pregnancy

Premature labour, malpresentations, transverse lie, obstructed labour and postpartum haemorrhage can occur. Red degeneration is very common in pregnancy and can cause severe pain. Fibroids should not be removed at Caesarean section as bleeding can be heavy. Pedunculated fibroids may tort postpartum.

Hormone replacement therapy (HRT) and fibroids

Hormone replacement therapy [→ p.90] can cause continued fibroid growth after the menopause. Treatment is as for premenopausal women or the HRT is withdrawn.

Investigations

To establish diagnosis: Ultrasound is helpful (Fig. 3.3) but laparoscopy may be required to distinguish the fibroid from the ovarian mass. Hysteroscopy is used to assess distortion of the uterine cavity.
To establish fitness: The haemoglobin concentration may be low as a result vaginal bleeding.

Treatment

Asymptomatic patients with small or slow-growing fibroids need no treatment. The risk of malignancy is small enough not to warrant routine removal. Larger fibroids that are not removed should be serially measured by examination or ultrasound because of the remote possibility of malignancy.

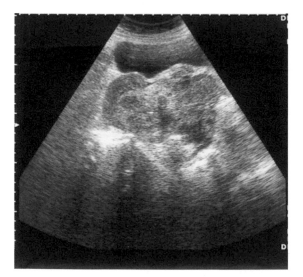
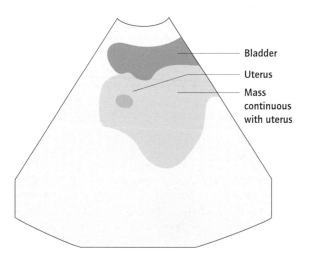

Bladder
Uterus
Mass continuous with uterus

Fig. 3.3 Ultrasound of fibroids on the uterus.

Is the fibroid malignant?

Uncommon but more likely if:
  Pain and rapid growth
  Growth in postmenopausal woman not on hormone
    replacement therapy (HRT)
  Poor response to gonadotrophin-releasing hormone
    (GnRH) agonists

Medical treatment

Tranexamic acid, non-steroidal anti-inflammatory drugs or *progestogens* are often ineffective when menorrhagia [→ p.10] is due to fibroids. Gonadotrophin-releasing hormone (GnRH) agonists cause temporary amenorrhoea and fibroid shrinkage by inducing a temporary menopausal state. Side effects and bone density loss restrict their use to only 9 months, usually near the menopause or to make surgery easier. However, concomitant use of ('add-back') HRT may prevent such effects without causing enlargement, allowing longer administration.

Surgical treatment

Hysteroscopic: The fibroid polyp or small submucous fibroid that is causing menstrual problems or subfertility can be resected at hysteroscopy [→ p.103].
Radical: Twenty per cent of all hysterectomies are performed because of fibroids. The fibroids can also be removed from the uterus: myomectomy (Fig. 3.4). Blood loss may be heavy and small fibroids can be missed, causing problems to recur. Myomectomy is performed if medical treatment has failed but preservation of reproductive function is required. Both operations are usually preceded by 3 months' treatment with GnRH analogues (*Cochrane* 2001: CD000547).
Embolization: Uterine artery embolization by radiologists has an 80% success rate and is an alternative to hysterectomy (*Radiology* 2003; **226**: 425). Symptoms such as pain may get worse, however, and hysterectomy may be required.

Adenomyosis

Definition and epidemiology

Previously called 'endometriosis interna', this is the presence of endometrium and its underlying stroma within the myometrium (Fig. 3.5). Its true incidence is unknown, but it occurs in up to 40% of hysterectomy specimens. It is most common around the age of 40 years and is associated with endometriosis and fibroids. Symptoms subside after the menopause.

Pathology and aetiology

The endometrium appears to grow into the myometrium to form adenomyosis. The extent is variable, but in severe cases pockets of menstrual blood can be seen in the myometrium of hysterectomy specimens. Occasionally, endometrial stromal tissue in the myometrium displays varying degrees of atypia or even invasion [→ p.24]. The condition is oestrogen dependent, but why it occurs is unknown.

Clinical features

History: Symptoms may be absent, but painful, regular, heavy menstruation is common.
Examination: The uterus is mildly enlarged and tender.

Investigations

Adenomyosis cannot be diagnosed by ultrasound but can be seen on magnetic resonance imaging (MRI).

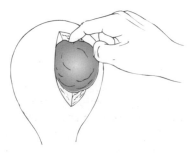

Fig. 3.4 Myomectomy.

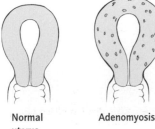

Endometrial tissue in myometrium causing moderate enlargement

Normal uterus

Adenomyosis

Fig. 3.5 Adenomyosis.

Treatment

Medical treatment with non-steroidals or progestogens may control the menorrhagia and dysmenorrhoea, but hysterectomy is often required. A trial of GnRH analogue therapy may determine if symptoms attributed to adenomyosis are likely to improve with hysterectomy.

Other benign conditions of the uterus

Endometritis [→ p.64]

This is often secondary to sexually transmitted infections, as a complication of surgery, particularly Caesarean section and intrauterine procedure (e.g. surgical termination) [→ p.97], or because of foreign tissue, particularly intrauterine devices (IUDs) [→ p.84] and retained products of conception. Infection in the postmenopausal uterus is commonly due to malignancy. The uterus is tender and pelvic and systemic infection may be evident. A pyometra is when pus accumulates and is unable to escape. Antibiotics and occasionally evacuation of retained products of conception (ERPC) [→ p.104] are required.

Intrauterine polyps

These are small, usually benign tumours that grow into the uterine cavity. Most are endometrial in origin (Fig. 3.6), but some are derived from submucous fibroids. They are common in women aged 40–50 years and when oestrogen levels are high. In the postmenopausal woman, they are often found in patients on tamoxifen for breast carcinoma. Occasionally they contain endometrial hyperplasia or carcinoma. Although sometimes asymptomatic, they often cause menorrhagia and intermenstrual bleeding and very occasionally prolapse through the cervix. They are normally diagnosed at ultrasound or when a hysteroscopy is performed because of abnormal bleeding. Resection of the polyp with cutting diathermy or avulsion normally cures bleeding problems.

Haematometra

This is menstrual blood accumulating in the uterus because of outflow obstruction. It is uncommon. The cervical canal is usually occluded by fibrosis after endometrial resection, cone biopsy or by a carcinoma. Congenital abnormalities, for example imperforate hymen or blind rudimentary uterine horn, present in adolescence.

Congenital uterine malformations

Abnormalities result from differing degrees of failure of fusion of the two müllerian ducts at about 9 weeks. These are common but are seldom clinically significant. Total failure of fusion leads to two uterine cavities and cervices; or one duct may fail, causing a 'unicornuate' uterus. If one duct develops better than the other one, a smaller 'rudimentary horn' is formed. Its cavity can be blind or continuous with the dominant horn. At the other end of the spectrum, there may simply be a small septum at the fundus.

About 25% cause pregnancy-related problems that lead to their discovery. These include malpresentations or transverse lie, premature labour, recurrent miscarriage (<5% of these) or retained placenta. Treatment for pregnancy-related problems, however, should not be undertaken lightly as congenital abnormalities may be incidental. Simple septa can be resected hysteroscopically; rudimentary horns need open removal.

Endometrial carcinoma

Epidemiology

This is now the most common genital tract cancer (Fig. 3.7). Prevalence is highest at the age of 60 years, with only 15% of cases occurring premenopausally and <1% in women under 35 years of age. Because it usually presents early, it is often incorrectly considered to be relatively

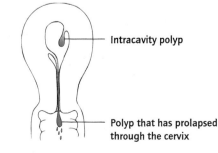

Intracavity polyp

Polyp that has prolapsed through the cervix

Fig. 3.6 Endometrial polyps.

benign, but stage for stage the prognosis is similar to ovarian malignancy.

Pathology

Adenocarcinoma of columnar endometrial gland cells accounts for >90%. Of the rest, the most common is adenosquamous carcinoma, which contains malignant squamous and glandular tissue and has a poorer prognosis.

Aetiology

The principal risk is a high ratio of oestrogen to progestogen. Malignancy therefore is most common when oestrogen production is high or when oestrogen therapy is used 'unopposed' by progestogens.

Risk factors

Exogenous oestrogens without a progestogen increase the rate sixfold. Obesity, polycystic ovary syndrome (PCOS), nulliparity and a late menopause, and ovarian granulosa and theca (oestrogen-secreting) tumours are all risk factors. Tamoxifen increases the risk of endometrial carcinoma (*Lancet* 1994; **343**: 448): although an oestrogen antagonist in the breast and used in the treatment of breast carcinoma, it is mainly an agonist in the postmenopausal uterus. Hypertension and diabetes are common, but probably not independent risk factors. The combined oral contraceptive and pregnancy are protective.

Premalignant disease: endometrial hyperplasia with atypia

Oestrogen acting unopposed or erratically can cause 'cystic hyperplasia' of the endometrium. Further stimulation predisposes to abnormalities of cellular and glandular architecture or 'atypical hyperplasia'. This may cause menstrual abnormalities or postmenopausal bleeding and is premalignant (dependent on the severity of atypia) but is seldom recognized prior to the diagnosis of malignancy. The discovery of atypia is unusual in women of reproductive age, but if the uterus must be preserved, progestogens in combination with 6-monthly endometrial biopsy are used. Otherwise hysterectomy is indicated.

Risk factors for endometrial carcinoma	
Endogenous oestrogen excess:	Polycystic ovary syndrome (PCOS) and obesity Oestrogen-secreting tumours Nulliparity and late menopause
Exogenous oestrogens:	Unopposed oestrogen therapy Tamoxifen therapy
Miscellaneous:	Diabetes; hypertension (not independent) History of breast or ovarian carcinoma Lynch type II syndrome (familial non-polyposis colonic carcinoma)

Clinical features

History: Postmenopausal bleeding (PMB; 10% risk of carcinoma) is the most common presentation [→ p.92]. Premenopausal patients have irregular or intermenstrual bleeding (IMB), or, occasionally, only recent-onset menorrhagia. A cervical smear may contain abnormal columnar cells (CGIN [→ p.30]).

Examination: The pelvis often appears normal and atrophic vaginitis may coexist.

Spread and staging

The tumour spreads directly through the myometrium to the cervix and upper vagina (Fig. 3.8). The ovaries

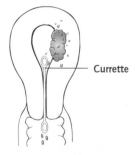

Fig. 3.7 Endometrial carcinoma.

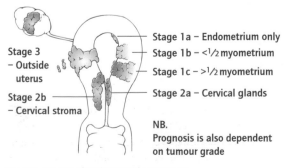

Fig. 3.8 Stages of endometrial carcinoma.

may be involved. Lymphatic spread is to pelvic and then para-aortic lymph nodes. Blood-borne spread occurs late. Staging is surgical and histological and, in contrast to cervical carcinoma, includes lymph node involvement.

Spread and staging for endometrial carcinoma	
Stage 1	*Lesions confined to uterus:*
1a	In endometrium only
1b	Deepest invasion $< \frac{1}{2}$ of myometrial thickness
1c	Deepest invasion $> \frac{1}{2}$ of myometrial thickness
Stage 2	*As above but in cervix also:*
2a	In endocervical glands only
2b	In cervical stroma
Stage 3	*Tumour invades through the uterus:*
3a	Invades serosa and/or adnexae and/or positive cytology
3b	Vaginal metastases
3c	Metastases to pelvic/para-aortic lymph nodes.
Stage 4	*Further spread:*
4a	In bowel or bladder
4b	Distant metastases

Histological grade: G1–3 is also included for each stage, G1 being a well-differentiated tumour.

Investigations

To confirm and help stage disease, endometrial biopsy at hysteroscopy (*JAMA* 2002; **288**:1610) and examination under anaesthetic (EUA) confirms the diagnosis. Uterine enlargement with immobility suggests advanced stage. A chest X-ray is required to exclude rare pulmonary spread. Ultrasound or MRI have also been used to assess spread.

To assess the patient's fitness, full blood count (FBC), renal function, glucose testing and an electrocardiogram (ECG) are normally required as most patients are elderly.

Treatment

Seventy-five per cent of patients present with Stage 1 disease. Unless the patient is unfit or has disseminated disease, a *laparotomy* is performed, with total abdominal hysterectomy (TAH) and bilateral salpingo-oöphorectomy (BSO). As staging is surgico-pathological, disease that appears to be Stage 1 at surgery may subsequently turn out to be Stage 3 if lymph nodes are involved. The role of lymphadenectomy in clinically

early stage disease is being assessed in a United Kingdom-based randomized clinical trial. If lymphadenectomy is not performed (these patients are often elderly), an estimate of stage and risk should be made to determine further management. Protocols are complicated and controversial: there are more prognostic factors than can be incorporated into a staging system and treatment must be individualized.

External beam radiotherapy is then used in patients with, or considered 'high risk' for, lymph node involvement. Risk factors are deep myometrial spread, poor tumour histology or grade, or cervical stromal involvement (Stage 2b). *Vaginal vault radiotherapy* is also used where these risk factors are present. Its usage reduces local recurrence but does not prolong survival. *Progestogens* are seldom used nowadays (*Cochrane* 2000: CD001040). *Chemotherapy* has a limited role, in advanced disease.

General indications for radiotherapy
High risk for, or proven, extrauterine disease
For inoperable and recurrent disease
Palliation for symptoms, e.g. bleeding

Prognosis

Recurrence is commonest at the vaginal vault, normally in the first 3 years. Poor prognostic features are older age, advanced clinical stage, deep myometrial invasion in Stage 1 and 2 patients, high tumour grade and adenosquamous histology.

Prognosis of endometrial carcinoma	
Stage	5-year survival rate (%)
1	85
2	70
3–4	50
4	25
Overall	75

Uterine sarcomas

These are rare tumours, accounting for only 150 cases per year in the United Kingdom. There are three categories. *Leiomyosarcomas* are 'malignant fibroids'. *Endometrial stromal tumours* are tumours of the stroma beneath the endometrium. Histological types vary from the benign endometrial stromal nodule, to the highly malignant endometrial stromal sarcoma. These are most common in the perimenopausal woman. The third group is the *mixed müllerian tumours*, derived from the embryological elements of the uterus, and these are more common in old age. They usually present with irregular or postmenopausal bleeding or, in the case of leiomyosarcomas, rapid painful enlargement of a fibroid. Treatment is with hysterectomy. Radiotherapy or chemotherapy can be used subsequently, but overall survival is only 30% at 5 years.

Further reading

Lawton F. Management of endometrial cancer. *The Obstetrician and Gynaecologist* 2003; **5**: 79–83.

Lethaby A, Vollenhoven B. Fibroids (uterine myomatosis, leiomyomas). *Clinical Evidence* 2002; **7**: 1666–78.

Matalliotakis IM, Kourtis AI, Panidis DK. Adenomyosis. *Obstetrics and Gynecology Clinics of North America* 2003; **30**: 63–82.

Fibroids at a Glance

Epidemiology	25% of women, older, Afro-Caribbean
Pathology	Benign tumours of myometrium
Aetiology	Oestrogen dependent
Clinical features	None (50%). Menstrual problems, dysmenorrhoea, pressure effects. Subfertility and pain (rare)
Complications	Torsion of pedunculated fibroid. Degenerations: red or hyaline degeneration. Sarcomatous change. Complicates pregnancy
Investigations	Full blood count (FBC), hysteroscopy, ultrasound. Laparoscopy if diagnosis unsure
Treatment	Observation or . . . *Conservative*: Symptomatic relief *Surgical*: Hysterectomy. Resection if polypoid; consider myomectomy and embolization

Endometrial Carcinoma at a Glance

Epidemiology	Commonest gynaecological carcinoma, usually over 60 years of age
Pathology	> 90% adenocarcinomas; also adenosquamous
Aetiology	High oestrogen : progesterone ratio. Nulliparity, late menopause, polycystic ovary syndrome (PCOS), obesity. Unopposed oestrogens and tamoxifen Combined pill protective
Clinical features	Postmenopausal bleeding. Premenopausal get a 'change': irregular, intermenstrual or heavier bleeding
Screening	Not routine. Presents early. Probably worthwhile if taking tamoxifen
Investigations	Hysteroscopy, biopsy and examination under anaesthetic (EUA) to diagnose. Full blood count (FBC), urea and electrolytes (U&E), chest X-ray, glucose, electrocardiogram (ECG)
Staging	**1** Uterus only. 1a: endometrium; 1b: $<\frac{1}{2}$ myometrial invasion; 1c: $>\frac{1}{2}$ myometrial invasion **2** Cervix also **3** Outside uterus, not outside pelvis **4** Bowel and bladder or distant spread
Treatment	Usually laparotomy with total abdominal hysterectomy (TAH) and bilateral salpingo-oöphorectomy (BSO) ± lymphadenectomy Radiotherapy if lymph nodes positive/likely to be positive
Prognosis	Dependent on clinical stage, histology, grade, patient's fitness Overall 75% 5-year survival

The Cervix and its Disorders

Anatomy and function of the cervix

Anatomy

The cervix is a tubular structure, continuous with the uterus, 2–3 cm long and made up predominantly of elastic connective tissue. It connects the uterus and vagina, allowing sperm in and menstrual flow out. In pregnancy it holds the fetus in the uterus and then dilates in labour to allow delivery. It is attached posteriorly to the sacrum by the uterosacral ligaments and laterally to the pelvic side wall by the cardinal ligaments. Lateral to the cervix is the parametrium, containing connective tissue, uterine vessels and the ureters.

Histology and the transformation zone

The endocervix (canal) is lined by columnar (glandular) epithelium. The ectocervix, continuous with the vagina, is covered in squamous epithelium. The two types of cell meet at the 'squamocolumnar junction' (Fig. 4.1). During puberty and pregnancy, partial eversion of the cervix occurs. The lower pH of the vagina causes the now exposed area of columnar epithelium to undergo metaplasia to squamous epithelium, producing a 'transformation zone' at the squamocolumnar junction (Fig. 4.1). Cells undergoing metaplasia are vulnerable to agents that induce neoplastic change, and it is from this area that cervical carcinoma usually originates.

Blood supply and lymph drainage

The blood supply is from upper vaginal branches and the uterine artery. Lymph drains to the obdurator and internal and external iliac nodes, and thence to the common iliac and para-aortic nodes. Cervical carcinoma characteristically spreads in the lymph.

Benign conditions of the cervix

Cervical ectopy (previously called erosion) is when the columnar epithelium of the endocervix is visible as a red area around the os on the surface of the cervix (Fig. 4.2a). This is due to eversion and is a normal finding in younger women, particularly those who are pregnant or taking the 'pill'.

Cervical ectropion appears as a more irregular redness and results from minor lacerations during childbirth (Fig. 4.2b). Normally asymptomatic, ectopy and ectropions occasionally cause vaginal discharge or postcoital bleeding (PCB). This can be treated by freezing (cryotherapy) without anaesthetic, but only after a smear and, ideally, colposcopy has excluded a carcinoma. Exposed columnar epithelium is also prone to infection.

Acute cervicitis is rare but often results from sexually transmitted disease [→ p.62]. Ulceration and infection are occasionally found in severe degrees of prolapse

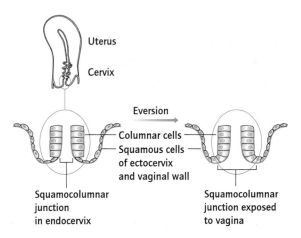

Fig. 4.1 The squamocolumnar junction.

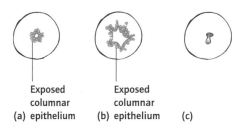

Fig. 4.2 (a) Cervical ectopy; (b) cervical ectropion; (c) cervical polyp.

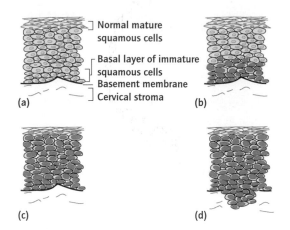

Fig. 4.3 The cervical epithelium and cervical intraepithelial neoplasia (CIN). (a) Normal cervical epithelium; proliferation in basal layer only with small nuclei. (b) CIN I–II: abnormal cells with larger nuclei proliferating in the lower $1/3$–$2/3$ of the epithelium. (c) CIN III: abnormal cells occupying the entire epithelium. (d) Microinvasion: abnormal cells have penetrated the basement membrane.

when the cervix protrudes or is held back with a pessary [→ p.48].

Chronic cervicitis is chronic inflammation or infection, often of an ectropion or ectopy. It is a common cause of vaginal discharge and may cause 'inflammatory' smears. Cryotherapy is used, with or without antibiotics, depending upon bacterial culture.

Cervical polyps are benign tumours of the endocervical epithelium (Fig. 4.2c). They are most common in women above the age of 40 years and are seldom larger than 1 cm. They may be asymptomatic or cause intermenstrual bleeding (IMB) or PCB. Small polyps are avulsed without anaesthetic and examined histologically, but bleeding abnormalities must still be investigated [→ p.14].

Nabothian follicles occur where squamous epithelium has formed by metaplasia over endocervical cells. The columnar cell secretions are trapped and form retention cysts, which appear as white or opaque swellings on the ectocervix. Symptoms are rare.

In *congenital malformations* the uterus and cervix may be absent or varying degrees of duplication may occur [→ p.23].

Premalignant conditions of the cervix: cervical intraepithelial neoplasia (CIN)

Definitions

Cervical intraepithelial neoplasia, or cervical dysplasia, is the presence of atypical cells within the squamous epithelium. These atypical cells are dyskaryotic, exhibiting larger nuclei with frequent mitoses. The severity of CIN is graded I–III and is dependent on the extent to which

these cells are found in the epithelium (Fig. 4.3). Cervical intraepithelial neoplasia is therefore a *histological* diagnosis.

CIN I (mild dysplasia): Atypical cells are found only in the lower third of the epithelium.
CIN II (moderate dysplasia): Atypical cells are found in the lower two-thirds of the epithelium.
CIN III (severe dysplasia): Atypical cells occupy the full thickness of the epithelium. This is carcinoma *in situ:* the cells are similar in appearance to those in malignant lesions, but there is no invasion. Malignancy ensues if these abnormal cells invade through the basement membrane.

Natural history

If untreated, about a third of women with CIN II/III will develop cervical cancer over the next 10 years. CIN I has the least malignant potential: it can progress to CIN II/III, but commonly regresses spontaneously (Fig. 4.4).

Pathology

As the columnar epithelium undergoes metaplasia to squamous epithelium in the transformation zone, exposure to certain human papilloma viruses (HPVs) results in incorporation of viral deoxyribonucleic acid

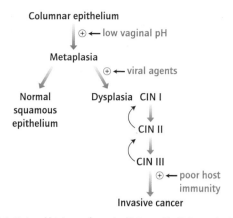

Columnar epithelium

⊕ ← low vaginal pH

Metaplasia

⊕ ← viral agents

Normal squamous epithelium   Dysplasia   CIN I

CIN II

CIN III

⊕ ← poor host immunity

Invasive cancer

Fig. 4.4 Natural history of cervical intraepithelial neoplasia (CIN).

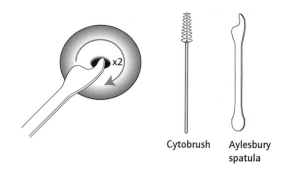

Cytobrush   Aylesbury spatula

Fig. 4.5 Taking a cervical smear.

(DNA) into cell DNA. If the body's immune system does not recognize or destroy such cells, malignancy may ensue.

Epidemiology

Cervical intraepithelial neoplasia is becoming more common. It is most prevalent in the 35–45 year age group and in lower socio-economic classes.

Aetiology

Human papilloma virus (HPV): The most important factor is the number of sexual contacts, particularly at an early age: CIN is almost unknown in virgins. This is because infection with a HPV (particularly types 16, 18, 31, 33) is sexually transmitted. Vaccination against individual viruses, and therefore potentially against cervical cancer, is under evaluation (*NEJM* 2002; **347**: 1645).

Other factors: Oral contraceptive usage (*Lancet* 2002; **359**: 1085) and smoking are associated with a slightly increased risk of CIN. Immunocompromised patients (e.g. human immunodeficiency virus (HIV), those on long-term steroids) are also at increased risk and of early progression to malignancy.

Diagnosis: screening for cervical cancer

Cervical intraepithelial neoplasia causes no symptoms and is not visible on the cervix. However, the diagnosis identifies women at high risk of developing carcinoma of the cervix, who could be treated before the disease develops. Identification of CIN is therefore the principal step in screening for cervical cancer.

Cervical smears

Screening is performed with cervical smears. These should be performed on all women at the age of 20 years, or after first intercourse if later, and then repeated every 3 years until the age of 64 years. The abnormal smear identifies women likely to have CIN and therefore at risk of subsequent development of invasive cancer.

Method

A spatula (or brush) is gently scraped around the external os of the cervix to pick up loose cells over the transformation zone (Fig. 4.5). The spatula is then smeared over a slide and the sample is fixed instantly and then examined with a microscope.

Results

Smears identify cellular, not histological, abnormalities as only superficial cells are sampled. Cellular abnormalities are called *dyskaryosis* and graded mild, moderate and severe. Dyskaryosis suggests the presence of CIN, and the grade partly reflects the severity of CIN. Smears are therefore often reported in histological terms: if severe dyskaryosis is seen, for instance, the report may read 'CIN III'. This does not mean that CIN III is present, merely that a biopsy would be likely to find it. Colposcopy is usually recommended (see box). Occasionally abnormal columnar cells are visible. Adenocarcinoma of the cervix or endometrium should then be excluded, using both colposcopy and endocervical curettage (sampling cells within the cervical canal) or with cone biopsy [→ p.31], in addition to hysteroscopy.

Management of the abnormal smear	
Smear result	Action
Normal	Repeat every 3 years
Mild dyskaryosis	Repeat in 6 months. If still present: colposcopy
BNA	Repeat in 6 months. If still present: colposcopy
Moderate dyskaryosis	Colposcopy
Severe dyskaryosis	Urgent colposcopy
CGIN (any grade)	Colposcopy, hysteroscopy

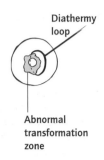

Fig. 4.6 Large loop excision of transformation zone (LLETZ).

Colposcopy

If a cervical smear is severely or persistently abnormal, a colposcopy is performed (see box above) to detect the presence and grade of CIN. The cervix is inspected with magnification 10–20-fold. Grades of CIN have characteristic appearances when stained with 5% acetic acid, although the diagnosis is only confirmed histologically and therefore biopsy is usual.

Treatment: prevention of invasive cervical cancer

If CIN II or III are present, the transformation zone is excised with cutting diathermy under local anaesthetic. This is called 'large loop excision of transformation zone' (LLETZ; Fig. 4.6), also sometimes called diathermy loop excision. The specimen is examined histologically. Occasionally an unsuspected malignancy is detected. Large loop excision of transformation zone enables diagnosis and treatment to be achieved at the same time and has replaced laser or diathermy treatment. The only major complication, postoperative haemorrhage, is rare, but the risk of subsequent preterm delivery is slightly increased (*JAMA* 2004; **291**: 2100).

Prevention of cervical cancer
Prevention of cervical intraepithelial neoplasia (CIN): sexual and (barrier) contraceptive education
Identification and treatment of CIN: cervical smear programmes

Results and problems with screening for cervical cancer

Cervical screening by 3-yearly smear reduces the cumulative incidence of cervical cancer by 91%: most women with cervical carcinoma have never had a smear, and those who have, tend to be identified at an earlier stage. Nevertheless, there is a significant false negative rate with cervical smears, dependent on both sampling and interpretation techniques. Furthermore, the distinctions between grades of dyskaryosis and CIN are blurred and spontaneous regression of CIN can occur. Some women do not have cervical smears through fear or ignorance.

Psychological aspects of cervical screening

The woman with an abnormal smear must be handled sensitively. The words 'early warning cells' are less alarming than 'pre-cancerous cells'. Discussion of sexual history and the papilloma virus is usually inappropriate because of feelings of guilt and recrimination. More even than discomfort or embarrassment, people fear cancer.

Malignant disease of the cervix

Epidemiology

The incidence of cervical carcinoma (9.3 per 100 000 women) is falling in the United Kingdom, largely due to the success of screening programmes. The disease can occur at any age after first intercourse, but is most common between the ages of 45 and 55 years.

Pathology

Ninety per cent of cervical malignancies are squamous cell carcinomas. Ten per cent are adenocarcinomas originating from the columnar epithelium: these have a worse prognosis.

Aetiology

Cervical intraepithelial neoplasia is the pre-invasive stage: causative factors are therefore the same. Cervical cancer is more common when screening has been inadequate. Immunosuppression (e.g. HIV) accelerates the process of invasion from CIN. Cervical cancer is not familial.

Clinical features

Occult carcinoma
This is when there are no symptoms, but the diagnosis is made by biopsy or LLETZ.

Clinical carcinoma
History: Postcoital bleeding, an offensive vaginal discharge and IMB or postmenopausal bleeding (PMB) are common. Pain is not an early feature. In the later stages of the disease, involvement of ureters, bladder, rectum and nerves causes uraemia, haematuria, rectal bleeding and pain respectively. Smears have usually been missed.
Examination: An ulcer or mass may be visible (Fig. 4.7) or palpable on the cervix. With early disease, the cervix may appear normal to the naked eye.

Spread and staging

The tumour spreads locally to the parametrium and vagina and then to the pelvic side wall. Lymphatic spread to the pelvic nodes is an early feature. Ovarian spread is rare with squamous carcinomas. Blood-borne spread occurs late. The International Federation of Gynaecology and Obstetrics (FIGO) classification is clinical (from examination), although divisions of Stage 1 are histological (from local excision). It is limited as a predictor of survival because it does not include whether or not there is lymph node (LN) involvement. Lymph node involvement is, however, more likely with advanced stages.

Spread and staging for cervical carcinoma	
Stage 1	*Lesions confined to the cervix:*
1a(i)	Microinvasion <3 mm from the basement membrane, <7 mm across, with no lymph/vascular space invasion
1a(ii)	Invasion >3 mm, <5 mm deep, <7 mm across
1b(i)	Tumour size <4 cm
1b(ii)	Tumour size >4 cm
Stage 2	*Invasion is into vagina, but not the pelvic side wall:*
2a	Invasion of upper two-thirds vagina but not parametrium
2b	Invasion of parametrium
Stage 3	*Invasion of lower vagina or pelvic wall, or causing ureteric obstruction*
Stage 4	*Invasion of bladder or rectal mucosa, or beyond the true pelvis*

Investigations

To confirm the diagnosis, the tumour is biopsied.
To stage the disease, vaginal and rectal examination are used to assess the size of the lesion and parametrial or rectal invasion. Unless it is clearly small, examination under anaesthetic (EUA) is performed. Cystoscopy detects bladder involvement; an intravenous pyelogram (IVP) is sometimes performed to exclude ureteric obstruction.
To assess the patient's fitness for surgery, a chest X-ray, full blood count (FBC) and urea and electrolytes (U&E) are checked. These may be abnormal with advanced disease. Blood is cross-matched before surgery.

Treatment of cervical malignancies
Microinvasive disease
Stage Ia(i) can be treated with cone biopsy (Fig. 4.8), as the risk of lymph node (LN) spread is 0.5%. Postopera-

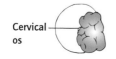

Fig. 4.7 Cervical carcinoma.

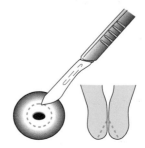

Fig. 4.8 Cone biopsy

tive haemorrhage and cervical incompetence are the main complications. Simple hysterectomy is preferred in older women.

All other Stage 1 and Stage 2a

Surgery can be used alone with radiotherapy and chemotherapy if LNs are involved. Or primary chemotherapy and radiotherapy are used instead of surgery.

Radical abdominal hysterectomy (Wertheim's hysterectomy) involves pelvic LN clearance, hysterectomy and removal of the parametrium and upper third of the vagina (Fig. 4.9). The ovaries are left only in the young woman with squamous carcinoma. This operation can also be performed vaginally, with laparoscopic LN dissection. *Specific complications* include haemorrhage, ureteric and bladder damage and fistulae, voiding problems and accumulation of lymph (lymphocyst).

Radical trachelectomy is a less invasive procedure for women who wish to conserve fertility. It involves removal of 80% of the cervix and the upper vagina, in combination with a laparoscopic pelvic lymphadenectomy (*BJOG* 2001; **108**: 882). It is appropriate within Stage 1a(ii)–1b(i) provided the tumour is <20 mm in diameter. A cervical suture is inserted to help prevent preterm delivery [→ p.159]. *Radiotherapy ± chemotherapy* is then used after surgery if histological examination shows LN involvement or the excision margins are incomplete.

Radiotherapy and chemotherapy with no surgery: This is often reserved for the older or medically unfit woman. However, most women with larger tumours, e.g. > 1b(ii), will require more treatment than surgery anyway, and surgery before chemo-radiotherapy is associated with more complications.

Stage 2b and worse

These should be treated with radiotherapy with chemotherapy, e.g. platinum agents, the usage of which reduces recurrence and increases survival (*Lancet* 2001; **358**: 7810). Palliative radiotherapy is used for bone pain or haemorrhage. Occasionally, pelvic exenteration, involving removal of the bladder and/or rectum, is tried in the young, fit woman, with a central recurrence.

Stages of cervical carcinoma and treatment	
Stage	Treatment
1a(i)	Cone biopsy or simple hysterectomy
1a(ii)–2a	Radical hysterectomy ± chemo-radiotherapy or chemo-radiotherapy alone if >1b(ii)
2b and above	Chemo-radiotherapy alone

Indications for radiotherapy for cervical carcinoma
After surgery: if resection margins close or lymph node (LN) involvement (with chemotherapy)
As alternative to surgery (with chemotherapy)
Palliation for bone pain or haemorrhage

Prognosis

Patients are reviewed at 3 and 6 months and then every 6 months for 5 years. Recurrent disease is commonly central. Poor prognostic indicators are LN involvement, advanced clinical stage, large primary tumour, a poorly differentiated tumour and early recurrence. Death is commonly from uraemia due to ureteric obstruction.

Prognosis of cervical carcinoma	
Indicator	5-year survival (%)
Stage 1a	95
Stage 1b	80
Stage 2	60
Stage 3–4	10–30
Lymph nodes (LNs) involved	40
LNs clear	80
Overall	65

Further reading

Green JA, Kirwan JM, Tierney JF *et al.* Survival and recurrence after concomitant chemotherapy and

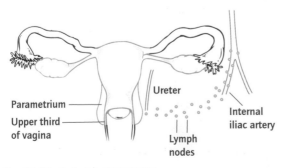

Fig. 4.9 Wertheim's hysterectomy.

Parametrium

Upper third of vagina

Ureter

Internal iliac artery

Lymph nodes

radiotherapy for cancer of the uterine cervix: a systematic review and meta-analysis. *Lancet* 2001; **358**: 781–6.

Nunns D, Symonds RP. Improving the prognosis in cervical cancer. In: Studd J, ed. *Progress in Obstetrics and Gynaecology* 2003; **15**: 317–31. RCOG Press.

Wright TC Jr, Cox JT, Massad LS, Twiggs LB, Wilkinson EJ. ASCCP-sponsored consensus conference: 2001 consensus guidelines for the management of women with cervical cytological abnormalities. *JAMA: the Journal of the American Medical Association* 2002; **287**: 2120–9.

Carcinoma of the Cervix at a Glance

Epidemiology	Becoming less common in the United Kingdom, deaths reducing
Pathology	90% squamous, also adenocarcinomas
Aetiology	Human papilloma virus (HPV), which is sexually transmitted, causing cervical intraepithelial neoplasia (CIN). Smoking, combined oral contraceptive, immunosuppression
Clinical features	None if occult. Postcoital (PCB) or intermenstrual bleeding (IMB), offensive discharge. Cervix initially appears normal, then ulcerated, then replaced by irregular mass
Screening	Routine use. Three-yearly cervical smears, colposcopy if abnormal
Investigations	Biopsy. Unless early, examination under anaesthetic (EUA), ± cystoscopy to stage. Chest X-ray, urea and electrolytes (U&E), full blood count (FBC), intravenous pyelogram (IVP)
Staging	**1** Cervix and uterus: 1a(i) <3 mm depth, <7 mm across; 1a(ii) <5 mm depth, <7 mm across; 1b rest **2** Upper vagina also: 2a not parametrium; 2b in parametrium **3** Lower vagina or pelvic wall, or ureteric obstruction **4** Into bladder or rectum, or beyond pelvis
Treatment	Depends on clinical stage: Microinvasion: Cone biopsy or simple hysterectomy Stage 1b–2a: Wertheim's hysterectomy then radiotherapy and chemotherapy if lymph nodes (LNs) positive or removal incomplete; consider radical trachelectomy *or* radiotherapy and chemotherapy without surgery Stage 2b–4: Radiotherapy and chemotherapy without surgery
Prognosis	Depends on LN involvement, clinical stage and histological grade Overall 65% 5-year survival

Cervical Intraepithelial Neoplasia (CIN) at a Glance

Definitions	Histological abnormality of the cervix in which abnormal epithelial cells occupy varying degrees of the squamous epithelium CIN I/mild dysplasia: Atypical cells in lower third CIN II/moderate dysplasia: Atypical cells in lower two-thirds CIN III/severe dysplasia: Atypical cells in full thickness (carcinoma *in situ*) Dyskaryosis: Describes cellular (nuclear) abnormality only from cervical smear. Suggests presence of CIN
Epidemiology	Becoming more common
Aetiology	As for cervical carcinoma
Diagnosis	No clinical features. Cervical smear abnormality and colposcopic abnormality suggests presence. Diagnosis confirmed histologically
Treatment	Rationale: to prevent progression to invasion CIN I usually observed; CIN II and III removed with large loop excision of transformation zone (LLETZ) This treats, and also identifies, hitherto unexpected invasion

Anatomy and function of the ovaries

The normal ovaries occupy the ovarian fossa on the lateral pelvic wall overlying the ureter, but are attached to the broad ligament by the mesovarium, to the pelvic side wall by the infundibulopelvic ligament and to the uterus by the ovarian ligament. Blood supply is from the ovarian artery, but there is an anastomosis with branches of the uterine artery in the broad ligament (Fig. 5.1).

The ovaries have an outer cortex covered by 'germinal' epithelium (*the most common carcinoma derives from this layer*). The inner medulla contains connective tissue and blood vessels. The cortex contains the follicles and theca cells. Oestrogen is secreted by granulosa cells in the growing follicles and also by theca cells. The rare tumours of these cells secrete oestrogens. A few follicles start to enlarge every month [→ p.9] under the influence of pituitary follicle-stimulating hormone (FSH), but only one will reach about 20 mm in size and rupture in mid-cycle to release its ovum (see Fig. 2.3). After ovulation, the collapsed follicle becomes a corpus luteum, which will continue to produce oestrogen and progesterone if fertilization occurs. Follicular and lutein cysts result from persistence of these structures.

Ovarian symptoms

Ovarian masses are often silent and detected either when they are very large and cause abdominal distension or on ultrasound scan. Acute presentation is associated with 'accidents'.

Ovarian cyst 'accidents'

Rupture of the contents of an ovarian cyst into the peritoneal cavity causes intense pain, particularly with an endometrioma or dermoid cyst (Fig. 5.2a). *Haemorrhage* into a cyst (Fig. 5.2b) or the peritoneal cavity often causes pain. Peritoneal cavity haemorrhage is occasionally so severe as to cause hypovolaemic shock. *Torsion* of the pedicle causes infarction and pain (Fig. 5.2c).

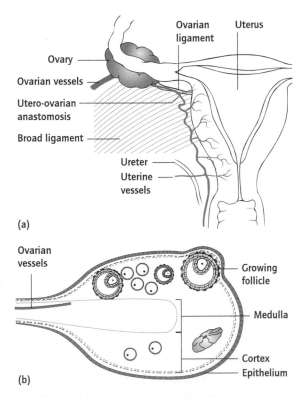

Fig. 5.1 Anatomy of the normal ovary. (a) Relations of the ovary; (b) transverse section of the normal ovary.

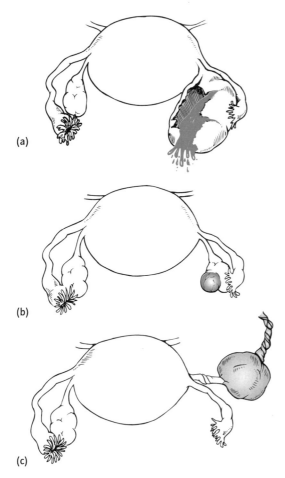

Fig. 5.2 (a) Rupture of an ovarian cyst. (b) Haemorrhage into an ovarian cyst (view from the abdomen). (c) Cyst twisting on its blood supply.

Disorders of ovarian function

Polycystic ovary syndrome (PCOS) is a common disorder that causes oligomenorrhoea, hirsutism and subfertility [→ p.70]. The 'cysts' are actually small multiple poorly developed follicles.

Premature menopause is when the last period is reached before the age of 45 years [→ p.88].

Problems of gonadal development include the gonadal dysgeneses, the most common of which is Turner's syndrome [→ p.15].

Classification of ovarian tumours

Primary neoplasms

These can be benign or malignant. They are classified together because a benign cyst may undergo malignant change. They fall into three main groups.

Epithelial tumours

Derived from the epithelium covering the ovary, these are most common in postmenopausal women. Uniquely, histology may demonstrate 'borderline' malignancy, when malignant histological features are present but invasion is not. Such tumours may become frankly malignant: surgery is advised but their optimum management is disputed.

Serous cystadenoma or adenocarcinoma: The malignant variety is the commonest malignant ovarian neoplasm (50% of malignancies). Benign and 'borderline' forms also exist.

Mucinous cystadenoma or adenocarcinoma can become very large and are less frequently malignant (10% of ovarian malignancies). A rare 'borderline' variant is pseudomyxoma peritonei, in which the abdominal cavity fills with gelatinous mucin secretions.

Endometrioid carcinoma: This malignant variant accounts for 25% of ovarian malignancies. It is similar histologically to endometrial carcinoma, with which it is associated in 20% of cases.

Clear cell carcinoma is a malignant variant that accounts for less than 10% of ovarian malignancies but has a particularly poor prognosis.

Brenner tumours are rare and usually small and benign.

Germ cell tumours

These originate from the undifferentiated primordial germ cells of the gonad.

Teratoma or dermoid cyst is a common benign tumour usually arising in young premenopausal women. It may contain fully differentiated tissue of all cell lines, commonly hair and teeth. They are commonly bilateral, seldom large and often asymptomatic. Rupture, however, is very painful. A malignant form, the solid teratoma, also occurs in this age group but is very rare.

Dysgerminoma is the female equivalent of the seminoma. Although rare, it is the commonest ovarian

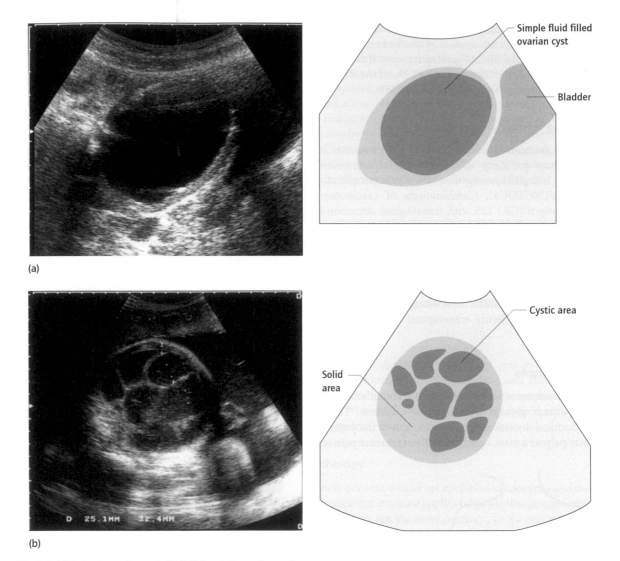

(a)

(b)

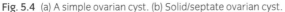

Fig. 5.4 (a) A simple ovarian cyst. (b) Solid/septate ovarian cyst.

monitoring tumour response to treatment. Liver function tests and a chest X-ray are performed. Paracentesis of ascites might spread the disease and is only used for palliation. Laparoscopy helps differentiate malignancy from other pelvic masses.

To establish fitness for surgery, blood is taken for full blood count (FBC), urea and electrolytes (U&E) and cross-match.

Management of suspected ovarian carcinoma

The diagnosis and histological type is only established with certainty after surgery, as prior biopsy is seldom practical. This disease is best managed in a cancer centre.

If malignancy is likely

Postmenopausal patients and premenopausal patients with almost certain malignancy undergo a *laparotomy* through a vertical incision (Fig. 5.5). The aim is to assess the stage and, if the disease is advanced, to remove as much tumour as possible (debulking). Total abdominal hysterectomy (TAH) with bilateral salpingo-oöphorectomy (BSO) and removal of the omentum should be performed. Bowel preparation is required.

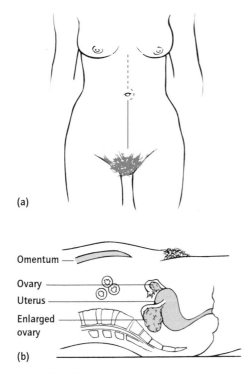

(a)

Omentum

Ovary

Uterus

Enlarged
ovary

(b)

Fig. 5.5 (a) Site of incision for suspected ovarian carcinoma (dotted line is potential extension if abdominal disease). (b) Laparotomy for ovarian carcinoma. The uterus, ovaries, omentum and as much of the affected tissue as possible are removed.

Ascites is sent for cytology, but peritoneal washing may spread early disease.

With very early stage or borderline disease in the woman who wants more children, the uterus and the unaffected ovary are preserved. This may be achieved laparoscopically. Meticulous follow up is required.

Chemotherapy is then normally given to all patients with epithelial carcinoma. In early stage disease, this increases survival from 74% to 82% at 5 years (*J Natl Cancer Inst* 2003; **95**: 125). Cisplatin or carboplatin are used, in conjunction with Taxol. Pegylated liposomal doxorubicin hydrochloride (PLDH) has a second-line role. A number of trials are currently assessing the value of different treatment options. If initially elevated, CA 125 levels can be used to monitor the response. The best results are seen when as little as possible of the tumour is left after surgery.

Radiotherapy is only used for dysgerminomas.

If malignancy is possible

This applies to premenopausal patients with a mass that warrants investigation because it is >5 cm or is persistent or growing. Laparoscopy is used. A simple functional cyst can be biopsied and drained laparoscopically; a dermoid cyst can be removed from the ovary (cystectomy). If the appearances prompt suspicions of malignancy a full laparotomy (as above) is needed.

Follow-up and prognosis

Levels of CA 125 are useful after as well as during chemotherapy. Computed tomography (CT) scanning aids detection of residual disease or relapse. Some centres perform a 'second look' laparoscopy or laparotomy to monitor response. Chemotherapy prolongs short-term survival and improves quality of life. Poor prognostic indicators are advanced stage, poorly differentiated tumours, clear cell tumours and poor response to chemotherapy. Death is commonly from bowel obstruction or perforation.

Prognosis of ovarian cancer	
Stage	5-year survival (%)
1a	80
1c	55
2	40
3 (most patients)	15
4	5
Overall	25

Palliative care

Only 30% of women are cured of their gynaecological carcinoma. Ovarian carcinoma causes the most deaths, but the principles outlined are applicable to all terminal disease.

Definition and aims

Palliative care is the active total care of the patient whose disease is incurable. The aim is to increase quality of life for the patient and her family. This involves addressing symptoms such as pain, nausea, bleeding and symptoms of intestinal obstruction, as well as meeting the patient's social, psychological and spiritual needs. Care therefore

6 Disorders of the Vulva and Vagina

Anatomy

The vulva is the area of skin that stretches from the labia majora laterally, to the mons pubis anteriorly and the perineum posteriorly. It overlaps with the vestibule, the area between the labia minora and the hymen, which surrounds the urethral and vaginal orifices. The vagina is 7–10 cm long. It is lined by squamous epithelium. Anteriorly lie the bladder and urethra. Posteriorly to the upper third is the pouch of Douglas (peritoneal cavity). The lower posterior wall is close to the rectum. Most lymph drainage occurs via the inguinal lymph nodes, which drain to the femoral and thence to the external iliac nodes of the pelvis (Fig. 6.1). This is a route for metastatic spread of carcinoma of the vulva.

Vulval symptoms

The most common vulval symptoms are *pruritus* (itching), *soreness*, *burning* and *superficial dyspareunia* (pain on sexual penetration). Symptoms can be due to local problems including infection, dermatological disease, malignant and premalignant disease, and the vulval pain syndromes. Skin disease affects the vulva, but rarely in isolation. Systemic disease may predispose to certain vulval conditions (e.g. candidiasis with diabetes mellitus).

Causes of pruritus vulvae

Infections:
Candidiasis (± vaginal discharge)
Vulval warts (condylomata acuminata)
Pubic lice, scabies

Dermatological disease:
Any condition, especially eczema, psoriasis, lichen simplex, lichen sclerosus, lichen planus, contact dermatitis

Neoplasia:
Carcinoma
Premalignant disease (vulvar intraepithelial neoplasia, VIN, III) [→ p.44]

Miscellaneous benign disorders of the vulva and vagina

Lichen simplex (Fig. 6.2)

There is a long history of vulval itching and soreness. The area, typically the labia majora, is inflamed and thickened with hyper- and hypo-pigmentation. Vulval biopsy is indicated if the diagnosis is in doubt. Irritants such as

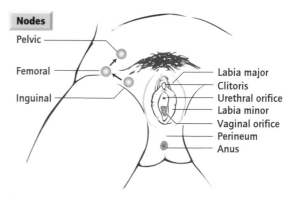

Fig. 6.1 Anatomy and lymph drainage of the vulva.

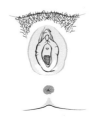

Fig. 6.2 Lichen simplex.

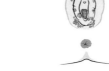

Fig. 6.3 Extensive vulval warts.

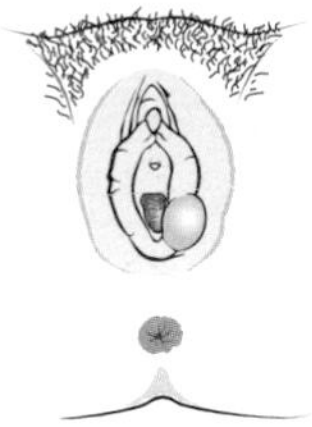

Fig. 6.4 Bartholin's abscess.

soap should be avoided; emollients, moderately potent steroid creams and antihistamines are used.

Lichen planus

Of unknown aetiology, this causes irritation with flat, papular purplish lesions in the anogenital area, but can affect hair, nails and mucous membranes. Treatment is with high potency steroid creams; surgery should be avoided.

Lichen sclerosus

The vulval epithelium is thin with loss of collagen. This may have an autoimmune basis and thyroid disease and vitiligo may coexist. The typical patient is postmenopausal, but much younger women are occasionally affected. Pruritus and soreness are usual. The appearance is of pink–white papules, which coalesce to form parchment-like skin with fissures. Atypical cells are found in 5% of cases. Biopsy is important to exclude atypia and to confirm the diagnosis. Treatment is with the ultra-potent topical steroids.

Vulvar dysesthesia or the vulval pain syndromes

These are diagnoses of exclusion, with no evidence of organic vulval disease. They are now divided into provoked or spontaneous vulvar dysesthesia and subdivided according to site: local (e.g. vestibular) or generalized. They are associated with many factors including a history of genital tract infections (*Infect Dis Obstet Gynecol* 2002; **10**: 193), former use of oral contraceptives and psychosexual disorders. Spontaneous generalized vulvar dysesthesia (formerly essential vulvodynia) describes a burning pain that is more common in older patients. Vulvar dysethesia of the vestibule causes superficial dyspareunia or pain using tampons and is more

common in younger women, in whom introital damage must be excluded. For both conditions, topical agents are seldom helpful and tricyclic antidepressants are sometimes used.

Infections of the vulva and vestibule

Herpes simplex, vulval warts (condylomata acuminata) (Fig. 6.3), syphilis and donovanosis may all affect the vulva [→ p.63]. Candidiasis may affect the vulva if there has been prolonged exposure to moisture. Candidiasis is common in diabetics, in pregnancy, when antibiotics have been used or when immunity is compromised.

Bartholin's gland cyst and abscess

The two glands behind the labia minora secrete lubricating mucus for coitus. Blockage of the duct causes cyst formation. If infection occurs, commonly with *Staphylococcus* or *Escherichia coli*, an abscess forms (Fig. 6.4). This is acutely painful and a large tender red swelling is evident. Treatment is with incision and drainage, and marsupialization, whereby the incision is sutured open to prevent re-formation.

Introital damage

This commonly follows childbirth. Overtightening, or

incorrect apposition at perineal repair, or extensive scar tissue commonly present with superficial dyspareunia. Symptoms often resolve with time. If the introitus is too tight, vaginal dilators or surgery (Fenton's repair) are used.

Vaginal cysts

Congenital cysts commonly arise in the vagina (Fig. 6.5). They have a smooth white appearance, can be as large as a golf ball, and are often mistaken for a prolapse. They seldom cause symptoms, but if there is dyspareunia they should be excised.

Vaginal adenosis

When columnar epithelium is found in the normally squamous epithelium of the vagina it is called vaginal adenosis. It commonly occurs in women whose mothers received diethylstilboestrol in pregnancy, when it is associated with genital tract anomalies. Spontaneous resolution is usual, but it very occasionally turns malignant (clear cell carcinoma of the vagina). It may also occur secondarily to trauma.

Vaginal wall prolapse and vaginal discharge are discussed in Chapters 7 and 10, respectively.

Premalignant disease of the vulva: vulvar intraepithelial neoplasia (VIN)

Vulvar intraepithelial neoplasia is the presence of atypical cells in the vulval epithelium. It is graded VIN I–III in a manner similar to cervical intraepithelial neoplasia (CIN) [→ p.28]. VIN III is carcinoma *in situ* (previously known as Bowen's disease) with atypical cells in the full epithelial thickness. It is becoming more common,

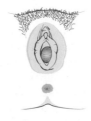

Fig. 6.5 Congenital vaginal cyst.

especially in young women, is often multifocal and can progress (in 5–10% of cases) to invasive cancer. It is associated with the oncogenic human papilloma viruses (HPVs) [→ p.62], with smoking, with lichen sclerosus and squamous hyperplasia of the vulva. Pruritus or pain are common; lesions can be seen by the naked eye as papular, usually white, areas. Colposcopy is helpful, but biopsy is essential to confirm the diagnosis.

Management is to alleviate symptoms and to exclude and observe for malignant change. Symptomatic VIN III is treated with local excision, laser therapy or topical chemotherapy (e.g. imiquimod), although the recurrence rate is 30%. In the long term, serial examination and biopsy of suspicious areas is required.

Carcinoma of the vulva

Epidemiology

Carcinoma of the vulva accounts for 5% of genital tract cancers, with up to 1000 new cases each year in the United Kingdom. It is most common after the age of 60 years.

Pathology

Ninety-five per cent of vulval malignancies are squamous cell carcinomas. Melanomas, basal cell carcinomas, adenocarcinomas and a variety of others, including sarcomas, account for the rest.

Aetiology

Although VIN III is a premalignant stage of squamous carcinoma, carcinoma often arises *de novo*.

Clinical features

History: The patient experiences pruritus, bleeding or a discharge, or may find a mass, but malignancy often presents late as lesions go unnoticed or cause embarrassment.

Examination: This will reveal an ulcer or mass, most commonly on the labia majora or clitoris (Fig. 6.6). The inguinal lymph nodes may be enlarged, hard and immobile.

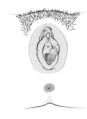

Fig. 6.6 Vulval carcinoma.

Spread and staging

Fifty per cent of patients present with Stage I disease. Vulval carcinoma spreads locally and via the lymph drainage of the vulva. Spread is to the superficial and then to the deep inguinal nodes, and thence to the femoral and subsequently external iliac nodes (see Fig. 6.1). Contralateral spread may occur.

Staging is surgical and histological (i.e. after surgery).

Spread and staging for carcinoma of the vulva	
Stage I	Tumour is <2 cm in diameter; no nodes are involved
Ia	Stromal invasion <1 mm
Ib	Stromal invasion >1 mm
Stage II	Tumour is >2 cm in diameter; no nodes are involved
Stage III	Tumour has spread beyond the vulva or perineum, to urethra, vagina or anus. Or nodes are involved on one side only
Stage IV	Tumour is in rectum, bladder, bone or distant metastases. And/or nodes are involved bilaterally

Investigations

To establish the diagnosis and histological type, a biopsy is taken.

To assess fitness for surgery, a chest X-ray, electrocardiogram (ECG), full blood count (FBC) and renal function are required, as these patients are usually elderly. Blood is cross-matched.

Treatment

For Stage Ia(i) disease, wide local excision is adequate.
For other stages, wide local excision and groin lymphadenectomy through separate 'skin sparing' incisions (Fig. 6.7) is performed. If the tumour does not extend to

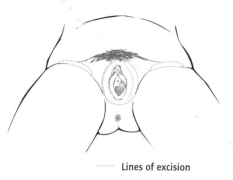

······· Lines of excision

Fig. 6.7 Skin sparing and separate incisions for a vulvectomy.

within 2 cm of the mid-line, unilateral excision and lymphadenectomy only are used. This approach has largely replaced the traditional 'radical vulvectomy'. Complications include wound breakdown, infection, leg lymphoedema, and sexual and body image problems. *Radiotherapy* instead of surgery has a lower morbidity but recurrence rates are increased (*Cochrane* 2001: CD002224); although seldom used as primary therapy, it is appropriate in those unfit for surgery. After surgery, however, it may reduce local recurrence risk and is also given if lymph nodes are positive.

Prognosis

Many of these patients die from other diseases related to their age. Survival at 5 years in Stage I is > 90%; in Stages III–IV the figure is 40%.

Malignancies of the vagina

Secondary vaginal carcinoma is common and arises from local infiltration from cervix, endometrium or vulva, or from metastatic spread from cervix, endometrium or gastrointestinal tumours.

Primary carcinoma of the vagina accounts for 2% of genital tract malignancies, affects older women and is usually squamous. Presentation is with bleeding or discharge and a mass or ulcer is evident. Treatment is with intravaginal radiotherapy or, occasionally, radical surgery. The average survival at 5 years is 50%.

Clear cell adenocarcinoma of the vagina is most common in the late teenage years. Most are a rare complication of maternal ingestion of diethylstilboestrol in pregnancy.

With radical surgery and radiotherapy, survival rates are good.

Further reading

De Hullu JA, Hollema H, Lolkema S *et al*. Vulvar carcinoma. The price of less radical surgery. *Cancer* 2002; **95**: 2331–8.

Edwards A, Wojnarowska F. The vulval pain syndromes. *International Journal of STD & AIDS* 1998; **9**: 74–8.

Powell JJ, Wojnarowska F. Lichen sclerosus. *Lancet* 1999; **353**: 1777–83.

Carcinoma of the Vulva at a Glance

Epidemiology	1000 cases per year in United Kingdom. Age >60 years
Aetiology	Vulvar intraepithelial neoplasia (VIN) III and oncogenic human papilloma viruses (HPVs)
Pathology	95% squamous cell carcinomas
Features	Pruritus, bleeding, discharge, mass
Spread	Local and lymph
Staging	I: <2 cm, no nodes: 1a stromal invasion <1 mm; 1b >1 mm II: >2 cm, no nodes III: Beyond vulva or unilateral nodes IV: In rectum/bone/bladder and/or bilateral nodes
Treatment	Biopsy, then wide local excision with separate groin node dissection, bilateral unless tumour >2 cm from mid-line Radiotherapy if lymph nodes involved
Prognosis	>90% 5-year survival in Stage I; 40% in Stages III–IV

Prolapse of the Uterus and Vagina

Prolapse is descent of the uterus and/or vaginal walls within the vagina. Behind the vaginal walls, other pelvic organs descend and therefore produce a form of hernia.

Anatomy and physiology of the pelvic supports

The transverse cervical (cardinal) ligaments and the *uterosacral ligaments* are the most important (Fig. 7.1). These attach to the cervix and suspend the uterus from the pelvic side wall and sacrum respectively; the upper vagina is also suspended. Laxity of these ligaments allows the uterus to prolapse and with it the upper vagina.

The levator ani muscle forms the floor of the pelvis from attachments on the bony pelvic walls and incorporates the perineal body in the perineum. The levator ani suspends the mid-vagina, urethra and rectum, which pass through it. Levator weakness allows prolapse of the vaginal walls and bladder or rectum. The round ligament has little role.

Types of prolapse

Uterine and vaginal prolapse often occur together as the causes are similar.

The uterus: Uterine prolapse (Fig. 7.2b) is graded 1–3. In first-degree prolapse, the cervix is still within the vagina. Second-degree prolapse is at the introitus, and in third-degree prolapse (procidentia) the entire uterus comes out of the vagina. If the uterus has been removed, the *vault*, or top of the vagina where the uterus used to be, can prolapse. This inverts the vagina.

The anterior vaginal wall: A *cystocoele* (Fig. 7.2c) is prolapse of the bladder forming a bulge in the anterior vaginal wall. A *urethrocoele* is when the 4 cm long urethra bulges in the lower anterior wall.

The posterior vaginal wall: A *rectocoele* (Fig. 7.2d) is a prolapse of the rectum forming a bulge in the middle of the posterior wall. An *enterocoele* (Fig. 7.2e) is a prolapse of the pouch of Douglas, i.e. peritoneal cavity, bulging into the posterior vaginal wall just behind the uterus. It usually contains small bowel. The perineum may

<table>
<tr><td>Gynaecological prolapses</td></tr>
<tr><td>Uterine
Anterior wall: bladder (cystocoele) and/or urethra (urethrocoele)
Posterior wall: rectum (rectocoele) and/or pouch of Douglas (enterocoele)
Vaginal vault</td></tr>
</table>

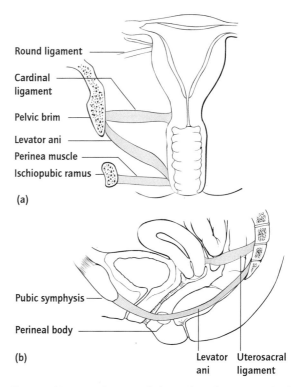

Fig. 7.1 (a) Coronal view of the pelvis showing cardinal ligaments and the levator ani. (b) Lateral view of the pelvis showing the uterosacral ligaments and levator ani.

also be deficient, in that the posterior vaginal opening is lax.

Epidemiology

Half of all parous women have some degree of prolapse and 10–20% seek medical attention.

Aetiology of prolapse
Weakened support of pelvic organs
Vaginal delivery is the most important. It can cause both mechanical and neurological (pudendal nerve) injury. Further deliveries often worsen the problem. Prolonged labour, forceps delivery, poor suturing of obstetric tears and bearing down before full dilatation are risk factors. *Oestrogen deficiency* after menopause causes partial atrophy of the pelvic supports and vaginal walls. *Iatrogenic* prolapse can follow hysterectomy as an inadequately supported vaginal vault will prolapse. *Genetic* predisposition to prolapse may be due to familial collagen weakness.

Increased strain on the supports
Obesity produces extra weight on the pelvic supports and they may weaken. *Pelvic masses* and a *chronic cough* have the same effect.

Causes of prolapse
Childbirth
Oestrogen deficiency
Obesity and chronic cough
Congenital weakness
Pelvic masses

Clinical features

History: Symptoms are often absent, but a dragging sensation or the sensation of a lump are common, usually worse at the end of the day or when standing up. Back pain is unusual. Severe prolapse interferes with intercourse, may ulcerate and cause bleeding or discharge. A cystocoele can cause urinary frequency and incomplete bladder emptying. Stress incontinence [→ p.52] is common, but it may be incidental. A rectocoele often causes no symptoms, but occasionally causes difficulty in defaecating.

Examination includes the chest and the abdomen. Bimanual examination will exclude pelvic masses. A large prolapse is visible from the outside (Fig. 7.3). A Sims' speculum [→ p.6] allows separate inspection of the anterior and posterior vaginal walls: the patient is asked to bear down to demonstrate prolapse. An enterocoele may be mistaken for a rectocoele, but a finger in the rectum will be seen to bulge into a rectocoele but not into an enterocoele, which does not contain rectum. Large polyps and vaginal cysts may be mistaken for a prolapse. Stress incontinence should be sought with the prolapse temporarily reduced.

Symptoms of prolapse
Often asymptomatic
General: Dragging sensation, lump
Cystocoele: Urinary frequency, incontinence
Rectocoele: Occasional difficulty in defaecating

Investigations

To look for a cause a pelvic ultrasound is often performed. Cystometry [→ p.52] is required if incontinence is the principal complaint.
To assess fitness for surgery (if appropriate) an electrocardiogram (ECG), chest X-ray, full blood count (FBC) and renal function may be required, as the women are often elderly.

Prevention

Prevention involves recognition of obstructed labour, adequate suturing of perineal lacerations and the avoidance of an excessively long second stage. Pelvic floor exercises after childbirth are encouraged.

Management

Treatment must be to alleviate symptoms and small prolapses often require no treatment. *Weight reduction* is often appropriate. Smoking is discouraged. *Physiotherapy* helps moderate degrees of prolapse and reduces the stress incontinence that may be associated.

Pessaries
These are used in the patient who is unwilling or unfit

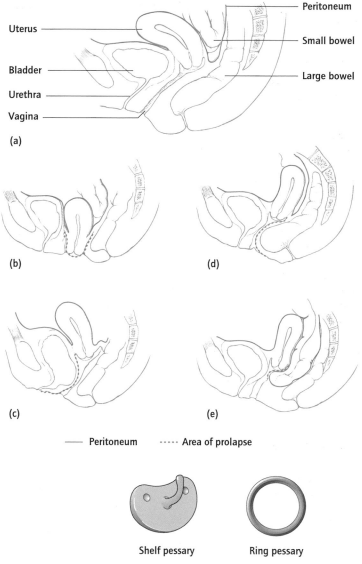

Fig. 7.2 Types of prolapse. (a) Normal pelvis, (b) uteric prolapse, (c) cystocoele, (d) rectocoele, (e) enterocoele.

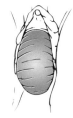

Fig. 7.3 Appearance of cystocoele.

Shelf pessary **Ring pessary**

Fig. 7.4 Pessaries for uterovaginal prolapse. (a) Shelf pessary; (b) ring pessary.

for surgery. They act like an artificial pelvic floor, placed in the vagina to stay behind the symphysis pubis and in front of the sacrum. The most commonly used is the ring pessary, but the shelf pessary is more effective for severe forms of prolapse (Fig. 7.4). They are changed every 9–12 months; topical oestrogen is used to prevent ulceration of the vagina. Occasionally

they cause pain, urinary retention or infection, or fall out.

Surgical treatment
Prolapse may kink the urethra, masking stress incontinence. As repair could precipitate incontinence, concomitant surgery for stress incontinence may be required. For major degrees of uterine descent, *vaginal*

hysterectomy will give the best results. A *sacrohysteropexy*, attaching the uterus to the sacrum, can be performed if the uterus is to be conserved (*BJOG* 2001; **108**: 629). Vaginal vault prolapse can be repaired vaginally with *sacrospinous suspension* by suspension to the sacrospinous ligament. Complications include nerve or vessel injury, infection and buttock pain. The abdominal route involves a *sacrocolpopexy*, by fixation to the sacrum using a mesh (*BJOG* 2000; **107**: 1371). Complications include mesh erosion and haemorrhage. *Anterior* and *posterior 'repairs'* are used for the relevant prolapse but, as several prolapses may occur in one patient, these operations are often combined. If genuine stress incontinence is present, the *Burch colposuspension* or the *tension-free vaginal tape* procedure [→ p.105] may be performed at the same time.

Prolapse: treatment options
Do nothing
Physiotherapy
Pessaries
Surgery

Further reading

Carey MP, Dwyer PL. Genital prolapse: vaginal versus abdominal route of repair. *Current Opinion in Obstetrics & Gynecology* 2001; **13**: 499–505.

Thakar R, Stanton S. Management of genital prolapse. *BMJ (Clinical Research Ed.)* 2002; **324**: 1258–62.

Genital Prolapse at a Glance

Definition	Descent of vaginal walls and pelvic organs within the vagina
Types	Anterior wall (bladder) is a cystocoele Posterior wall is a rectocoele (rectum) or enterocoele (pouch of Douglas) Uterine prolapse graded 1–3, depending on descent Vault prolapse after hysterectomy
Epidemiology	Very common; older multiparous women
Aetiology	Pregnancy and vaginal delivery, oestrogen deficiency, obesity, chronic cough, pelvic masses, surgery, iatrogenic (vault)
Features	Dragging sensation or lump coming down Bulge of vaginal wall visible from outside or with Sims' speculum
Prevention	Improved management of labour
Treatment	General: Lose weight, treat chest problems inc. smoking Pessaries: Ring or shelf, if frail. Change 9–12 monthly Surgery: Vaginal hysterectomy for uterine prolapse, anterior repair for cystocoele, posterior repair for rectocoele. Consider surgery for genuine stress incontinence

Disorders of the Urinary Tract

Anatomy and function of the female urinary system

Voluntary control of urine release is achieved by the bladder and urethra. The ureters bring urine to the bladder from the kidneys and enter the bladder obliquely. The bladder has a smooth muscle wall (detrusor muscle) and can normally 'store' about 400 mL of urine, although the normal first urge to void is at about 200 mL. It is drained by the urethra. This is about 4 cm long and has a muscular wall and an external orifice in the vestibule just above the vaginal introitus.

Neural control of the bladder and urethra

Parasympathetic nerves aid voiding; sympathetic nerves prevent it. The voiding reflex consists of afferent fibres, which respond to distension of the bladder wall and pass to the spinal cord. Efferent parasympathetic fibres pass back to the detrusor muscle and cause contraction. They also enable opening of the bladder neck. Meanwhile, efferent sympathetic fibres to the detrusor muscle are inhibited. This 'micturition reflex' is controlled at the level of the pons. The cerebral cortex modifies the reflex and can relax or contract the pelvic floor and the striated muscle of the urethra.

Continence

Continence is dependent on the pressure in the urethra being greater than that in the bladder (Fig. 8.1). Bladder pressure is influenced by detrusor pressure and external (intra-abdominal) pressure. Urethral pressure is influenced by the inherent urethral muscle tone and also by external pressure, namely the pelvic floor and, normally, intra-abdominal pressure. The detrusor muscle is expandable: as the bladder fills, there is no increase in pres-

sure. Increases in abdominal pressure such as coughing will be transmitted equally to the bladder and upper urethra because both lie within the abdomen. Normally, therefore, coughing does not alter the pressure difference and does not lead to incontinence.

Micturition

Micturition results when bladder pressure exceeds urethral pressure. This is achieved voluntarily by a simultaneous drop in urethral pressure (partly due to pelvic floor relaxation) and an increase in bladder pressure due to a detrusor muscle contraction.

Incontinence

This can be due to:
1 Uncontrolled increases in detrusor pressure increasing bladder pressure beyond that of the normal urethra. 'Overactive bladder', previously called 'detrusor instability' is the most common cause of this mechanism.

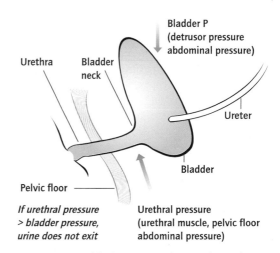

Fig. 8.1 Anatomy of the lower urinary tract and contributors to bladder and urethral pressure.

2 Increased intra-abdominal pressure transmitted to bladder but not urethra, because the upper urethra neck has slipped from the abdomen. Bladder pressure therefore exceeds urethral pressure when intra-abdominal pressure is raised, for example when coughing. 'Genuine stress incontinence' (GSI) is the most common cause of this mechanism.

3 Urine may bypass the sphincter mechanism altogether through a fistula.

Urinary symptoms	
Urgency:	A severe desire to void
Frequency:	Micturition more than six times a day
Nocturia:	Micturition more than once a night
Nocturnal enuresis:	Incontinence during sleep
Stress incontinence:	Incontinence with raised intra-abdominal pressure
Urge incontinence:	Incontinence with urgency

Investigation of the urinary tract

Urine microscopy, culture and sensitivity (MC&S). A midstream urine (MSU) sample is essential whenever a patient presents with urinary symptoms. Microscopy will detect white blood cells and organisms quickly. Culture will confirm infection and the type of organism. Sensitivity of the organism to different antibiotics is tested.

Urinalysis. Leucocytes, and particularly nitrites, suggest the presence of infection. Glycosuria and haematuria can be detected: diabetes and bladder carcinoma or calculi can cause urinary symptoms.

Urinary diary. The patient keeps a record for a week of the time and volume of fluid intake and micturition. This gives invaluable information about drinking habits, frequency and bladder capacity.

Post-micturition ultrasound or catheterization. These exclude chronic retention of urine.

Urodynamic studies. These are necessary prior to surgery for GSI. Urodynamics may be performed with or without video imaging and includes the following tests:

Cystometry. This measures detrusor pressure whilst the bladder is filled and provoked with coughing. Transducers are placed in the rectum to measure abdominal pressure and in the bladder to measure intravesical pressure (Fig. 8.2). As bladder pressure is the sum of abdominal pressure and detrusor pressure, detrusor activity can be automatically calculated by subtracting the abdominal pressure from the bladder pressure.

The detrusor pressure does not normally alter with filling or provocation (raised intra-abdominal pressure). If leaking occurs with coughing in the absence of a detrusor contraction, then the problem is likely to be GSI. If an involuntary detrusor contraction occurs, 'overactive bladder' is diagnosed. Initially the patient experiences urgency and then incontinence if bladder pressure is increased beyond that of the urethra. As both these conditions (see below) cause the *symptom* of stress incontinence, but their treatments are very different, cystometry is essential to the management of incontinence.

Urethral pressure profile. Measurement of maximum urethral closure pressure with a urethral tranducer identifies women with a low pressure for whom retropubic surgery for GSI will be less successful.

Uroflowmetry. Poor voiding rates identify women likely to develop voiding problems after surgery for GSI.

Intravenous pyelogram (IVP). This is useful for assessment and localization of fistulae and filling defects, and in women with recurrent infections or haematuria.

Methylene dye test. Blue dye is instilled into the bladder. Dye leakage from places other than the urethra, i.e. fistulae, can be seen.

Cystoscopy. Inspection of the bladder cavity is useful to exclude tumours, stones and fistulae but gives little indication of bladder performance.

Genuine stress incontinence

Definition

This is defined as involuntary loss of urine when bladder pressure exceeds maximum urethral pressure in the absence of a detrusor (bladder muscle) contraction. The diagnosis can only be made with certainty after excluding an overactive bladder using cystometry (Fig. 8.2).

Epidemiology

Genuine stress incontinence accounts for almost 50% of causes of incontinence in the female and occurs to varying degrees in more than 10% of all women.

Aetiology

Important causes of GSI include pregnancy and vaginal delivery, particularly prolonged labour and forceps de-

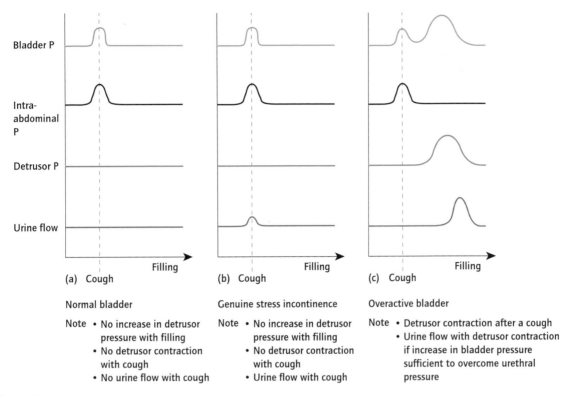

Fig. 8.2 Cystometry.

---

livery, obesity and age (particularly postmenopausal). Prolapse commonly coexists but is not always related.

Mechanism of incontinence

When there is an increase in intra-abdominal pressure ('stress'), the bladder is compressed and its pressure rises. In the normal woman, the bladder neck is equally compressed so that the pressure difference is unchanged. If, however, the bladder neck has slipped below the pelvic floor because its supports are weak, it will not be compressed and its pressure remains unchanged (Fig. 8.3). If the rest of the urethra and the pelvic floor are unable to compensate, the bladder pressure exceeds urethral pressure and incontinence results.

Clinical features

History: This must assess the degree to which the patient's life is disrupted. Stress incontinence predominates, but many patients also complain of frequency, urgency or urge incontinence. It is important to have

the patient prioritise her symptoms as the treatment for GSI differs from that for the overactive bladder. Faecal incontinence [→ p.228], also due to childbirth injury, may coexist.

Examination with a Sims' speculum often, but not invariably, reveals a cystocoele and urethrocoele. Leakage of urine with coughing will be seen. The abdomen is palpated to exclude a distended bladder.

Investigations

Urine culture is important to exclude infection. Cystometry (Fig. 8.2b) is required to exclude overactive bladder if surgery is contemplated.

Management

If obese, the patient is encouraged to lose weight. Causes of a chronic cough (e.g. smoking) are addressed.

Conservative
Conservative treatment is aimed at strengthening the

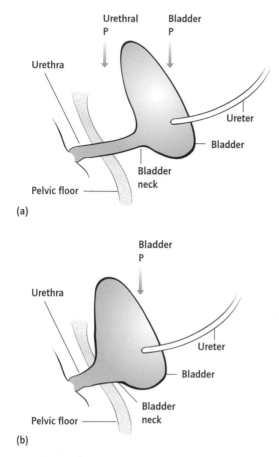

Fig. 8.3 (a) Normal bladder neck. (b) Bladder neck in genuine stress incontinence (GSI).

pelvic floor. Physiotherapy (pelvic floor exercises) or vaginal 'cones' or sponges alleviate incontinence adequately in more than half of patients. The 'cones' are inserted into the vagina and held in position by voluntary muscle contraction. Increasing sizes are used as muscle strength increases.

Surgery

This is only performed after cystometry has excluded an overactive bladder. The primary aim is to allow transmission of raised intra-abdominal pressure to the bladder neck as well as the bladder. The best procedures are the *Burch colposuspension* and the *tension-free vaginal tape (TVT)* [→ p.105], with up to 90% cure rates. The latter is newer, and therefore long-term data are lacking. However, the TVT procedure is less invasive and can be performed under spinal or local anaesthesia and requires

a shorter hospital stay. Both operations can cause bleeding, infection, voiding difficulty and *de novo* overactive bladder, although these are less common after the TVT (*Neurourol Urodyn* 2000; **19**: 386). With low urethral pressures, or in the very elderly, periurethral injections of collagen have a limited role. Operations such as the anterior repair and the Stamey procedure are no longer recommended for GSI.

Distinction between genuine stress incontinence (GSI) and stress incontinence

Genuine stress incontinence (GSI) is a *disorder* diagnosed only after cystometry, of which stress incontinence is the major symptom

Stress incontinence is a *symptom*: 'I leak when I cough'. It can be due to GSI, but it may also be the result of overactive bladder or overflow incontinence

---

Overactive bladder (previously detrusor instability)

Definition

This is involuntary urine loss due to uninhibited detrusor contractions either on provocation or spontaneously (Fig. 8.2c) when the patient is trying to inhibit micturition.

Epidemiology

Overactive bladder causes 35% of cases of female incontinence.

Aetiology

It is most commonly idiopathic. The condition can follow operations for GSI and is then probably the result of bladder neck obstruction. It is common in patients with multiple sclerosis. If a neurological disorder is present, the term neurogenic detrusor overactivity or detrusor hyper-reflexia is used: interference with cortical inhibition of the reflex arc causes uninhibited detrusor contractions.

Mechanism of incontinence

The detrusor contraction is normally felt as urgency. If strong enough, it causes the bladder pressure to overcome the urethral pressure and the patient leaks: urge incontinence. This can occur spontaneously or with provocation, for example, with a rise in intra-abdominal pressure or a running tap. Coughing may therefore lead to incontinence.

Clinical features

History: Urgency and urge incontinence, frequency and nocturia are usual. Stress incontinence is common. Some patients leak at night or at orgasm. A history of childhood enuresis is common, as is faecal urgency.
Examination is often normal, but an incidental cystocoele may be present.

Investigations

The urinary diary will show frequent passage of small volumes of urine, particularly at night. Cystometry demonstrates detrusor contractions on filling or provocation (Fig. 8.2c). Occasionally, the bladder pressure merely rises steadily with filling.

Treatment of overactive bladder

Tolterodine and *oxybutynin* relax smooth muscle in the bladder and are anticholinergic. Equally effective (*Cochrane* 2002: CD003781), the side-effect profile, principally a dry mouth, is better with tolterodine. *Bladder drill* involves retraining of the bladder. Instead of voiding at first desire, the patient voids by the clock at increasing intervals. Evidence regarding its effectiveness is poor (*Cochrane* 2000: CD001308). *Synthetic antidiuretic hormone* reduces urine production and can be used for nocturnal symptoms. Very severe and resistant symptoms may be helped by surgery: by *clam augmentation ileocystoplasty*.

Causes of incontinence

Genuine stress incontinence (GSI)	50%
Overactive bladder	35.0%
Mixed	10.0%
Overflow incontinence	1.0%
Fistulae	0.3%
Unknown	4.0%

Causes of urgency and frequency

Urinary infection
Bladder pathology
Pelvic mass compressing the bladder
Sensory urgency
Overactive bladder
Genuine stress incontinence (GSI)

Other urinary disorders

'Mixed' GSI and overactive bladder

This accounts for about 10% of all cases of incontinence. The diagnosis is made at cystometry. The overactive bladder is treated first.

Acute urinary retention

The patient is unable to pass urine for 12 h or more, catheterization producing as much or more urine than the normal bladder capacity. It is painful, except when due to epidural anaesthesia or failure of the afferent pathways. Causes include childbirth, particularly with an epidural, vulval or perineal pain (e.g. herpes simplex), surgery, drugs such as anticholinergics, the retroverted gravid uterus, pelvic masses and neurological disease (e.g. multiple sclerosis or cerebrovascular accident). Catheterization is maintained for 48 h whilst the cause is treated.

Chronic retention and urinary overflow

This accounts for only 1% of cases of incontinence. Leaking occurs because bladder overdistension eventually causes overflow. It can be due to either urethral obstruction or detrusor inactivity. Pelvic masses and incontinence surgery are common causes of urethral obstruction. Autonomic neuropathies (e.g. diabetes) and previous overdistension of the bladder (e.g. unrecognised acute retention after epidural anaesthesia) [→ p.203] cause detrusor inactivity. Presentation may mimic stress incontinence or urinary loss may be continuous. Examination reveals a distended nontender bladder. The diagnosis is confirmed by ultrasound or catheterization after micturition. Intermittent self-catheterization is commonly required.

Sensory urgency

The patient experiences urgency, frequency and nocturia and has a reduced bladder capacity, but the detrusor muscle is not overactive. It is seldom associated with incontinence, but is common in postmenopausal women. Bladder stones, infections and tumours, interstitial cystitis (frequency, urgency and pain, a low-capacity hypersensitive bladder, mucosal haemorrhages and tearing on bladder distention) or psychological factors may be implicated. Cystometry (to exclude overactive bladder), cystoscopy, urinalysis and sometimes an IVP are indicated. Treatment is of any underlying disorder: if none is found, hormone replacement therapy and the bladder drill have been used. Repair of a cystocoele may help.

Fistulae

These are abnormal connections between the urinary tract and other organs (Fig. 8.4). The most common are the vesico- and urethro-vaginal fistulae. In the developing world they are common as a result of obstructed labour: in the West they are rare and usually due to surgery, radiotherapy or malignancy. Whilst small fistulae may resolve spontaneously, surgery is usually required, the timing depending on the site and the cause.

Further reading

Bidmead J, Cardozo L. What's new in urogynaecology?

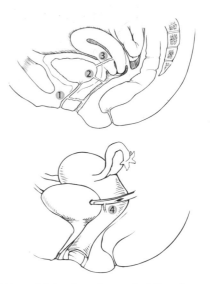

Fig. 8.4 Urinary fistulae: 1, urethro-vaginal; 2, vesico-vaginal; 3, vesico-terine; 4, uretero-vaginal.

Trends in Urology Gynaecology and Sexual Health 2003; **8**: 24–7.

Dwyer PL, Rosamilia A. Evaluation and diagnosis of the overactive bladder. *Clinical Obstetrics and Gynecology* 2002; **45**: 193–204.

Thakar R, Stanton S. Regular review: management of urinary incontinence in women. *BMJ (Clinical Research Ed.)* 2000; **321**: 1326–31.

www.continence-foundation.org.uk

Genuine Stress Incontinence (GSI) at a Glance	
Definition	Leakage of urine with raised bladder pressure in the absence of a detrusor contraction
Epidemiology	10% of women, varying severity. More common with age
Aetiology	Childbirth and the menopause
Clinical features	Stress incontinence, also frequency and urgency. Prolapse common
Investigations	Mid-stream urine (MSU); diary; cystometry essential for definitive diagnosis
Treatment	Conservative: Physiotherapy
	Surgical: Colposuspension or tension-free vaginal tape (TVT)

9 Endometriosis and Chronic Pelvic Pain

Endometriosis

Definition and epidemiology

Endometriosis is the presence and growth of tissue similar to endometrium outside the uterus. Some 1–2% of women are diagnosed as having endometriosis, but endometriotic lesions may occur in 1–20% of all women, albeit asymptomatically in most. It is more common in nulliparous women, particularly between the age of 30 and 45 years.

Pathology

Endometriosis, like normal endometrium, is oestrogen dependent: it regresses after the menopause and during pregnancy. It can occur throughout the pelvis, particularly in the uterosacral ligaments, and on or behind the ovaries (Fig. 9.1). Occasionally it affects the umbilicus or abdominal wound scars, the vagina, bladder, rectum and even the lungs. Accumulated altered blood is dark brown and can form a 'chocolate cyst' or endometrioma in the ovaries. Endometriosis causes inflammation, with progressive fibrosis and adhesions. In its most severe form, the entire pelvis is 'frozen', the pelvic organs rendered immobile by adhesions. Symptoms, particularly pain, correlate poorly with the extent of the disease.

Aetiology

Endometriosis in the pelvis is probably a result of retrograde menstruation. More distant foci may result from mechanical, lymphatic or blood-borne spread. As retrograde menstruation is common, but is not always associated with endometriosis, unknown individual factors appear to determine whether the retrograde menstrual endometrium implants and grows. A currently less pop-ular theory is that endometriosis is the result of metaplasia of coelomic cells. It is also not understood why symptoms correlate poorly with the extent of the disease.

Clinical features

History: Symptoms are often absent, but endometriosis is an important cause of chronic pelvic pain. This is usually cyclical. Presenting complaints include dysmenorrhoea before the onset of menstruation, deep dyspareunia, subfertility and, occasionally, menstrual problems. Rupture of a chocolate cyst causes acute pain, and this may be the first symptom. Cyclical haematuria, rectal bleeding or bleeding from the umbilicus are rare.

Examination: Common findings on vaginal examination are tenderness and/or thickening behind the uterus or in the adnexa. In advanced cases, the uterus is retroverted and immobile. With mild, asymptomatic endometriosis the pelvis often feels normal.

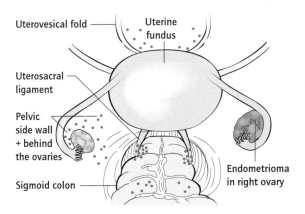

Fig. 9.1 Common sites of endometriosis in the pelvis.

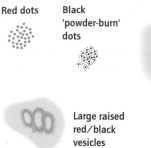

Red dots

Black
'powder-burn'
dots

Large raised
red/black
vesicles

White area
of scarring
with surrounding
abnormal blood vessels

Fig. 9.2 Appearances of endometriosis.

Common symptoms of endometriosis
None
Dysmenorrhoea
Chronic pelvic pain
Deep dyspareunia
Subfertility

Investigations

The diagnosis is only made with certainty after visualisation ± biopsy, usually at laparoscopy. Active lesions are red vesicles or punctate marks on the peritoneum. White scars or brown spots ('powder burn') represent less active endometriosis, while extensive adhesions and endometriomata indicate severe disease (Fig. 9.2). Serum CA 125 levels [→ p.37] are sometimes raised but have little diagnostic value.

Differential diagnosis of endometriosis
Chronic pelvic inflammatory disease [→ p.66]
Pelvic pain syndrome [→ p.59]
Other causes of pelvic masses
Irritable bowel syndrome

Treatment

Endometriosis is a common incidental finding at laparoscopy. In more than 50% of women the disease regresses or does not progress (*BMJ* 1987; **294**: 272). The management of asymptomatic endometriosis is controversial: treatment is warranted in a young woman with more than minimal disease because of possible progression and subfertility. Mild disease in an older woman who has completed her family does not warrant treatment. Symptoms should be ascribed to endometriosis

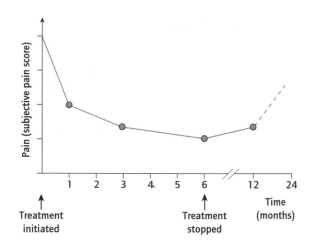

Fig. 9.3 Effect of gonadotrophin-releasing hormone (GnRH) analogue on pain score in patients with endometriosis.

with caution and the diagnosis reviewed if treatment does not relieve the patient's symptoms.

Medical treatment

This is based upon the observations that symptoms regress during pregnancy, in the postmenopausal period and under the influence of androgens. Treatment therefore mimics pregnancy (e.g. the 'pill' or progestogens) or the menopause (e.g. gonadotrophin-releasing hormone, GnRH, analogues) or is androgenic (e.g. danazol).

The combined oral contraceptive is useful for mild symptoms (*Cochrane* 2000: CD001019) and may limit progression in the younger patient with mild disease.

Progestogen preparations are used on a cyclical or continuous basis. Though generally well tolerated, the side effects of fluid retention, weight gain, erratic bleeding and premenstrual syndrome-like symptoms are severe in a few patients.

Gonadotrophin-releasing hormone analogues act by inducing a temporary menopausal state: overstimulation of the pituitary leads to down-regulation of its GnRH receptors (Fig. 9.3). Pituitary gonadotrophin and therefore ovarian hormone production are inhibited. Side effects mimic the menopause [→ p.88]: reversible bone demineralization limits therapy to 6 months, although it can be extended using 'add-back' hormone replacement therapy (HRT) [→ p.90], which prevents bone loss and reduces menopausal side effects.

Danazol and *gestrinone*, synthetic compounds with androgenic effects, are seldom used now because of their severe side effects.

Treatment of endometriosis	

Medical:	The 'pill'
	Progestogens
	Gonadotrophin-releasing hormone (GnRH)
	    analogues ± hormone replacement therapy
	    (HRT)

Surgical:	Laparoscopic laser ablation/diathermy Total abdominal hysterectomy (TAH) and bilateral salpingo-oöphorectomy (BSO)

Surgical treatment

The *laser* or bipolar diathermy can be used laparoscopically at the time of diagnosis to destroy endometriotic lesions. In expert hands, symptomatic improvement is seen in 70% of patients: this may be longer term than with medical therapy. It also improves fertility rates. More *radical surgery* involves dissection of adhesions and removal of endometriomata, or even a total abdominal hysterectomy with bilateral salpingo-oöphorectomy (TAH + BSO). Hysterectomy should be considered a 'last resort'; it is usually only appropriate in the woman whose family is complete, and it may be technically difficult. Hormone replacement therapy will be required, and only exceptionally causes a reactivation.

Endometriosis and fertility [→p.75]

The more severe the endometriosis, the greater the chance of subfertility. Endometriosis is found in 25% of laparoscopies for investigation of subfertility. If the fallopian tubes are unaffected, medical treatment will not increase fertility, but laparoscopic ablation may, particularly when adhesions are present (*Cochrane* 2002: CD001398).

Chronic pelvic pain syndrome

Definition

This syndrome is when chronic pelvic pain, often with deep dyspareunia, occurs in the absence of a known organic cause. It accounts for about 5% of gynaecological referrals.

Assessment

This needs time. A full history will prevent non-gynaecological diagnoses being missed. Psychological evaluation is helpful with some patients. Laparoscopy is used to exclude organic gynaecological pathology. It is obvious, but essential to remember, that just because no cause can be found for pain does not mean that it does not exist.

Possible causes of pain

Oestrogen activity appears to be important as postmenopausal pain is rare (and more likely to be due to malignancy) and suppression of ovarian activity appears to cure two-thirds of cases. *Undetected disease* is relatively common. There may be gynaecological or pelvic adhesions, although these may be incidental findings. The criteria used for diagnosis of *irritable bowel syndrome* are found in many patients (*Gut* 1989; **30**: 996). Pain may be of *renal origin*. *Psychological factors* are important: many patients have neurotic tendencies, but this may be the effect rather than cause of the pain. A substantial number give a history of childhood sexual or physical abuse. *Other possible theories* include the 'pelvic congestion syndrome', in which venous congestion in the pelvis is said to cause chronic pain and the 'myofascial syndrome', in which, it is said, the pain originates in muscle trigger points.

Management

The diagnosis is only made after finding a normal pelvis at laparoscopy. Further invasive investigation is usually counterproductive. Irritable bowel syndrome should be treated by a gastroenterologist. Counselling and psychotherapy are useful and pain management programmes involve relaxation techniques, sex therapy, diet and exercise. Laser uterosacral nerve ablation (LUNA) has been used. Suppression of ovarian activity with progestogens or GnRH analogues is helpful for some: it is these patients who are likely to benefit from a TAH + BSO, which should nevertheless be regarded as a last resort.

Further reading

Farquhar C. Endometriosis. *Clinical Evidence* 2002; **8**: 1864–74.

Gelbaya TA, El-Halwagy HE. Focus on primary care: chronic pelvic pain in women. *Obstetrical & Gynecological Survey* 2001; **56**: 757–64.

Moore J, Kennedy S, Prentice A. Modern combined oral contraceptives for pain associated with endometriosis. *Cochrane Database System Review (Online: Update Software)* 2000; **2**: CD001019.

Olive DL, Pritts EA. Treatment of endometriosis. *The New England Journal of Medicine* 2001; **345**: 266–75.

Stones RW, Mountfield J. Interventions for treating chronic pelvic pain in women. *Cochrane Database System Review (Online: Update Software)* 2000; **4**: CD000387.

Endometriosis at a Glance

Definition	Endometrium outside the uterus
Epidemiology	Common. More prevalent in nulliparous women, aged 35–40 years
Aetiology	Poorly understood. Probably retrograde menstruation that implants
Pathology	Peritoneal inflammation causes fibrosis, adhesions, 'chocolate cysts'
Clinical features	Pelvic pain, dysmenorrhoea, dyspareunia, subfertility
Investigations	Laparoscopy, biopsy
Medical treatment	The combined pill, progestogens, gonadotrophin-releasing hormone (GnRH) analogues ± hormone replacement therapy (HRT)
Surgical treatment	Laser vaporization; total abdominal hysterectomy and bilateral salpingo-oöphorectomy (TAH + BSO) if severe in older woman
Prognosis	Disease usually recurs after cessation of medical treatment

10 Genital Tract Infections

The normal vagina is lined by squamous epithelium. It is richly colonized by a bacterial flora, predominantly *Lactobacillus*, and has an acidic pH (<4.5). This normal flora plays a significant role in defence against infection by pathogens. In prepubertal girls and postmenopausal women, lack of oestrogen results in a thin, atrophic epithelium, a higher pH (6.5–7.5) and reduced resistance to infection.

Genital infections, several of which are sexually transmitted, are a common cause of gynaecological symptoms, but may also be asymptomatic. In recent years the incidence of major sexually transmitted infections (STIs) has risen in the United Kingdom as a result of changes in sexual behaviour, particularly frequent partner change, among young people.

Infections of the vulva and vagina

Non-sexually transmitted infections (STIs)

Candidiasis (thrush)

Infection with *Candida albicans*, a yeast-like fungus (Fig. 10.1), is the commonest cause of vaginal infection and is found in up to 20% of women, often without symptoms. Pregnancy, diabetes and the use of antibiotics are risk factors. There is little evidence that it is sexually transmitted. If symptomatic, there is a 'cottage cheese' discharge with vulval irritation and itching. Superficial dyspareunia and dysuria may occur. The vagina and/or vulva are inflamed and red. The diagnosis is established by culture and treatment is with topical imidazoles (e.g. Canesten) or oral fluconazole. Recurrent candidiasis is more common and more severe in the immunocompromised.

Bacterial vaginosis (formerly *Gardnerella* or anaerobic vaginosis)

This is when the normal lactobacilli are overgrown by a mixed flora including anaerobes, *Gardnerella* and *Mycoplasma hominis*. It is found in 12% of women, but why it occurs is poorly understood. A grey–white discharge is present, but the vagina is not red or itchy. There is a characteristic fishy odour from amines released by bacterial proteolysis. The diagnosis is established by a raised vaginal pH, the typical discharge, a positive 'whiff' test (fishy odour when 10% potassium hydroxide, KOH, is added to the secretions) and the presence of 'clue cells' (epithelial cells studded with Gram-variable coccobacilli) on microscopy. Treatment of symptomatic women is with metronidazole or clindamycin cream. These bacteria can cause secondary infection in pelvic inflammatory disease (PID; [→ p.64]). There is also an association with preterm labour [→ p.158].

Infection associated with foreign bodies

Infection and discharge in children is often due to a foreign body. Sexual abuse must also be considered, but discharge is more often due to atrophic vaginitis due to low oestrogen levels. *Toxic shock syndrome* usually occurs as a rare complication of the retained, particularly hyperabsorbable tampon. A toxin-producing *Staphylococcus aureus* is responsible: a high fever, hypotension and

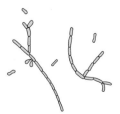

Fig. 10.1 *Candida albicans* showing budding hyphae and oval spores.

multisystem failure can occur. Treatment is with antibiotics and intensive care.

Sexually acquired infections

Principles in the management of STIs

Screening for concurrent disease is important because more than one STI may be present.

The regular sexual partner should be treated and screened for other infections.

Contact tracing involves identification and contacting recent sexual contacts, for screening and treatment. This is usually performed by the patient.

Confidentiality should be maintained. The doctor is breaching confidentiality if he/she informs sexual contacts of his/her patient of her diagnosis without her permission. Sexually transmitted infections can occur within monogamous relationships (e.g. genital herpes following orogenital sex). The diagnosis of an STI is emotive and patients need to be handled sensitively and with adequate explanation.

Education: Frequently changing partners increases the risk of acquiring STIs, including human immunodeficiency virus (HIV).

Barrier methods of contraception greatly reduce the risk of acquiring STIs, including HIV.

Chlamydia

Chlamydia trachomatis is a small bacterium (Fig. 10.2) and is now the commonest sexually transmitted bacterial organism in the developed world. Some 5–10% of women aged 20–30 years have been infected. This is usually asymptomatic, but urethritis and a vaginal discharge can occur. The principal complication is pelvic infection, which may also be silent. This can cause tubal damage leading to subfertility and/or chronic pelvic pain. *Chlamydia* infection also causes Reiter's syndrome, characterized by a triad of urethritis, conjunctivitis and arthritis. Enzyme-linked immunosorbent assay (ELISA) is often used but not highly sensitive; nucleic acid amplification tests (NAATs), e.g. polymerase chain reaction (PCR), are best and can be used on urine for screening purposes. Treatment is with doxycycline or azithromycin.

Gonorrhoea

This is caused by *Neisseria gonorrhoeae*, a Gram-negative diplococcus (Fig. 10.3). It is common, particularly so in the developing world. It is commonly asymptomatic in women, although vaginal discharge, urethritis, bartholinitis and cervicitis can occur and the pelvis is commonly infected. Men usually develop urethritis. Systemic complications include bacteraemia and acute, usually monoarticular, septic arthritis. Diagnosis is from culture of endocervical swabs. In the United Kingdom, penicillin and even ciprofloxacin resistance is increasing: ceftriaxone may be required, particularly for 'imported' infections. Contact tracing and treatment of partners is essential.

Genital warts (condylomata acuminata)

These are caused by the human papilloma virus (HPV). They are extremely common. Appearances vary from tiny flat patches on the vulval skin to small papilliform (cauliflower-like) swellings. Warts are usually multiple and may affect the cervix, where certain oncogenic types (16 and 18) are associated with the development of cervical intraepithelial neoplasia (CIN; [→ p.28]) (*Nature* 1985; **314**: 111). Treatment is with topical podophyllin or imiquimod cream (external warts only). Cryotherapy or electrocautery is used for resistant warts. There is a high recurrence rate (up to 25%).

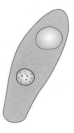

Fig. 10.2 *Chlamydia trachomatis*.

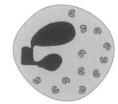

Fig. 10.3 Gram-negative *Neisseria gonorrhoeae* in pairs in a human neutrophil.

Genital herpes

Genital infection is mostly with the herpes simplex virus (HSV) type 2, although type 1, the cause of cold sores, is increasingly implicated (Fig. 10.4). The primary infection is the worst, with multiple small painful vesicles and ulcers around the introitus. Local lymphadenopathy, dysuria and systemic symptoms are common; secondary bacterial infection, aseptic meningitis or acute urinary retention are rarer. The virus then lies dormant in the dorsal root ganglia: in about 75% of patients reactivations occur. These attacks are less painful and often preceded by localized tingling. The diagnosis is established from examination and with viral swabs. Aciclovir (also valaciclovir or famciclovir) is used in severe infections and will also reduce the duration of symptoms if started early in a reactivation. Neonatal herpes has a high mortality and can be prevented [→ p.133].

Syphilis

Infection by the spirochaete *Treponema pallidum* (Fig. 10.5) is now rare in developed countries but is still common in the developing world. *Primary syphilis* is characterized by a solitary painless vulval ulcer (chancre). Untreated, *secondary syphilis* may develop weeks later,

often with a rash, influenza-like symptoms and warty genital or oral growths (condylomata lata). At this stage the spirochaete infiltrates other organs and can cause a variety of symptoms. *Latent syphilis* follows as this phase resolves spontaneously. Primary or secondary syphilis during pregnancy carries a high risk of *congenital infection*. *Tertiary syphilis* is now very rare. It develops many years later and virtually any organ can be affected. Aortic regurgitation, dementia, tabes dorsalis and gummata in skin and bone are the best-known complications. A variety of diagnostic tests are used (including Venereal Disease Research Laboratories, VDRL, testing). Treatment of all stages is with penicillin.

Trichomoniasis (TV)

Trichomonas vaginalis is a flagellate protozoan (Fig. 10.6) that is common worldwide but relatively rare in the United Kingdom. Typical symptoms are an offensive grey–green discharge, vulval irritation and superficial dyspareunia, but it can be asymptomatic. Cervicitis has a punctate erythematous ('strawberry') appearance. Diagnosis is from wet film microscopy, special staining or culture of vaginal swabs. Treatment is with metronidazole.

Other STIs causing genital ulcers

Other than herpes and syphilis, chancroid (*Haemophilus ducreyi*), lymphogranuloma venereum (subtypes of *Chlamydia trachomatis*) and donovanosis (*Calymmatobacterium granulomatis*) —formerly called granuloma inguinale —all cause genital ulceration. They are rare in the United Kingdom but not in the tropics and are occasionally seen as 'imported' diseases.

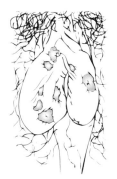

Fig. 10.4 Genital herpes.

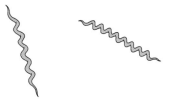

Fig. 10.5 *Treponema pallidum.*

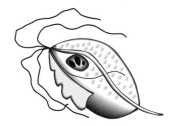

Fig. 10.6 *Trichomonas vaginalis.*

Human immunodeficiency virus (HIV)

Infection with this retrovirus (Fig. 10.7) is the cause of the clinical syndrome acquired immune deficiency syndrome (AIDS). It is increasing more among women than among men. In the United Kingdom in 2002, 42.2% of new diagnoses were in women. Heterosexual contact is numerically the most important mode of infection. Risk factors are multiple sexual partners, migration from high prevalence countries (e.g. sub-Saharan Africa), failure to use barrier contraception and the presence of other STIs, as well as intravenous drug abuse and sexual contact with high-risk males. Seroconversion is often accompanied by an influenza-like illness with a rash, but most HIV-positive women are asymptomatic. The development of opportunistic infections or malignancy (including cervical carcinoma) or a CD4 count <200 (US) are diagnostic of AIDS. Cervical intraepithelial neoplasia [→ p.28] is more common in HIV-infected women, affecting one third. Yearly smears are recommended as progression to malignancy is more rapid. Genital infections, particularly candidiasis and menstrual disturbances, are more common. Vertical transmission to the fetus [→ p.134] is reduced by antiretroviral therapy, elective Caesarean and avoidance of breastfeeding.

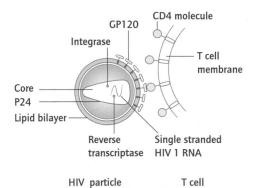

HIV particle   T cell

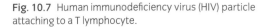

Fig. 10.7 Human immunodeficiency virus (HIV) particle attaching to a T lymphocyte.

Infections of the uterus and pelvis

Endometritis

This is infection confined to the cavity of the uterus alone. Untreated, spread of infection to the pelvis is common. Endometritis is often the result either of *instrumentation of the uterus* or as a *complication of pregnancy*, or *both*. Infecting organisms include *Chlamydia* and gonococcus if these are present in the genital tract. However, the organisms of bacterial vaginosis and organisms such as *Escherichia coli*, staphylococci and even clostridia may be implicated. It is common after Caesarean section; it is also common after miscarriage or abortion, particularly if some 'products of conception' are retained. Illegal abortions are rare in the West but are particularly prone to sepsis.

Endometritis presents with persistent and often heavy vaginal bleeding, usually accompanied by pain. The uterus is tender and the cervical os is commonly open. A fever may initially be absent but septicaemia can ensue. Investigations include vaginal and cervical swabs and a full blood count (FBC); pelvic ultrasound is not very reliable. Broad-spectrum antibiotics are given. An evacuation of retained products of conception (ERPC; [→ p.104]) is then performed if symptoms do not subside or if there are 'products' in the uterus at ultrasound examination.

Acute pelvic infection and pelvic inflammatory disease (PID)

Definition and epidemiology

Pelvic inflammatory disease or salpingitis traditionally describes sexually transmitted pelvic infection, but pelvic infection is best considered as a single entity. Endometritis usually coexists. The incidence is increasing: 2% of women will be affected. Younger, poorer, sexually active nulliparous women are at most risk. Pelvic infection almost never occurs in the presence of a viable pregnancy.

Aetiology

Ascending infection of bacteria in the vagina and cervix:
Sexual factors account for 80%. These are more common

in women with multiple partners, not using barrier contraception. The combined oral contraceptive is partly protective. Spread of previously asymptomatic STIs to the pelvis is usually spontaneous but can be the result of *uterine instrumentation* (e.g. termination of pregnancy, ERPC and dilatation and curettage (D&C), the laparoscopy and dye test and the intrauterine contraceptive device) and/or *complications of childbirth and miscarriage*. In these latter instances, infection is often due to introduction of non-sexually transmitted bacteria.

Descending infection from local organs such as the appendix can also occur.

Pathology and bacteriology

Infection is frequently polymicrobial. *Chlamydia* (up to 60%) and gonococcus are the principal sexually transmitted culprits. The latter causes an acute presentation; the former is often asymptomatic and symptoms, if present, may be due to secondary infection. Endometritis and a bilateral salpingitis and parametritis occur; the ovaries are rarely affected. Perihepatitis (Fitz–Hugh–Curtis syndrome) affects 10% and causes right upper quadrant pain.

Clinical features

History: Many have no symptoms and present later with subfertility or menstrual problems. Bilateral lower abdominal pain with deep dyspareunia is the hallmark, usually with abnormal vaginal bleeding or discharge (Fig. 10.8).

Examination: In severe cases examination reveals a tachycardia and high fever, signs of lower abdominal peritonism with bilateral adnexal tenderness and cervical excitation (pain on moving the cervix). A mass (pelvic abscess) may be palpable vaginally. More frequently, the diagnosis is less clear and may be confused with appendicitis and ovarian cyst accidents (pain usually unilateral) or ectopic pregnancy (pregnancy test positive).

Investigations

Separate swabs must be taken from the cervix and vagina, with blood cultures if there is a fever. The white blood cell count (WBC) and C-reactive protein (CRP) may be raised. Pelvic ultrasound helps to exclude an

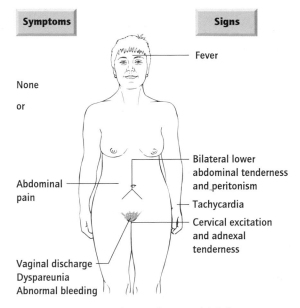

Fig. 10.8 Symptoms and signs of acute pelvic inflammatory disease (PID).

abscess or ovarian cyst. Laparoscopy with fimbrial biopsy and culture is the 'gold standard'.

Treatment

Analgesics and either a parenteral cephalosporin followed by doxycycline and metronidazole, or ofloxacin with metronidazole are most effective (*BMJ* 2001; **322**: 251). Febrile patients should be admitted for intravenous therapy. The diagnosis should be reviewed after 24h if there is no significant improvement and a laparoscopy performed.

Complications

The main early complication is the formation of an abscess or pyosalpinx. Later, many women develop tubal obstruction and subfertility, chronic pelvic infection or chronic pelvic pain [→ p.59]. Ectopic pregnancy is six times more common after pelvic infection.

Features of pelvic inflammatory disease (PID)
Silent (particularly chlamydial)
Bilateral pain
Vaginal discharge
Cervical excitation
Adnexal tenderness
Fever
White blood cell count (WBC) and C-reactive protein (CRP) raised

Late complications of pelvic inflammatory disease (PID)
Subfertility
Chronic PID
Chronic pelvic pain
Ectopic pregnancy

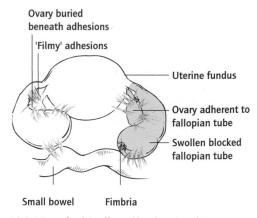

Fig. 10.9 View of pelvis affected by chronic pelvic inflammatory disease (PID).

Chronic PID

This is a persisting infection and is the result of non-treatment or inadequate treatment of acute PID. Typically, there are dense pelvic adhesions and the fallopian tubes may be obstructed and dilated with fluid (hydrosalpinx) or pus (pyosalpinx) (Fig. 10.9). Common symptoms are chronic pelvic pain or dysmenorrhoea, deep dyspareunia [→ p.3], heavy and irregular menstruation, chronic vaginal discharge and subfertility. Examination may reveal features similar to endometriosis: abdominal and adnexal tenderness and a fixed retroverted uterus. Laparoscopy is the best diagnostic tool; culture is often negative. Treatment is with analgesics and antibiotics if there is evidence of active infection. Severe cases occasionally respond to cutting of the adhesions (adhesiolysis), but often only a total abdominal hysterectomy with bilateral salpingo-oöphorectomy (TAH + BSO) will help.

Vaginal discharge: causes and treatment

Discharge from the vagina is a common complaint which, despite often being labelled as 'intractable', can usually be treated if properly evaluated:

Physiological discharge is usually non-offensive. It is common around ovulation, during pregnancy and in women taking the combined oral contraceptive. Exposure of columnar epithelium in cervical eversion and

Differential diagnosis of vaginal discharge						
Cause	Itching	Discharge	pH	Redness	Odour	Treatment
Ectropion/eversion	No	Clear	Normal	No	Normal	Cryotherapy
Bacterial vaginosis	No	Grey–white	Raised	No	Fishy	Antibiotics
Candidiasis	Yes	White	Normal	Yes	Normal	Imidazoles
Trichomoniasis	Yes	Grey–green	Raised	Yes	Yes	Antibiotics
Malignancy	No	Red–brown	Variable	No	Yes	Biopsy
Atrophic	No	Clear	Raised	Yes	No	Oestrogen

ectropion [→ p.27] may cause discharge and can be treated by cryotherapy or diathermy once infection (cervicitis) has been excluded with swabs.

Infection. Bacterial vaginosis and candidiasis are the most common; chlamydial infection, gonorrhoea and TV all can cause a discharge, particularly with cervicitis [→ p.27] and PID. Many other organisms can be present in the presence of a foreign body.

Atrophic vaginitis. This is due to oestrogen deficiency and is common before the menarche, during lactation and after the menopause. Treatment of symptomatic discharge is with oestrogen cream; systemic hormone replacement therapy (HRT) may be preferred in the postmenopausal woman.

Foreign body. Retained tampons or swabs after childbirth are all too common. Foreign bodies are not uncommon in the young child. Discharge is usually very offensive.

Malignancy. A bloody and offensive discharge is suggestive of cervical carcinoma, but any genital tract malignancy can be responsible. The very rare fallopian tube carcinoma typically presents with a watery discharge in the postmenopausal women.

Common causes of vaginal discharge
Candidiasis
Bacterial vaginosis
Atrophic vaginitis
Cervical eversion and ectropion

Further reading

Holmes KK, Sparling PF, Mardh P-A *et al.*, eds. *Sexually Transmitted Diseases*, 3rd edn. New York: McGraw-Hill, 1999.

Pisani E, Garnett GP, Grassly NC *et al.* Back to basics in HIV prevention: focus on exposure. *BMJ (Clinical Research Ed.)* 2003; **326**: 1384–7.

Taylor-Robinson D. *Chlamydia trachomatis* and sexually transmitted disease. *BMJ (Clinical Research Ed.)* 1994; **308**: 150–1.

UK national guidelines on sexually transmitted infections (clinical effectiveness guidelines) http://www.mssvd.org.uk/CEG/ceguidelines.htm

Whitely RJ, Roizman B. Herpes simplex virus infections. *Lancet* 2001; **357**: 1513–8.

Acute Pelvic Inflammatory Disease (PID) at a Glance	
Definition	Infection of the pelvis, usually sexually transmitted
Epidemiology	2% lifetime risk, younger, multiple partners
Aetiology	Ascending: Sexually transmitted infections (STIs): *Chlamydia* and gonorrhoea spontaneous or after childbirth/uterine instrumentation. Non-STIs: seldom spontaneous
	Descending: Rarer; from other organs or blood
Clinical features	Chlamydial PID often silent. Bilateral abdominal pain, vaginal discharge, fever, erratic menstrual bleeding
Investigations	Swabs, full blood count (FBC), C-reactive protein (CRP). Laparoscopy if doubt or poor response to treatment. Pregnancy test
Treatment	Analgesia and antibiotics, e.g. metronidazole and ofloxacin
Complications	Pelvic abscess, chronic PID, chronic pelvic pain, subfertility, ectopic pregnancy

Fertility and Subfertility

Definitions

A couple are 'subfertile' if conception has not occurred after a year of regular unprotected intercourse. Fifteen per cent of couples are affected. Infertility is an absolute term and should be avoided. Failure to conceive may be *primary*, meaning that the female partner has never conceived, or *secondary*, indicating that she has previously conceived, even if the pregnancy culminated in a miscarriage or abortion.

Conditions for pregnancy

Four basic conditions are required for pregnancy:
1 An egg must be produced. Failure is 'anovulation' (30% of cases). Management of subfertility involves finding out if ovulation is occurring and, if not, why.
2 Adequate sperm must be released. 'Male factor' problems contribute to 25% of cases. The history, examination and investigations should involve the male, or at least examination of his semen.
3 The sperm must reach the egg. Most commonly the fallopian tubes are damaged (25% of cases). Sexual (5%) and cervical (<5%) problems may also prevent fertilization.
4 The fertilized egg must implant. The incidence of defective implantation is unknown but may be as high as 30%.

Contributors to subfertility	
Anovulation	30%
Male problems	25%
Tubal problems	25%
Coital problems	5%
Cervical problems	<5%
Unexplained	25%

N.B. Because more than one cause may be present, the percentage total is more than 100%.

Counselling and support for the subfertile couple

A trained counsellor should be available in every subfertility clinic. Reproduction is a fundamental body function that these patients have not achieved and over which they have little control. One partner may feel responsible, or guilty about past abortions or sexually transmitted disease. Many men feel disempowered and less 'male'. The relationship may suffer and intercourse becomes clinical. Counsellors allow couples to talk about these problems. They can also educate the couple and may even uncover a hidden (e.g. sexual) problem.

Disorders of ovulation

Anovulation is a contributory cause in 30% of subfertile couples. Fertility declines with increasing age.

The physiology of ovulation

At the beginning of each cycle, *low* oestrogen levels exert a positive feedback to cause hypothalamic gonadotrophin-releasing hormone (GnRH) pulses to stimulate the anterior pituitary gland to produce gonadotrophins: follicle-stimulating hormone (FSH) and luteinizing hormone (LH) (Fig. 11.1). These cause growth and initiate maturation of several of the follicles of the ovary, each of which contains an immature ovum. These follicles also start producing oestradiol. The resulting *intermediate* oestradiol level has a negative feedback effect on the hypothalamus, such that less FSH and LH is produced. Therefore, the maturing follicles compete for less stimulating hormones, and usually only one is able to survive. The development of one dominant follicle is co-regulated by inhibin B, which also suppresses FSH. As this follicle matures, its oestradiol output increases considerably. When a *high* 'threshold' level of

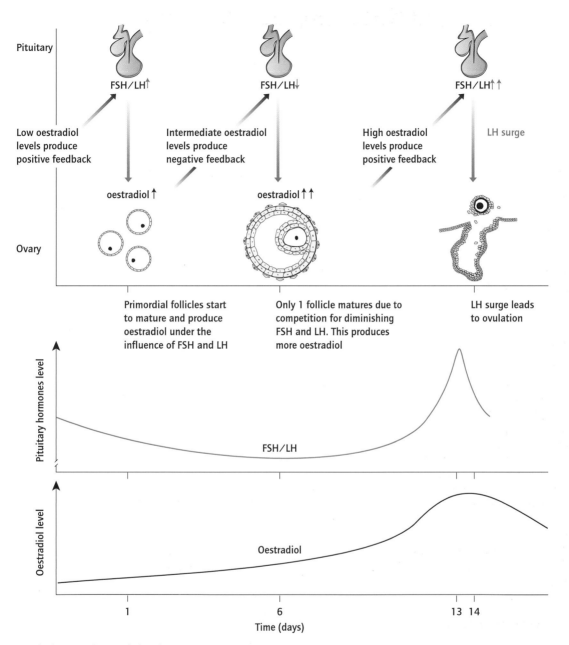

Fig. 11.1 The hormonal control of ovulation.

oestradiol is attained, the negative feedback is reversed and positive feedback now causes LH and FSH levels to again increase and dramatically so: it is the peak of the former that ultimately leads to rupture of the now ripe follicle. This is ovulation and the egg spills onto the ovarian surface where it can be picked up by the fallopian tube.

Detection of ovulation

History: The vast majority of women with regular cycles are ovulatory. Some experience an increase in vaginal discharge or pelvic pain around the time of ovulation.

Examination: Cervical mucus pre-ovulation is normally

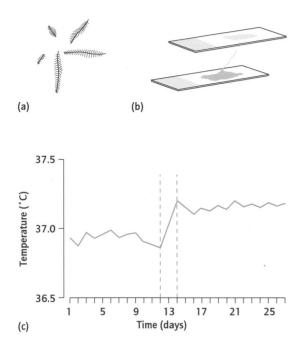

(a)   (b)

(c)

Fig. **11.2** Evidence of ovulation: (a) cervical mucus showing fern-like pattern; (b) spinnbarkeit formation of mucus between two glass slides; (c) temperature chart.

acellular, will 'fern' (form fern-like patterns) when on a dry slide (Fig. 11.2a) and will form 'spinnbarkeit' (elastic-like strings) of up to 15 cm (Fig. 11.2b). The body temperature normally drops some 0.2°C pre-

ovulation and then rises 0.5°C in the luteal phase. If the woman is asked to record her temperature every day, the pattern can be seen on a temperature chart (Fig. 11.2c).

Investigations are more reliable and are used more frequently:

1 Elevated progesterone levels in the mid-luteal phase (usually day 21) usually indicate that ovulation has occurred.

2 Ultrasound scans can serially monitor follicular growth and demonstrate the fall in size that should occur after ovulation.

3 Over-the-counter predictor kits will indicate if the LH surge has taken place.

Detection of ovulation
Temperature charts
Luteinizing hormone (LH) -based predictor kits
Luteal-phase progesterone

Causes of anovulation: polycystic ovary syndrome (PCOS)

Definitions and epidemiology

Polycystic ovary (PCO) describes a characteristic appearance of multiple small (<10 mm) follicles on the ovarian epithelium, which are found in about 20% of women (Fig. 11.3). Patients have, or are at risk of developing, PCOS (*Hum Reprod* 2002; **17**: 2495).

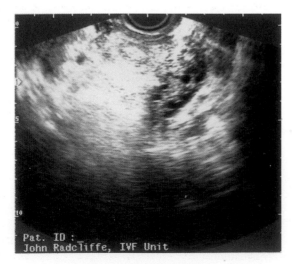

Fig. 11.3 Ultrasound of a polycystic ovary (PCO).

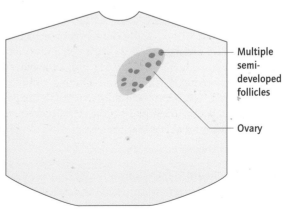

Multiple semi-developed follicles

Ovary

Polycystic ovary syndrome: polycystic ovaries coexist with a spectrum of biochemical ± clinical abnormalities, characterized by hypersecretion of LH and androgens. Polycystic ovary syndrome accounts for up to 60% of anovulatory women. The Stein–Leventhal syndrome describes the most severe end of the disease spectrum.

Pathology/aetiology

Susceptibility to polycystic ovaries is mainly genetic. Development of the syndrome is poorly understood. Endocrine factors, particularly increased insulin secretion and insulin resistance, and increased LH and adrenal and ovarian androgen production, are involved in a breakdown of the normal feedback mechanisms between the ovary and the pituitary. Anovulation, if present, is closely related to increased LH secretion.

Clinical features

Polycystic ovaries without the syndrome are generally asymptomatic. The typical patient with the syndrome is obese, has acne, hirsutism and oligomenorrhoea or amenorrhoea: these may therefore be the presenting symptoms (Fig. 11.4). Miscarriage is more common if there are increased LH levels. Some woman have none of these features and indeed may ovulate; nevertheless, they have some or all of the characteristic laboratory findings.

Investigations

Polycystic ovaries have a typical ultrasound appearance: there is a 'necklace' of multiple small follicles on the surface of the ovaries (Fig. 11.3). Biochemical abnormalities found in PCOS include an elevated LH : FSH ratio, elevated testosterone levels (particularly with anovulatory patients) and reduced sex hormone-binding globulin. Prolactin (PRL) levels may be mildly elevated. If the patient is anovulatory, luteal-phase progesterone levels are low. Screening for diabetes is also advised.

Clinical features of polycystic ovary syndrome (PCOS)
None
Subfertility
Oligomenorrhoea or amenorrhoea
Hirsutism and/or acne
Obesity
Recurrent miscarriage

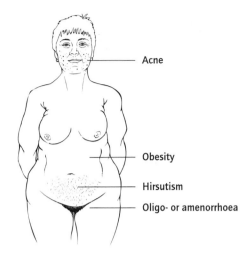

Fig. 11.4 Typical features of severe polycystic ovary syndrome (PCOS).

Complications of PCOS

Forty to fifty per cent of women with PCOS develop diabetes in later life. Cardiovascular disease and endometrial and breast carcinoma are also more common.

Treatment of symptoms other than infertility

Advice regarding diet and exercise are given, and lipid and triglyceride levels should be assessed. If fertility is not required, treatment with the combined oral contraceptive will usually regulate menstruation and prevent endometrial hyperplasia. Cyproterone acetate is particularly useful for acne; it and finasteride will also reduce hirsutism (*Gynecol Endocrinol* 2003; **17**: 57).

Other causes of anovulation

These may originate in the ovary, the pituitary or hypothalamus, or in other parts of the endocrine system (Fig. 11.5).

Hypothalamic causes

Hypothalamic hypogonadism. A reduction in hypothalamic GnRH release causes amenorrhoea, because reduced stimulation of the pituitary reduces FSH and LH levels, which in turn reduces oestradiol levels. This is usual with anorexia nervosa (Fig. 11.6) and common in women on diets, athletes and those under stress.

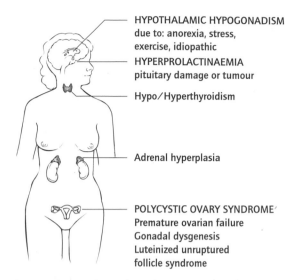

HYPOTHALAMIC HYPOGONADISM
due to: anorexia, stress,
exercise, idiopathic

HYPERPROLACTINAEMIA
pituitary damage or tumour

Hypo/Hyperthyroidism

Adrenal hyperplasia

POLYCYSTIC OVARY SYNDROME
Premature ovarian failure
Gonadal dysgenesis
Luteinized unruptured
follicle syndrome

Fig. 11.5 Causes of anovulation (common causes shown in capital letters).

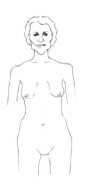

Fig. 11.6 Anorexia nervosa causes amenorrhoea and subfertility.

Restoration of body weight, if appropriate, restores hypothalamic function. *Kallmann's syndrome* occurs when GnRH secreting neurons fail to develop; in other patients, the cause is obscure. Exogenous gonadotrophins or a GnRH pump will induce ovulation.

Pituitary causes

Hyperprolactinaemia is excess PRL secretion, which reduces GnRH release. It is usually caused by benign tumours (adenomas) or hyperplasia of pituitary cells, but is also associated with PCOS and the use of psychotropic drugs. It accounts for 10% of anovulatory women, who commonly have oligomenorrhoea or amenorrhoea,

galactorrhoea and, if a pituitary tumour is enlarging, headaches and a bitemporal hemianopia. Prolactin levels are elevated. Computed tomography (CT) imaging is indicated if neurological symptoms occur. Treatment with a dopamine agonist (bromocriptine or cabergoline) usually restores ovulation, because dopamine inhibits PRL release. Surgery is needed if this fails or neurological symptoms warrant it.

Pituitary damage can reduce FSH and LH release. Production of GnRH is normal. This results from pressure from tumours, or infarction following severe postpartum haemorrhage (Sheehan's syndrome).

Ovarian causes of anovulation (in addition to PCOS)

The luteinized unruptured follicle syndrome is present when a follicle develops but the egg is never released.
Premature ovarian failure [→ p.88]: As the ovary fails, oestradiol levels are low, so reduced negative feedback on the pituitary causes FSH and LH levels to be raised. Exogenous gonadotrophins are of no use and donor eggs are required for pregnancy.
Gonadal dysgenesis: These rare conditions present with primary amenorrhoea [→ p.15].

Other causes

Hypo or *hyperthyroidism* reduces fertility. Menstrual disturbances are usual.
Androgen-secreting tumours [→ p.17] cause amenorrhoea and virilization.

Common causes of anovulation
Polycystic ovary syndrome (PCOS)
Hypothalamic hypogonadism
Hyperprolactinaemia

Induction of ovulation

Lifestyle changes and treatment of associated disease

Treatment of fertility involves health advice regarding pregnancy, the risks of multiple pregnancy with ovulation and induction and the use of folic acid [→ p.127].

Restoration of normal weight is advised and this may restore ovulation. Treatment of specific causes, such as a thyroid abnormality or hyperprolactinaemia, usually leads to restoration of ovulation. Smoking should cease.

Treatment of PCOS

Clomiphene (*Cochrane* 2000: CD000056) is the traditional drug in PCOS and will induce ovulation in about half of women. Clomiphene is an anti-oestrogen, blocking oestrogen receptors in the hypothalamus. As gonadotrophin release is normally inhibited by oestrogen, its effect is to increase the release of FSH and LH. Effectively, therefore, it 'fools' the pituitary into 'believing' there is no oestrogen. As it is only given at the start of the cycle, from day 2–6, it can initiate the process of follicular maturation that is thereafter self-perpetuating. Clompihene cycles should be monitored by ultrasound to reduce the risk of multiple follicle maturation and multiple pregnancy; its use is limited to 6 months.

Gonadotrophins (see below) are traditionally used where clomiphene has failed.

Metformin, an insulin sensitizing drug, is a relatively new treatment and appears to be superior to clompihene. Additional benefits include a reduction in early miscarriage and the development of gestational diabetes, both of which are more common with PCOS (*Fertil Steril* 2003; **79**: 1).

Laparoscopic ovarian diathermy is as effective as gonadotrophins (*Cochrane* 2001: CD001122) and with a lower multiple pregnancy rate.

Gonadotrophin induction of ovulation

These are used when clomiphene has failed, but also in hypothalamic hypogonadism if the weight is normal. Purified FSH ± LH acts as a substitute for the normal pituitary production. Given at regular intervals or as a pump in the follicular phase, this stimulates follicular growth. The result is often maturation of more than one follicle. Follicular development is monitored with ultrasound. Once a follicle is the size adequate for ovulation (about 17 mm), the process can be artificially stimulated by an injection of human chorionic gonadotrophin (HCG). Structurally similar to LH, this therefore imitates the pre-ovulatory LH surge.

Inducing ovulation	
If polycystic ovary syndrome (PCOS):	Weight loss and lifestyle changes. If inappropriate/fails . . . Clomiphene or metformin. If fails . . . Gonadotrophins Consider ovarian diathermy
If hypothalamic hypogonadism:	Restore weight Gonadotrophins if weight normal
If hyper-prolactinaemia:	Bromocriptine or cabergoline

Side effects of ovulation induction

Multiple pregnancy is more likely with drug therapy as more than one follicle may mature. Multiple pregnancy increases perinatal complication rates [→ p.182].

Ovarian hyperstimulation syndrome: Gonadotrophin (and occasionally clomiphene) stimulation 'overstimulates' the follicles, which can get very large and painful (Fig. 11.7). The severity varies, but, in all forms, the incidence is 4%. In severe cases, hypovolaemia, electrolyte disturbances, ascites and pulmonary oedema may develop. Prevention involves ultrasound monitoring and use of the lowest possible doses. Treatment is initially with 'coasting': withdrawing gonadotrophins but continuing down-regulation (*Cochrane* 2002: CD002811). More severe cases require restoration of intravascular volume, electrolyte monitoring and correction, analgesia and thromboprophylaxis [→ p.151]. Drainage of fluid is occasionally necessary to increase comfort and breathing.

Ovarian carcinoma: The evidence is conflicting, but prolonged ovulation induction may increase the lifetime risk of this (*NEJM* 1994; **331**: 771).

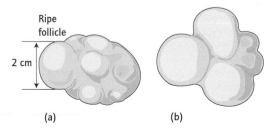

Fig. 11.7 Ovarian hyperstimulation. (a) Normal ovary pre-ovulation. (b) Mildly hyperstimulated ovary.

Male subfertility

Male factors contribute in 25% of subfertile couples.

The physiology of sperm production

Spermatogenesis in the testis is dependent on pituitary LH and FSH, the former largely acting via testosterone production in the Leydig cells of the testis. Follicle-stimulating hormone and testosterone control Sertoli cells, which are involved in synthesis and transport of sperm. Testosterone and other steroids inhibit the release of LH, completing a negative feedback control mechanism with the hypothalamic–pituitary axis. It takes about 70 days for sperm to develop fully.

Detection of adequate sperm production: semen analysis

The most important factor is 'progressive motility' of the sperm. A normal semen analysis result virtually excludes a male cause for infertility. An abnormal analysis result must be repeated after 70 days. If persistently abnormal, examination and investigation of the male must follow (Fig. 11.8).

Normal semen analysis

Normal semen analysis	
Volume	>2 mL
Sperm count	>20 million/mL
Progressive motility	>50%
Abnormal forms	<30%

Definitions of terms describing abnormal semen

Definitions of terms describing abnormal semen	
Azoospermia:	No sperm present
Oligospermia:	<20 million/mL
Severe oligospermia:	<5 million/mL
Asthenozoospermia:	Absent or low motility
Teratozoospermia:	Excess of abnormal forms

Common causes of abnormal semen analysis

Common causes of abnormal semen analysis
Unknown
Smoking/alcohol/drugs/chemicals/inadequate local cooling
Varicocoele
Antisperm antibodies

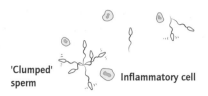

Fig. 11.8 Semen analysis. Antisperm antibodies causing clumping.

Common causes of abnormal/absent sperm release

Idiopathic oligospermia and *asthenozoospermia* are common. Sperm numbers and/or motility are low but not absent.

Drug exposure: Alcohol, smoking and exposure to industrial chemicals, particularly solvents, can impair male fertility.

Varicocoele: This refers to varicosities of the pampiniform venous plexus and usually occurs on the left side. It is present in about 25% of infertile men (but 15% of all men). It is not fully understood how it impairs fertility.

Antisperm antibodies are present in about 5% of infertile men and are common after vasectomy reversal. Poor motility and 'clumping' together of the sperm are evident on the semen analysis.

Other causes include infections (e.g. epididymitis), mumps orchitis, testicular abnormalities (e.g. in Klinefelter's syndrome), obstruction to delivery (e.g. congenital aplasia of the vas), hypothalamic problems, Kallmann's syndrome and hyperprolactinaemia, retrograde ejaculation and drugs (e.g. sulfasalazine or anabolic steroids).

Management of male factor subfertility

General advice: Lifestyle changes and drug exposures are addressed. The testicles should be below body temperature: advice on wearing loose clothing and testicular cooling is given.

Specific measures: Ligation of a varicocoele slightly improves fertility (*Lancet* 2003; **361**: 1849). Gonadaotrophin treatment of pituitary disease may be required.

Assisted conception techniques: Intrauterine insemination (IUI) may help. Sperm can be extracted direct from the testis (testicular sperm extraction: testicular sperm aspiration, TESA, or from the epididymis: microsurgical epididymal sperm aspiration, MESA) and then used for intracytoplasmic sperm injection (ICSI) (*Cochrane* 2001: CD002807). Or, donor sperm may be used after appropriate counselling; this is called donor insemination (DI).

Disorders of fertilization

The egg and sperm are unable to meet in 30% of subfertile couples.

The physiology of fertilization

At ovulation, the fallopian tube moves so that the fimbrial end collects the ovum from the ovary. The tube must have adequate mobility to move onto the ovary to achieve this. Peristaltic contractions and cilia in the tube help sweep the ovum along toward the sperm. Blockage or ciliary damage will impair this. At ejaculation, millions of sperm enter the vagina. The cervical mucus helps them get through the cervix.

Why the sperm might not meet the egg	
Tubal damage:	Infection
	Endometriosis
	Surgery
Cervical problems	
Sexual problems	

Causes of failure to fertilize: tubal damage

This contributes in 25% of subfertile couples.

Infection

Pelvic inflammatory disease (PID) [→ p.64], particularly due to sexually transmitted infections (e.g. *Chlamydia*), causes adhesion formation within and around the fallopian tubes (Fig. 11.9). It is the main cause of tubal damage and 12% of women will be infertile after one episode of infection. Intrauterine contraceptive devices and appendicitis may also be responsible. Most women will have had no symptoms, but some give a previous history of pelvic pain, vaginal discharge or abnormal menstruation.

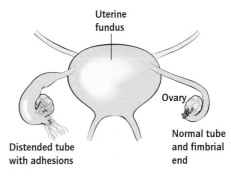

Fig. 11.9 Tubal blockage.

Microsurgery is often used for mild disease and is best performed laparoscopically. The principal techniques are adhesiolysis of peritubal adhesions, reanastomosis after removal of a tubal blockage and reopening of distal tubal blockage (salpingostomy). Ectopic pregnancy rates are increased. It is still important to eradicate active infection.

In vitro fertilization (IVF) is an alternative and is the treatment of choice if tubal damage is severe or if surgery fails.

Endometriosis [→p.57]

This is found in 25% of subfertile women, but is probably contributory in many fewer. Its role in subfertility is more than simply mechanical (*Obstet Gynecol Clin North Am* 2003; **30**: 181), but this is poorly understood. Laparoscopic surgery improves fertility even in mild cases; medical treatment is not used (*Cochrane* 2002: CD001398). *In vitro* fertilization is the next step if this fails.

Previous surgery

Any pelvic surgery may cause adhesion formation. The now obsolete 'wedge resection' of the ovaries in PCOS patients was notorious for this. Treatment is as for infectious causes but IVF is often needed.

Other causes of failure to fertilize

Cervical problems

'Cervical factors' rarely contribute to subfertility and the postcoital test is no longer recommended. Cervical problems can be due to *antibody production* by the woman, whereby antibodies agglutinate or kill the sperm, *infection* in the vagina or cervix that prevents adequate mucus production or *cone biopsy* for cervical intraepithelial neoplasia (CIN) [→ p.105]. Intrauterine insemination is often used.

Sexual problems

These occur in about 5% of subfertile couples. Impotence can be psychological or organic. Ignorance or discomfort can also prevent coitus. Counselling is required, after exclusion of organic disease.

Detection of problems with fertilization

Detection of tubal damage

As pelvic infection and endometriosis are often symptomless, only limited information can be gained from the history and examination. One or other of the following tests is always necessary for full assessment of subfertility.

Laparoscopy and dye test [→ p.103] allows visualization and assessment of the fallopian tubes. Methylene blue dye is injected through the cervix from the outside. Whether it enters or spills from the tubes can then be seen, demonstrating whether the tubes are patent. *Hysteroscopy* is performed first to assess the uterine cavity for abnormalities.

Hysterosalpingogram: Without anaesthetic, radio-opaque contrast is injected through the cervix. Spillage from the fimbrial end (and filling defects) can be seen on X-ray. A variant of this test can be performed using transvaginal ultrasound (HyCoSy).

Assisted conception

Recent advances have greatly increased the success of fertility treatment. The current methods are IVF, gamete intrafallopian transfer (GIFT) and intrauterine insemination (IUI). They are often unavailable on the National Health Service. Success is best measured by the live birth rate: this declines after 35 years, and considerably after 40 years, of age. Sperm quality is important but ICSI has rendered this less significant. Ovum donation is now possible with resistant anovulation or premature ovarian failure.

Whether anovulation is present or not, ovulation is induced with gonadotrophins after GnRH down-regulation [→ p.58] to abolish endogenous FSH and LH and allow more predictable and safer ovarian stimulation. The aim is to produce more than one ovum: '*superovulation*'. The procedure of choice is then started. Screening ± treatment for *Chlamydia* is also performed.

Indications for assisted conception
When any/all other methods have failed
Unexplained subfertility
Male factor subfertility (intracytoplasmic sperm injection, ICSI)
Tubal blockage (standard *in vitro* fertilization, IVF)

Intrauterine insemination (IUI): superovulation

Method: At the time of ovulation, washed sperm are injected directly into the cavity of the uterus.

Criteria: The tubes should be patent, as the ovum still needs to travel from the ovary to the sperm. This is suitable for couples with unexplained subfertility, cervical and sexual, and some male factors, and is much cheaper than IVF. It is common for it to be tried whilst awaiting IVF.

Results: The live birth rate is about 15% per stimulated cycle.

In vitro fertilization (IVF)

Method: The eggs are collected under local anaesthetic by aspirating follicles under ultrasound control. They are then incubated with washed sperm and transferred to a growth medium. Transfer into the uterus takes place some 3–5 days later. Transferring no more than two embryos is mandatory (except under exceptional circumstances) to reduce the obstetric complications associated with high order multiples. Other embryos can be frozen for future transfer. Luteal phase support, using progesterone or HCG, usually given until 12 weeks, increases pregnancy rates (*Hum Reprod* 2002; **17**: 2287).

Criteria: The fallopian tubes need not be patent.

Results: The live birth rate in younger women in the best centres is about 25% per stimulated cycle.

Intracytoplasmic sperm injection (ICSI)

This is the injection, with a very fine needle, of one sperm right into the oöplasma (Fig. 11.10). It is therefore useful for male factor infertility, allowing use of poor-quality sperm that would normally be unable to penetrate the ovum. Indeed, sperm can now be recovered directly from the testis (TESA) or epididymis (MESA).

Gamete intrafallopian transfer (GIFT)

Method: The eggs are collected laparoscopically, mixed with sperm and transferred back to the fallopian tube straight away.
Criteria: This technique requires that at least one tube is functional and the use of an operating theatre.
Results are similar to IVF, but the procedure is seldom used nowadays. It is not subject to regulation under the Human Fertilization and Embryology Authority (HFEA).

Complications of assisted conception

Superovulation: Multiple pregnancy (25% of live births from IVF) and ovarian hyperstimulation are discussed above. The former are producing a significant impact on obstetric and neonatal services.
Egg collection: Intraperitoneal haemorrhage and reactivation of pelvic infection may complicate the ultrasound-guided aspiration of mature follicles necessary for IVF.
Pregnancy: In addition to the multiple pregnancy rates, miscarriage and ectopic pregnancy rates are also higher, as is the perinatal mortality and morbidity, and long-term morbidity (*Lancet* 2002; **359**: 461), even allowing for multiple pregnancies. A small increase in chromosomal and gene abnormalities is reported with ICSI (*Hum Reprod* 2003; **18**: 925).

Ethics and regulation of assisted conception

The many ethical and practical problems in subfertility treatment are regulated by the HFEA (www.hfea.gov.uk). All centres offering IVF must be licensed and their data are collected.

Rapid advances have occurred in reproductive medicine in the last 25 years and ethical dilemmas have followed. These include those of surrogacy, ovum donation, embryo selection, storage of and research on embryos and their use after divorce or death. In the future, the practical possibilities of genetic testing, manipulation and even human cloning are likely to pose even greater problems.

Further reading

Al-Shawaf T, Grudzinskas JG. Prevention and treatment of ovarian hyperstimulation syndrome. *Best Practice & Research. Clinical Obstetrics & Gynaecology* 2003; **17**: 249–61.

Evers JL. Female subfertility. *Lancet* 2002; **360**: 151–9.

Garceau L, Henderson J, Davis LJ *et al*. Economic implications of assisted reproductive techniques: a systematic review. *Human Reproduction (Oxford, England)* 2002; **17**: 3090–109.

Jacobson TZ, Barlow DH, Koninckx PR, Olive D, Farquhar C. Laparoscopic surgery for subfertility associated with endometriosis. *Cochrane Database System Review (Online: Update Software)* 2002; **4**: CD001398.

Ludwig M, Westergaard LG, Diedrich K, Andersen CY. Developments in drugs for ovarian stimulation. *Best Practice & Research. Clinical Obstetrics & Gynaecology* 2003; **17**: 231–47.

Mortimer D. The future of male infertility management and assisted reproduction technology. *Human Reproduction (Oxford, England)* 2000; **15** (Suppl. 5): 98–110.

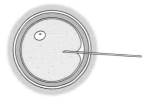

Fig. 11.10 Intracytoplasmic sperm injection (ICSI).

Subfertility at a Glance

Definition	Failure to conceive after a year Primary: female never conceived. Secondary: previously conceived	
Epidemiology	15% of couples	
Aetiology	Anovulation (30%):	Polycystic ovary syndrome (PCOS), hypothalamic hypogonadism, hyperprolactinaemia
	Male factor (25%):	Idiopathic, varicocoele, antibodies, drug/chemical exposure, many others
	No fertilization:	Tubal factor (25%): infection, endometriosis, surgery Cervical factor (<5%) Sexual factor (5%)
	Unexplained (25%)	
Investigations	Detect ovulation:	Luteal phase progesterone, ultrasound scan
	Cause of anovulation:	Follicle-stimulating hormone (FSH), luteinizing hormone (LH), oestradiol, testosterone, prolactin (PRL)
	Detect male factor:	Semen analysis
	Detect tubal factor:	Laparoscopy and dye or hysterosalpingogram
Treatment	General:	Ensure correct weight. Give folic acid
	If anovulation:	Treat specific disorder PCOS: clomiphene, metformin, gonadotrophins, ovarian diathermy
	If male factor:	Treat specific disorder. intracytoplasmic sperm injection (ICSI)
	If tubal factor:	Laparoscopic surgery if mild/endometriosis *In vitro* fertilization (IVF) if fails or with severe disease
	If unexplained:	Intrauterine insemination (IUI)/IVF

Polycystic ovary syndrome (PCOS) at a Glance

Definition	Polycystic ovary (PCO) is multiple small follicles on the surface of ovaries PCOS is PCO in conjunction with biochemical ± clinical evidence of hyperandrogenism and raised luteinizing hormone (LH) secretion	
Epidemiology	20% of women have PCO; 70% of anovulation due to PCOS	
Aetiology	PCO is genetic. Development of the syndrome is poorly understood	
Features	Asymptomatic, anovulatory infertility, oligo/amenorrhoea, obesity, hirsutism, acne	
Investigations	Ultrasound scan of ovaries	
	Blood:	Often raised testosterone and luteinizing hormone to follicle-stimulating hormone (LH : FSH) ratio Low luteal phase progesterone if anovulatory
Treatment	None if chance finding. Weight loss if appropriate	
	If infertility:	Clomiphene, ovarian diathermy, metformin; gonadotrophins if failed
	If menstrual problems:	Combined oral contraceptive
	If acne/hirsutism:	Cyproterone acetate or finasteride
Complications	Infertility, obesity, miscarriage Long-term risks: diabetes, endometrial/breast carcinoma, cardiovascular disease	

12 Contraception

Contraception is the prevention of pregnancy. On an individual basis it is important to ensure that all pregnancies are wanted or intended (www.fpa.org.uk). It is also important on a global scale because the world population is rapidly increasing. Contraceptive methods may help reduce the spread of disease, e.g. human immunodeficiency virus (HIV) [→ p.64] and *Chlamydia* [→ p.62].

Efficacy of contraception

This is measured as the risk of pregnancy per 100 woman years of using the given method, and is called the Pearl index (PI). If the PI of a contraceptive is 2 then, of 100 women using it for a year, two will be pregnant by the end. The effectiveness of a contraceptive is also determined by the user's compliance.

Safety of contraception

Most methods of contraception have been the subject of adverse publicity. Some are less safe than others, or are contraindicated in particular women. By taking a full medical history, the doctor can decide what is medically appropriate. It is important that measurements of safety are compared with the safety of pregnancy; for instance, the diabetic woman is at increased risk of complications with 'the pill', but pregnancy risks more complications. Similarly, smoking is considerably more hazardous than using the pill.

Compliance with contraception

This is a major problem. Contraception must be appropriate to the woman's lifestyle; if it is disliked or misunderstood it will not be used. The woman must be fully counselled about any proposed contraceptive: its major problems and minor side effects. This will enable the woman to know what to expect, and may prevent discontinuation of the chosen method.

Media 'scares' over the 'pill' have led to inappropriate discontinuation.

Contraception for the adolescent

One in 100 of 13–15-year olds become pregnant every year in the United Kingdom, and this figure has only fallen by 10% since 1998. The current Department of Health target aims to reduce the under 18 years of age conception rate by 50% by the year 2010. Sex education and public awareness of family planning services will need to increase. It may be too late to prevent intercourse, but the implications, including sexually transmitted disease and unwanted pregnancy, should be discussed. The combined oral contraceptive or depot preparations are usually indicated, but should be used in conjunction with a condom to prevent sexually transmitted disease.

It is acceptable to prescribe contraception to sexually mature girls <16 years, and there is no obligation to tell the parents, if she cannot be persuaded to do so. The General Medical Council guidelines permit a doctor to breach the young woman's confidentiality where it is essential to her medical interests, but she must be told before information is disclosed.

Contraception in later life

Although fertility is reduced after 40 years of age, most women with regular cycles still ovulate. All methods of contraception can be used; including a low-dose combined oral contraceptive (e.g. Mercilon) in non-smoking women with no other risk factors. The intrauterine device (IUD) is particularly appropriate and, if fitted after the age of 40 years, does not need to be replaced. The hormone-releasing intrauterine system (IUS) [→ p.13] will, in addition, greatly reduce menstrual loss. Despite this, many women seek sterilization.

Contraception in the developing world

Where education and access to health care is poor, the practical requirements of a contraceptive are different. Minimal medical supervision, prevention of sexually transmitted disease, cost and duration of treatment are important. This means reversible depot methods, such as Implanon and vaccines have more potential. Breast-feeding has important contraceptive benefits where contraception is scarce, although around 2% of women will fall pregnant in the first 6 months if no additional contraception is used.

The organization and planning of family planning services

In the United Kingdom, contraception is available from general practitioners and family planning clinics. In addition, emergency contraception [→ p.83] can be purchased over-the-counter from pharmacies.

The concept of the 'sexual health clinic' has developed, with contraception, genitourinary medicine, and even colposcopy and menopause services alongside each other.

Hormonal contraception

Oestrogens and progestogens can be used for contraception in the following ways:

1 Progestogen as a tablet: the progestogen-only pill ('mini pill').

2 Progestogen as a depot: Implanon, Depo-Provera or in the levonorgestrel-containing intrauterine device (IUD), now called the frameless IUS.

3 Oestrogen and progestogen: the combined oral contraceptive (the 'pill'): mono/bi/triphasic.

4 Novel methods include patch combinations of oestrogen and progestogen.

Combined oral contraceptives (COCs or the 'pill')

Combined oral contraceptives act mainly by exerting a negative feedback effect [→ p.9] on gonadotrophin release and thereby inhibiting ovulation. A single tablet, containing both an oestrogen and a progestogen, is taken

every day for 3 weeks and then stopped for 1 week (Fig. 12.1). Vaginal bleeding then occurs as a result of withdrawal of the hormonal stimulus on the endometrium. The cycle is then restarted.

Types

Monophasic pills deliver the same dose of oestrogen and progestogen every day. The oestrogen (ethinyloestradiol) content may range from 20 to 50 µg. The usual preparations of choice are the 30-µg pills (e.g. Microgynon 30). In *biphasic* or *triphasic pills*, the doses of both hormones alter two and three times respectively. Better regulation of menstruation may occur, but they are more complex to use.

Contraceptive efficacy

Taken properly, the combined pill is highly effective, with a failure rate of 0.2 per 100 woman years. If less care is taken, failure rates are much higher.

Common side effects of sex hormones	
Progestogenic	Oestrogenic
Depression	Nausea
Postmenstrual tension-like symptoms	Headaches
Bleeding; amenorrhoea	Increased mucus
Acne	Fluid retention and weight gain
Breast discomfort	Occasionally hypertension
Weight gain	Breast tenderness and fullness
Reduced libido	Bleeding

Indications

All women without major contraindications may use it. It is suitable for the teenager (in conjunction with

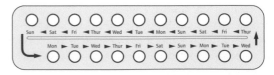

Fig. 12.1 The combined oral contraceptive.

condoms) and the older woman with no cardiovascular risk factors. It is also useful for menstrual cycle control, menorrhagia, premenstrual symptoms, dysmenorrhoea, mild endometriosis and prevention of recurrent simple ovarian cysts.

The 'pill' in practice

Reduced absorption of the 'pill' often occurs with oral antibiotics and with diarrhoea and vomiting. Additional precautions should be taken for the duration of illness or therapy, and afterwards for a week. If liver enzyme inducing drugs (e.g. anticonvulsants) are used, the oestrogen dose may need to be increased.

The missed 'pill': If the pill is missed by less than 12 h, it should be taken and further tablets continued. No additional precautions are required. If the pill is missed by more than 12 h, the last missed pill should be taken and the packet finished as usual, with no break before the next packet if there were less than seven pills left. A barrier method should be used for the next 7 days. Women should be warned that if they have to start the next packet immediately they will not menstruate, but they may have irregular bleeding during the next packet.

The 'pill' and surgery: The pill is normally stopped 4 weeks before major surgery because of its prothrombotic risks, but the risks of pregnancy should also be considered. The pill is not discontinued prior to minor surgery.

Counselling the woman starting on the 'pill'

Advise of major complications and benefits

Advise to stop smoking

Advise to see doctor if symptoms suggestive of major complications

Advise about poor absorption with antibiotics and sickness and what to do about missed pill(s) (give leaflet)

Stress the importance of follow-up and blood pressure measurement

---

Disadvantages

Major: complications

These are very rare. *Venous thrombosis* and *myocardial infarction* are the most important (*Drug Saf* 2000; **22**: 361). The risk is further multiplied by smoking and increased age.

Thromboembolic disease is marginally more common with third-generation progestogen pills, but these are less likely to increase cardiovascular risk (*BMJ* 1996; **312**: 88). In older women, where cardiovascular problems are more likely, the new pills are more appropriate; in younger women, where thromboembolism is relatively a greater risk, first-line use should usually be a second-generation pill. Other problems include a slightly increased risk of *cerebrovascular accidents, focal migraine, hypertension, jaundice,* and *liver, cervical and breast carcinoma* (Fig. 12.2).

Minor: side effects

Both oestrogenic and progestogenic side effects may occur. The most common are weight gain, nausea, headaches and breast tenderness. Breakthrough bleeding is common in the first few months, but has usually settled after 3 months. Lactation is partly suppressed.

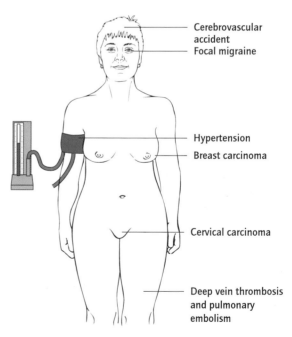

Fig. 12.2 Major complications of the combined oral contraceptive.

Contraindications to the combined oral contraceptives (COCs)	
Absolute:	History of venous thrombosis
	History of cerebrovascular accident, ischaemic heart disease
	Severe/focal migraine
	Active breast/endometrial cancer
	Inherited thrombophilia
	Pregnancy
	Smokers >35 years
	Active/chronic liver disease
Relative:	Smokers
	Obesity
	Chronic inflammatory disease
	Renal impairment, diabetes
	Age >35 years
	Breastfeeding

Advantages

Contraceptive: Despite the rare complications, the 'pill' is a very effective and acceptable method of contraception: it has been the subject of considerable research and in appropriate women it is very safe (*Drug Saf* 2002; **25**: 893).

Risk of non-fatal venous thromboembolism for users of combined oral contraceptives (COCs)	
User category	Incidence per 100 000 women per year
All women not using 'pill'	5
Pregnant women	60
Women using older 30 µg 'pill'	15
Women using new 30 µg 'pill'	25
Women smoking and using 'pill'	60

Non-contraceptive benefits: Useful effects include more regular, less painful and lighter menstruation. There is protection against simple ovarian cysts, benign breast cysts, fibroids and endometriosis: the pill need not be prescribed merely for contraception. The risk of pelvic inflammatory disease (PID), but not HIV, is reduced possibly because of thicker cervical mucus. Longer term, there is protection against ovarian cancer.

Progestogen-only pill (the 'mini pill')

This contains a small dose of progestogen (e.g. 350 mg of norethisterone: Micronor). It must be taken every day without a break and at the same time (±3 h). It makes cervical mucus hostile to sperm and in some women inhibits ovulation too. Failure rates are 1 per 100 woman years: higher than the combined pill. Side effects are progestogenic: vaginal spotting (breakthrough bleeding), weight gain, mastalgia and premenstrual-like symptoms are most common. It is less effective than the combined pill, and the need for meticulous timing can spell failure, particularly in younger women. It is particularly suitable for older women and those in whom the combined pill is contraindicated. It is also used for lactating mothers. There is no increased risk of thrombosis and it can be used in almost all the situations where the combined pill is contraindicated.

Counselling before using the 'mini pill'
Advise woman about bleeding patterns
Emphasize the importance of meticulous timekeeping

Depot contraception

In depot administration methods, progestogens are slowly released, bypassing the portal circulation. The mode of action is similar to that of the 'mini pill', but ovulation is normally also prevented.

Depo-Provera and Noristerat

Depo-Provera, containing medroxyprogesterone acetate (150 mg), is administered by injection every 3 months. The failure rate is <1.0 per 100 woman years. It often causes irregular bleeding in the first weeks, but this is usually followed by amenorrhoea. Other progestogenic side effects may occur. Prolonged amenorrhoea may follow its cessation and women should be warned of this. Osteoporosis may occur. It is useful during lactation and when compliance is a problem. An alternative depot preparation is Noristerat, containing norethisterone, which is given every 8 weeks.

Implanon

This consists of a single 60-mm rod containing progestogen (etonogestrel) (*Hum Reprod* 1999; **14**: 976–81), which is inserted in the upper arm subder-

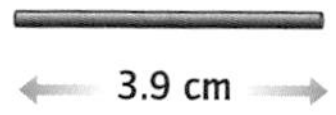

← 3.9 cm →

Fig. 12.3 Implanon.

mally with local anaesthetic (Fig. 12.3). The failure rate is <1.0 per 100 woman years. It will last 3 years and female satisfaction is high. Side effects include progestogenic symptoms, particularly irregular bleeding in the first year. Removal is usually easy and there is a rapid resumption of fertility. Because it is simple and long acting, it may have a particular role in the developing world.

Progestogen-impregnated intrauterine device (IUD)

This is discussed on page 13.

Emergency contraception

The 'morning-after pill'

If unprotected intercourse occurs, the chances of conception can be reduced by taking the 'morning-after pill'. A single dose of 1.5 mg of levonorgestrel (Levonelle) is taken, preferably within 12 h, and no later than 72 h after unprotected intercourse (*Lancet* 2002; **360**: 1803). This has a 95% success rate if used within 24 h, reduced to 58% if delayed until 72 h. Vomiting and menstrual disturbances in the following cycle can occur.

Others

An alternative is to insert an IUD within 5 days of intercourse, which will usually prevent implantation. Mifepristone [→ p.97] may be taken orally but is more likely to cause cycle disturbance.

Barrier contraception

Barrier methods physically prevent the sperm from getting through the cervix. A principal advantage, especially with condoms, is the protection against sexually transmitted infections (STIs).

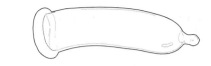

Fig. 12.4 The male condom.

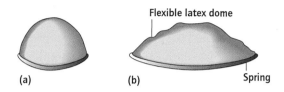

Flexible latex dome

(a)   (b)   Spring

Fig. 12.5 (a) The cervical cap. (b) The diaphragm.

Male condom

This consists of a sheath (latex or not) that fits onto the erect penis (Fig. 12.4). The failure rate is 2–15 per 100 woman years; this is dependent on using it properly. It affords the best protection against disease, including HIV, and should always be used for casual intercourse, even if in conjunction with other methods.

Female condom

This fits inside the vagina. Failure rates are similar to the condom but it is less well accepted. It too protects against STIs.

Diaphragms and caps

These are fitted before intercourse and must remain *in situ* for at least 6 h afterwards. Cervical caps fit over the cervix (Fig. 12.5a), whilst the spring of the latex dome of the diaphragm holds it between the pubic bone and the sacral curve, covering the cervix (Fig. 12.5b). Types and sizes vary, and selection should be determined by trained personnel. Failure rates are about 5 per 100 woman years and dependent on the type used (*Cochrane* 2002: CD003551). Although some protection against PID is gained, there is less protection against HIV. Some women find them inconvenient, and they are best suited to a woman with good motivation.

Spermicides

Barrier methods are used in conjunction with a spermicide, in the form of a jelly, cream or pessary. Spermicides are not recommended for use on their own.

Intrauterine devices (IUDs or 'the coil')

These devices are inserted into the uterine cavity. Thin plastic strings protrude through the cervix and are pulled to remove the device. They are normally changed every 5–10 years. They prevent pregnancy by effects on fertilization and implantation depending on the type used.

Types of IUDs

Copper-containing devices (Fig. 12.6a,c) can be small, and copper has the additional benefits of being spermicidal and bactericidal.

Hormone-containing devices contain the progestogen levonorgestrel, which is slowly released locally (Fig. 12.6b). This is now called the frameless IUS. It has the additional benefit of reducing menstrual loss with few side effects [→ p.13].

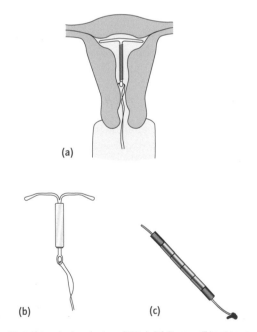

Fig. 12.6 Intrauterine devices (IUDs). (a) Copper T in uterus, (b) intrauterine system (IUS), (c) Gynefix.

Contraceptive efficacy

With high copper content and progestogen-releasing devices, the failure rate is <0.5 per 100 woman years.

Indications

The IUD is usually used when the woman finds it difficult to use other methods, is older and has finished her family. It is normally inserted during the first half of the cycle, but can be used straight after delivery of the placenta or 6 weeks post-delivery (*Hum Reprod* 2002: **17**: 549), or at termination of pregnancy. The progestogen-releasing IUS is also used for its effect on menstrual loss.

Complications

Pain or cervical shock (due to increased vagal tone) can complicate insertion. The device can be *expelled*, usually within the first month. *Perforation* of the uterine wall (0.5–1.0%) can occur at insertion, or the device may migrate through the wall afterwards. Expulsion or perforation will cause the threads to disappear, but they may also have been cut too short. *Heavier or more painful menstruation* can occur (except with progestogen devices). Women with asymptomatic STIs in the cervix are at increased risk of PID. The risk of *infection* (10%) is therefore mainly limited to younger women with multiple partners and is reduced by screening for infection first. If pregnancy occurs despite the presence of an IUD, it is more likely to be *ectopic*, but the overall ectopic rate is still lower than in a woman using no contraception. If ectopic pregnancy has been excluded, the IUD should be removed early so as to lower the risk of miscarriage.

Contraindications to the intrauterine device (IUD)	
Absolute:	Endometrial or cervical cancer
	Undiagnosed vaginal bleeding
	Active/recent pelvic infection
	Pregnancy
Relative:	Previous ectopic pregnancy
	Excessive menstrual loss (unless hormone releasing)
	Multiple sexual partners
	Young/nulliparous
	Immunocompromised, including human immunodeficiency virus (HIV) -positive

Advantages

The IUD is extremely safe. The woman does not need to remember to use other contraception. Menstrual loss is reduced if progestogen-containing devices are used. The IUD can be used as emergency contraception if inserted within 5 days of unprotected intercourse.

Counselling before inserting an intrauterine device (IUD)	
Advise of the major risks	
Advise to inform her doctor if:	She bleeds intermenstrually
	She experiences pelvic pain or a vaginal discharge, or if she feels she might be pregnant
Advise about checking for strings after each period	

Female sterilization

Twenty-five per cent of couples rely on male or female sterilization. The minimum that needs to be done for female sterilization is interruption of the fallopian tubes so that sperm and egg cannot meet. More radical procedures such as hysterectomy should only be performed if specific indications are present. The most common technique uses clips (e.g. Filshie clip; Fig. 12.7). These are applied to the tubes laparoscopically [→ p.103], com-

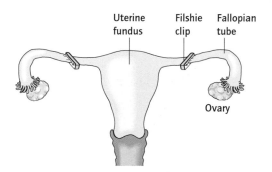

Fig. 12.7 Female sterilization. View of uterine fundus with Filshie clips on tubes.

pletely occluding the lumen. This normally involves a general anaesthetic.

Contraceptive efficacy

The Filshie clip has a failure rate of 0.5%: i.e. about 1 in 200 women will become pregnant at some time.

Indications

Both doctor and woman must be satisfied that there will be no regret: therefore it is usually used in an older woman whose family is complete, or when disease contraindicates pregnancy.

Complications

Laparoscopic sterilization is a safe procedure (*Cochrane 2003*: CD003034), but perioperative complications include the risks of laparoscopy (primarily visceral damage) and inadequate access to the tubes (0.5%, both of which warrant a laparotomy. Postoperative pain is reduced by using local anaesthetic on the tubes and in the skin incisions. If pregnancy does occur, it is more likely to be ectopic. Requests for reversal should be rare with adequate woman selection and counselling.

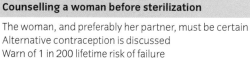

Counselling a woman before sterilization
The woman, and preferably her partner, must be certain
Alternative contraception is discussed
Warn of 1 in 200 lifetime risk of failure
Risk of ectopic if pregnancy
Reversal not always successful and unavailable on the National Health Service (NHS)
Risks of surgery [→ p.103] and of possible laparotomy

Male sterilization

Vasectomy is more effective than female sterilization (1 in 2000 lifetime risk after two negative semen analyses) and involves ligation and removal of a small segment of the vas deferens, thereby preventing release of sperm. It can be performed under local anaesthetic. Sterility is not assured until azoospermia is confirmed by two semen analyses and may take up to 6 months to achieve. Complications (5%) include failure, postoperative haematomas and infection. Successful reversal is often (50%) prevented by antisperm antibody formation [→ p.74].

Natural contraception

This is less reliable than most methods and offers no protection against STIs. It is only suitable for monogamous women who would not be concerned by pregnancy. *Lactation* has a major contraceptive role in the developing world. The *'rhythm' method* avoids the fertile period around ovulation and over-the-counter kits can help this. *'Withdrawal'* involves removal of the penis just be-fore ejaculation, but is not recommended because sperm can be released before orgasm.

Further reading

Contraception in teenagers. *Drug and Therapeutics Bulletin* 2002; **40**: 92–5.

Hormonal contraception: what is new? *Human Reproduction Update* 2002; **8**: 359–71.

Kubba A, Guillebaud J, Anderson RA, MacGregor EA. Contraception. *Lancet* 2000; **356**: 1913–9.

Rivera R, Best K. Current opinion: consensus statement on intrauterine contraception. *Contraception* 2002; **65**: 385–8.

Vandenbroucke JP, Rosing J, Bloemenkamp KW *et al.* Oral contraceptives and the risk of venous thrombosis. *The New England Journal of Medicine* 2001; **344**: 1527–35.

Contraception at a Glance

Combined oral contraceptive

Women:	Any, except smoker >35 years, history of venous thromboembolism, cerebrovascular disease and cerebrovascular accident, hypertension or inherited thrombophilia.
Failure:	Pearl index (PI) 0.2
Mode of action:	Inhibits ovulation
How to use:	Start on day 1 of cycle, 3 weeks, then 1 week's break
Rare major problems:	Deep vein thromboses, ischaemic heart disease, cerebrovascular accident, hypertension, breast and cervical carcinoma
Common side effects:	Breast tenderness, weight gain, bleeding, headaches, nausea
Benefits:	Good contraception, cycle control, well accepted
Drawbacks:	Major side effects and contraindications

Progestogen-only pill

Women:	Any. Need to be well motivated
Failure:	PI 1.0
Mode of action:	Cervical mucus and sometimes inhibition of ovulation
How to use:	Continuous, every day at same time
Side effects:	Vaginal spotting, other progestogenic effects
Benefits:	Few contraindications, lactation
Drawbacks:	Compliance and failure rate

Depot progestogens

Women:	Any. When compliance a problem
Failure:	PI <1.0
Mode of action:	As above, and ovulation usually inhibited
How to use:	Depo-Provera intramuscularly every 3 months, Noristerat every 8 weeks, Implanon every 3 years
Side effects:	Progestogenic; prolonged amenorrhoea and osteoporosis with Depo-Provera
Benefits:	Woman can 'forget about it'
Drawbacks:	Progestogenic side effects

Intrauterine devices (IUDs)

Women:	Older, multiparous, monogamous
Failure:	PI 0.2–2.0 depending on type
Mode of action:	Prevents implantation/fertilization
How to use:	Insert into uterus, change every 5–10 years
Side effects:	Pelvic infection, menstrual disturbance, perforation
Benefits:	Woman can 'forget about it', intrauterine system (IUS) reduces blood loss
Drawbacks:	Pelvic infection

Condoms

Person:	Any, essential for casual intercourse
Failure:	PI about 5
Benefits:	Non-hormonal, safe, protection against sexually transmitted infection (STIs)
Drawbacks:	Inconvenience, poor technique

Caps/diaphragms

Woman:	Any, well motivated, usually monogamous
Failure:	PI about 5
How to use:	Insert before intercourse, with spermicide, remove 6 h later
Benefits:	Non-hormonal, woman has control
Drawbacks:	Failure rates, inconvenience, limited protection against STIs

Sterilization

Person:	Older, multiparous, family finished
Failure:	1 in 200 (female); 1 in 2000 (male) lifetime risk
How to do:	Female: laparoscopic clip occlusion of fallopian tubes
	Male: ligation and removal of segment of vas deferens (vasectomy)
Side effects:	Peri-operative complications
Benefits:	Permanent
Drawbacks:	Permanent, common source of litigation

13 The Menopause and Hormone Replacement Therapy

Definitions

The *menopause* is the last menstruation. It is a natural phenomenon of age, occurring at the average age of 51 years.

The *climacteric* precedes it and is a time of transition from reproductive to non-reproductive state.

A '*premature*' menopause occurs before the age of 45 years.

Postmenopausal bleeding [→ p.92] is that which occurs at least 12 months after cessation of menstruation.

Physiology

The response of the ovaries to pituitary hormones becomes increasingly irregular as the number of follicles declines. Ovulation and menstruation become erratic and the first symptoms of this oestrogen deficiency state may occur (Fig. 13.1). As the menopause is reached, the ovaries 'fail': there is no response to pituitary hormones (Fig. 13.2b). Oestrogen production diminishes, so the negative feedback effect on pituitary hormone production is reduced and luteinizing hormone (LH) and follicle-stimulating hormone (FSH) (>30 iu/mL) levels rise.

Premature menopause

The menopause occurs before the age of 45 years in only 1% of women. Those undergoing bilateral salpingo-oöphorectomy (BSO) will also be affected. It is important to recognize because of the increased risks of heart disease and osteoporosis. In most women no cause is found, but infections such as mumps and pelvic tuberculosis, autoimmune disorders, chemotherapy, ovarian dysgenesis and metabolic diseases such as myotonic dystrophy have been implicated. Hormone replacement therapy (HRT) [→ p.90] is indicated at least until the age of 51 years.

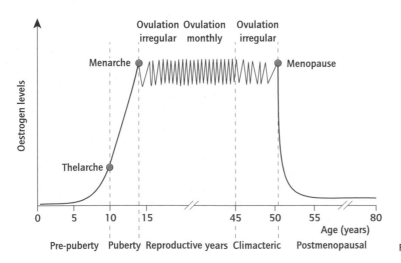

Fig. 13.1 Oestrogen levels in a lifetime.

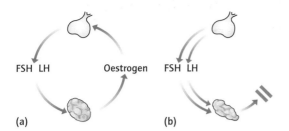

Fig. 13.2 Ovarian responsiveness to pituitary hormones. (a) Reproductive years: feedback control between ovary and hypothalamic–pituitary axis. (b) Postmenopausal years: unresponsive ovaries produce no oestrogen. Lack of feedback on hypothalamus–pituitary axis causes high levels of follicle-stimulating hormone (FSH) and luteinizing hormone (LH).

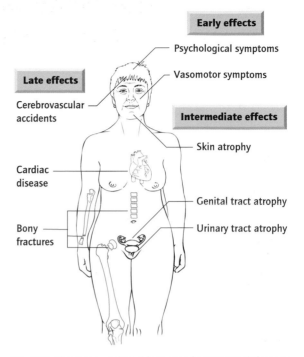

Fig. 13.3 Changes and clinical features of oestrogen deficiency.

Symptoms and consequences of the menopause (Fig. 13.3)

Early menopausal changes

Vasomotor changes: The 'hot flush', whereby a woman experiences a feeling of intense heat, sweats profusely and blushes, occurs in 70% of women. Its mechanism is not fully understood. *Psychological* symptoms such as insomnia, poor concentration, anxiety and lethargy, and reduced libido are common after the menopause. *Female sexual dysfunction*, consisting of decreased desire and arousal, dyspareunia and failure to achieve orgasm, is common.

Longer term changes

Skin and breasts: Collagen is lost from the skin, which becomes drier and more wrinkled. Hair loss may occur. Breast tissue is replaced by fatty tissue and the breasts shrink.
Genital tract: Cessation of menstruation may be welcome if it has been heavy or irregular during the climacteric. However, the vagina becomes drier and the walls thinner. It is more liable to infection as its pH rises. Prolapse may occur as the pelvic floor becomes more lax.
Urinary tract: Sensory urgency [→ p.56], with frequency and the inability to fill the bladder completely, may occur as the bladder wall atrophies. Incontinence is common.

Bone: Oestrogen deficiency causes calcium loss such that, after 20 years, more than a third of bone density may have been lost. This causes osteoporosis: 'characterised by low bone mass and micro-architectural deterioration of bone tissue, leading to enhanced bone fragility and a consequent increase in fracture risk' (World Health Organization definition). It affects 1 in 3 women. In the spine this causes height loss; in the long bones, Colles' fractures and fractured neck of femur occur. About 40% of 80-year-old women have had an osteoporotic fracture. Osteoporosis can be treated and prevented with biphosphanates, calcium supplementation and selective oestrogen receptor modulators (SERMs) in older women or with HRT in younger women.
Cardiovascular system: Strokes and heart attacks are rare in the premenopausal woman. This changes after the menopause as the risk approaches that of a man of similar age, and in women aged over 60 years cardiovascular disease is the leading cause of mortality.

Investigations

Endocrine tests: LH and FSH are only helpful if the diagnosis is in doubt as they fluctuate daily in the climacteric (*JAMA* 2003; **289**: 895). Levels of FSH > 30 iµ/mL are characteristic postmenopausally. Other hormonal tests are of little value in the diagnosis of the menopause. *Mammography* is advised 3-yearly after the menopause. *Endometrial biopsy* [→ p.92] is required for postmenopausal bleeding. *Bone density assessment* is performed in women at increased risk for osteoporosis. Methods include dual-energy X-ray absorptiometry (DXA) and quantitative ultrasound.

Treatment of the menopause — hormone replacement therapy (HRT)

Drug treatment of the menopause is controversial. A woman's decision to use it should be helped by individual risk assessment of its advantages and disadvantages. In practice, <50% of women prescribed HRT are using it after a year. Other risk factors for heart disease and osteoporosis, such as smoking and lack of exercise, should be addressed. Irregular or intermenstrual bleeding should be investigated as for a postmenopausal bleed [→ p.92]. There is no consensus as to how long women should stay on HRT: the risks of breast cancer and venous thromboembolism need to be balanced, both mathematically and emotionally, against the alleviation of postmenopausal symptoms and prevention of osteoporosis.

Preparations (Fig. 13.4)

Hormone replacement therapy is usually a combination of oestrogens and progestogens or a synthetic compound with properties of both (e.g. tibolone). Oestro-

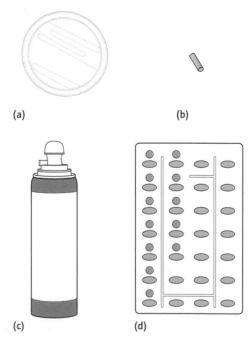

Fig. 13.4 Preparations of hormone replacement therapy (HRT): (a) patch, (b) implant, (c) gel and (d) pills.

gen, either from plants or animals, is used to replace the natural oestrogens that the ovaries no longer produce. Synthetic progestogens are used because oestrogen alone ('unopposed') increases the risk of endometrial carcinoma (*NEJM* 1975; **293**: 1164). Progestogens are not therefore required if the woman has had a hysterectomy. *Oral* preparations are taken in 28-day cycles, the oestrogens continuously and the progestogens for 12 days of the 28. Shortly after stopping the progestogen, a withdrawal bleed will occur. The result will be regular monthly 'periods'. Preparations using longer courses of progestogens now allow 3-monthly or even no menses. *Implant* preparations are inserted subcutaneously under local anaesthetic, usually in the abdominal wall. An implant will last up to a year, depending on the dose given. Progestogens still need to be taken if the woman has her uterus. Testosterone implants are occasionally used as well to improve libido.

Other: *Transdermal* patches are self-adhesive and contain oestrogens, which are absorbed transdermally. They are normally changed twice a week. Alternatively *gel* is rubbed into the skin daily. *Nasal sprays* and *vaginal rings* can also be used. If progestogens are needed too (intact uterus), they can be included in a patch or may be taken orally.

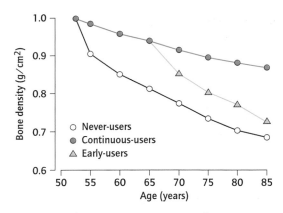

Fig. 13.5 Bone density in oestrogen users and non-users.

Contraindications to the use of hormone replacement therapy (HRT)	
Absolute:	Current breast or endometrial cancer Undiagnosed irregular vaginal bleeding Acute phase venous or arterial thrombosis Undiagnosed breast mass Severe active liver disease
Relative:	Endometriosis Fibroids Past/family history of breast cancer Past/family history of thrombotic disease Liver/gall bladder disease

Preparations of hormone replacement therapy (HRT)
Combined oral oestrogen and progestogen in a pill Combined oestrogen and progestogen in a patch Oestrogen patch/gel/implant plus oral progestogen N.B. Progestogen is omitted if post-hysterectomy

Benefits

Short-term: symptom relief

Hormone replacement therapy will cure early symptoms of the menopause. It may be successful in regulating erratic bleeding during the climacteric, so long as a biopsy has been taken to exclude endometrial cancer. Mood is improved (*BJOG* 1995; **102**: 735).

Long-term

Osteoporosis: HRT reduces bone density loss (Fig. 13.5), pathological fractures and partly reverses established osteoporosis. These effects are lost after cessation of therapy.

Other long-term benefits: HRT reduces collagen loss in the skin and may preserve a 'younger' appearance. It reduces bladder dysfunction, may increase libido, protects against bowel carcinoma (*JAMA* 2002; **288**: 321), tooth loss and may prevent Alzheimer's disease, macular degeneration and cataracts.

Disadvantages

Short-term: side effects

Hormone replacement therapy simply replaces the oestrogens that the body itself produced formerly. Side effects can be due to either the oestrogen or the progestogen [→ p.80]. Most women dislike menstruation, although more 'period-free' preparations are now available. Irregular bleeding warrants endometrial biopsy. Other common effects are headaches, breast tenderness, fluid retention and premenstrual symptoms, although most diminish after about 3 months. Weight gain is unusual.

Long-term: complications

Breast cancer: The risk of a diagnosis is slightly increased (*JAMA* 2002; **288**: 321), by 2.3% per year of use, and disappears after about 5 years. Risk is related to lifetime exposure to oestrogens and progestogens, and HRT does not increase the risk of breast cancer in women with a premature menopause beyond what would have occurred naturally. Curiously, the prognosis of breast cancer in women taking HRT is better than in those who are not. The use of HRT in women with a past history of breast cancer is disputed, but seldom recommended.

Thromboembolic disease: There is a two- to fourfold increase in the risk of thromboembolic disease (*JAMA* 2002; **288**: 58).

Other long-term disadvantages: Unopposed oestrogen increases the risk of endometrial carcinoma. Progestogens are used to prevent this: oestrogen with cyclical usage of progestogens is still associated with small increase in risk. When progestogens are used continuously the risk is reduced. The effect of cardiovascular disease remains disputed, but, in older women, HRT may actually increase the risk where once it was thought to be protective (*JAMA* 2002; **288**: 321).

Postmenopausal bleeding (PMB)

Definition

Vaginal bleeding occurring at least 12 months after cessation of menstruation.

Causes

Carcinoma of the endometrium and atypical hyperplasia [→ p.24] account for about 20% of cases. Cervical and ovarian cancer may also present with PMB. Bleeding may also occur from a poorly oestrogenized vaginal wall: 'atrophic vaginitis'. Sometimes no cause is found. Withdrawal bleeds occur with many forms of HRT and, so long as they are regular, do not warrant investigation.

Causes of postmenopausal bleeding (PMB)
Endometrial carcinoma
Endometrial hyperplasia ± atypia and polyps
Cervical carcinoma
Atrophic vaginitis
Cervicitis
Ovarian carcinoma
Cervical polyps
N.B. Normal only if patient on hormone replacement therapy (HRT) *and* regular

Management

Endometrial biopsy is imperative, even if atrophic vaginitis is evident. This is best achieved at hysteroscopy [→ p.103] because polyps will be visualized and the detection of malignancy is better than 'blind' methods. The pelvic organs are palpated, the cervix is inspected and a smear is taken. Other methods of investigation include endometrial sampling with a Pipelle [→ p.12]. Transvaginal ultrasound can be used to measure endometrial thickness: if <4 mm in the postmenopausal woman, biopsy may even be unneccessary. Its use as a first-line alternative to biopsy remains disputed. If malignancy is excluded, atrophic vaginitis can be treated with HRT or topical oestrogen.

Further reading

Nelson HD, Humphrey LL, Nygren P *et al*. Postmenopausal hormone replacement therapy: scientific review. *JAMA: the Journal of the American Medical Association* 2002; **288**: 872–81.

Rees M, Purdie DW, eds. *Management of the Menopause*. BMS Publications, 2002.

www.the-bms.org for information on the menopause and HRT.

The Menopause at a Glance

Definition	The last menstrual period
Average age	51 years. Premature if <40 years
Climacteric	Time preceding menopause, menstruation often erratic
Features	Early changes: Hot flushes, insomnia, psychological
	Later changes: Skin and breast atrophy, hair loss, atrophic vaginitis, prolapse, urinary symptoms, osteoporosis, cardiovascular disease
Investigations	Follicle-stimulating hormone (FSH) raised, but these may be normal initially
Treatment	Not mandatory or universal. Hormone replacement therapy (HRT) to alleviate symptoms and prevent osteoporosis, but beware of risks
Bleeding	Postmenopausal bleeding is 1+ years after last period, unless it is regular *and* patient is taking HRT. Is always abnormal: endometrial biopsy is required

Hormone Replacement Therapy (HRT) at a Glance

Definition	Use of exogenous oestrogens when endogenous secretion is absent
Preparations	Progesterone used with oestrogen or as synthetic combination (oestrogen alone if patient has had hysterectomy) Oral, patch, gel, implant, spray or vaginal ring
Advantages	Short-term relief from menopausal symptoms May regulate erratic bleeding during climacteric Protects against and partly reverses osteoporosis Reduces sensory urgency; improved skin and hair appearance Protects against tooth loss, Alzheimer's disease and bowel carcinoma
Disadvantages	Menstruation unless 'period-free' preparation Oestrogenic and progestogenic side effects Increased risk of breast cancer, venous thromboembolism, possibly cardiovascular disease

Disorders of Early Pregnancy

Physiology of early pregnancy

The ovum is fertilized in the ampulla of the fallopian tube. Mitotic division occurs as the zygote is swept toward the uterus by ciliary action and peristalsis (Fig. 14.1a). Tubal damage will impair movement and render tubal implantation and ectopic pregnancy more likely. The zygote normally enters the uterus on day 4, at the eight-cell (morula) stage. The morula becomes a blastocyst by developing a fluid-filled cavity within. Its outer layer becomes trophoblast, which will form the placenta, and from the sixth to twelfth day, this invades the endometrium to achieve implantation (Fig. 14.1b). Fifteen per cent of embryos are lost at this stage and so many miscarriages go unnoticed.

The trophoblast produces hormones almost immediately, notably human chorionic gonadotrophin (HCG) (detected in pregnancy tests), which will peak at 12 weeks. This ability to invade and produce HCG is reflected in gestational trophoblastic disease. Nutrients are gained from the secretory endometrium, which turns deciduous (rich in glycogen and lipids) under the influence of oestrogen and progesterone from the corpus luteum and trophoblast. Trophoblastic proliferation leads to formation of chorionic villi. On the endometrial surface of the embryo, this villous system proliferates (chorion frondosum) and will ultimately form the surface area for nutrient transfer, in the cotyledons of the placenta. Placental morphology is complete at 12 weeks. A heartbeat is established at 4–5 weeks and is visible on ultrasound a week later.

Spontaneous abortion or miscarriage

Definition and epidemiology

The fetus dies or delivers dead before 24 completed

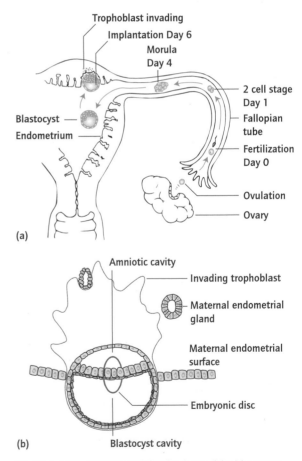

Fig. 14.1 (a) Fertilization and development of the blastocyst. (b) Implantation: day 6.

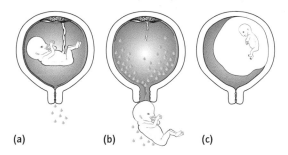

Fig. 14.2 (a) Threatened miscarriage. (b) Incomplete miscarriage. (c) Missed miscarriage.

weeks of pregnancy. The majority occur before 12 weeks. Fifteen per cent of clinically recognized pregnancies spontaneously abort; more will be so early as to go unrecognized. Miscarriage is more common in older women.

Types of miscarriage

Threatened miscarriage: There is bleeding but the fetus is still alive, the uterus is the size expected from the dates and the os is closed (Fig. 14.2a). Only 25% will go on to miscarry.

Inevitable miscarriage: Bleeding is usually heavier. Although the fetus may still be alive, the cervical os is open. Miscarriage is about to occur.

Incomplete miscarriage: Some fetal parts have been passed, but the os is usually open (Fig. 14.2b).

Complete miscarriage: All fetal tissue has been passed. Bleeding has diminished, the uterus is no longer enlarged and the cervical os is closed.

Septic miscarriage: The contents of the uterus are infected, causing endometritis [→ p.64]. Vaginal loss is offensive and the uterus is tender. A fever can be absent. If pelvic infection occurs there is abdominal pain and peritonism.

Missed miscarriage: The fetus has not developed or died *in utero*, but this is not recognized until bleeding occurs or ultrasound scan is performed. The uterus is smaller than expected from the dates and the os is closed (Fig. 14.2c).

Aetiology of sporadic miscarriage

Isolated non-recurring chromosomal abnormalities account for >60% of 'one-off' or sporadic miscarriages.

However, if three or more miscarriages occur, then the rarer causes are more likely [→ p.96]. Exercise, intercourse and emotional trauma do not cause miscarriage.

Clinical features

History: Bleeding is usual unless a missed miscarriage is found incidentally at ultrasound examination. Pain from uterine contractions can cause confusion with an ectopic pregnancy.

Examination: Uterine size and the state of the cervical os are dependent on the type of miscarriage. Tenderness is unusual.

Investigations

An *ultrasound scan* will show if a fetus is in the uterus and if it is viable (Fig. 14.3), and it may detect retained fetal tissue (products). If there is any doubt, the scan should be repeated a week later as non-viable pregnancies can be confused with a very early pregnancy, especially where the date of the last menstrual period is uncertain. Ultrasound does not always allow visualization of an ectopic pregnancy, but if a fetus is seen in the uterus, ectopic pregnancy is extremely unlikely. *Human chorionic gonadotrophin beta-subunit* (β-HCG) levels in the blood normally increase by >66% in 48 h with a viable intrauterine pregnancy. This helps differentiate between ectopic and viable intrauterine pregnancies at early gestations when ultrasound is less helpful. The *full blood count* (FBC) and *rhesus group* should also be checked.

Management

Admission is necessary if ectopic pregnancy is not excluded, if the miscarriage is inevitable, incomplete or septic, or if the patient's social circumstances warrant it. Bed rest does not prevent miscarriage.

Resuscitation is occasionally required as bleeding can be heavy. Products of conception in the cervical os cause pain, bleeding and vasovagal shock and are removed. Intramuscular *ergometrine* will reduce bleeding by contracting the uterus, but is only used if the fetus is non-viable. If there is a fever, swabs for bacterial culture are taken and intravenous antibiotics are given. *Anti-D* is usually given to women who are rhesus negative, but is not required with threatened miscarriages before 12 weeks.

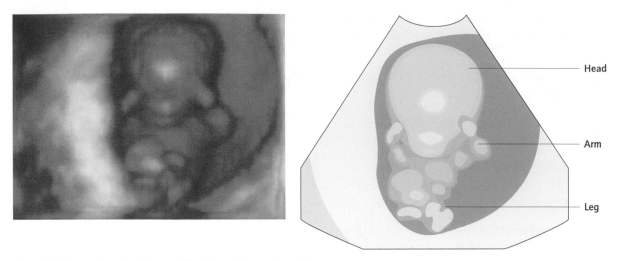

Fig. 14.3 Three-dimensional image of live fetus at 11 weeks gestation.

Evacuation of retained products of conception (ERPC) under anaesthetic using vacuum aspiration (*Cochrane* 2001: CD001993) is normally performed unless the miscarriage is complete. Tissue is examined histologically to exclude molar pregnancy. Alternatively, misoprostol can be given (*Fertil Steril* 1999; **71**: 1054) or spontaneous resolution simply awaited.

Complications

Haemorrhage and infection can occur if fetal tissue is retained, particularly after inadequately performed ERPC. If infection becomes systemic, endotoxic shock occasionally ensues, with hypotension, renal failure, adult respiratory distress syndrome and disseminated intravascular coagulation. In addition, curettage can partially remove the endometrium causing Asherman's syndrome [→ p.16] or even perforate the uterus.

Counselling after miscarriage

Patients should be told that the miscarriage was not the result of anything they did and could not have been prevented. Reassurance as to the high chance of successful further pregnancies is important and intensive support is offered for these. Referral to a support group may be useful. Because miscarriage is so common, further investigation is usually reserved for women who have had three miscarriages.

Recurrent miscarriage

Definition and epidemiology

Recurrent miscarriage is when three or more miscarriages occur in succession; 1% of couples are affected. The chance of miscarriage in a fourth pregnancy is still only 40%, but a recurring cause is more likely and investigations and support should be arranged. In practice, investigation is often requested and performed after only two miscarriages.

Causes and their management

Whilst investigation may reveal a possible cause, few treatments are of proven value. These patients are often extremely distressed and support is vital. Serial ultrasound scans are used in early pregnancy for reassurance. In later pregnancy, 'high-risk' monitoring is important because perinatal mortality is higher.

Autoimmune disease [→ p.150] can cause recurrent miscarriage (*Lancet* 2003; **361**: 901). Thrombosis in the uteroplacental circulation is likely to be the mechanism. Treatment is with aspirin and low-dose heparin (*BMJ* 1997; **314**: 253).

Chromosomal defects are found in 4% of couples. Karyotyping is therefore necessary.

Polycystic ovary syndrome and *luteinizing hormone hypersecretion*. This is common, but the mechanism of pregnancy failure is unknown. The use of metformin may reduce this but good evidence is limited (*Lancet* 2003; **361**: 1894).

Anatomical factors: Uterine abnormalities are more common with late miscarriage. Many, however, are incidental findings and surgical treatment could lead to uterine weakness or adhesion formation. Cervical incompetence [→ p.158] is a recurrent cause of late miscarriage as well as preterm labour, but cerclage is not performed before 12 weeks.

Infection: This is implicated in preterm labour and late miscarriage only, where treatment of bacterial vaginosis reduces the incidence and recurrence of fetal loss [→ p.158].

Others: Obesity, smoking and higher maternal age have been implicated.

Investigation of recurrent miscarriage

Autoimmune and thrombophilia screen (repeat at 6 weeks if positive)
Karyotyping of both parents and of products of conception
Pelvic ultrasound

Unwanted pregnancy and therapeutic abortion

Definition

A therapeutic abortion is when abortion is artificially induced before the 24th completed week of gestation. Approximately 170 000 abortions are performed in the United Kingdom every year, 90% before the 12th week, and most commonly for social reasons.

Methods of abortion

Screening for *Chlamydia* [→ p.62] and/or anti-chlamydial treatment is usually offered.

Medical: Up to the ninth completed week, oral mifepristone followed by vaginal prostaglandin or misoprostol is used. Complete abortion occurs in more than 95% of cases obviating the need for an anaesthetic or surgery. Surgical termination remains slightly more effective and is less painful (*Cochrane* 2002; CD003037).

Suction curettage: Up to the 12th completed week, the uterus can be evacuated by suction after dilatation of the cervix. The latter is achieved with dilators, often after cervical 'ripening' with vaginal prostaglandins or misoprostol.

Prostaglandin induction: After the 12th week, surgery is less safe: expulsion is achieved with vaginal prostaglandins ± oxytocin, usually 48 h after administration of mifepristone. Late (beyond 20 weeks) abortion may be performed where a fetal abnormality is diagnosed. Feticide using potassium chloride (KCl) into the umbilical vein or fetal heart is performed first.

Selective abortion is occasionally performed with high-order multiple pregnancies or where one fetus of a twin pregnancy is abnormal [→ p.184].

Complications of therapeutic abortion

Medical termination may be incomplete, necessitating a surgical procedure. Complications of surgery include infection, uterine perforation and visceral damage and cervical trauma. Illegal methods of abortion increase mortality 500-fold, accounting for approximately 70 000 death worldwide per annum. There is often long-lasting psychological morbidity after termination of pregnancy.

The law, ethics and therapeutic abortion

In the United Kingdom, two doctors must agree to the patient's request for an abortion. This involves ethical conflict of the physician's duties to the unborn fetus with both his/her duties to the mother and her right to autonomy. In practice, 90% are performed under (c), effectively recognizing a maternal right to autonomy: although performed so as not to 'endanger the mental health' of the woman, these are predominantly social abortions. The grounds for abortion in the United Kingdom are:

(a) That the continuance of the pregnancy would involve risk to the life of the pregnant woman greater than if the pregnancy were terminated.

(b) That the termination is necessary to prevent grave permanent injury to the physical or mental health of the pregnant woman.

(c) That the pregnancy has not exceeded its 24th week and that the continuance of the pregnancy would involve risk, greater than if the pregnancy were terminated, of injury to the physical or mental health of the pregnant woman.

(d) That the pregnancy has not exceeded its 24th week and that continuance of the pregnancy would involve risk, greater than if the pregnancy were terminated, of injury to the physical or mental health of any existing child(ren) of the family of the pregnant woman.

(e) There is a substantial risk that if the child were born it would suffer from such physical or mental handicap as to be seriously handicapped.

Effectively, therefore, abortion to prevent maternal death or serious morbidity, or to prevent serious handicap in the child, is legal at any time in pregnancy.

After therapeutic abortion

The woman may need counselling and contraceptive advice should always be given. This must take into account the reasons why the unwanted pregnancy occurred. Anti-D should be given if she is rhesus negative.

Ectopic pregnancy

Definition and epidemiology

An ectopic pregnancy is when the embryo implants outside the uterine cavity. This is becoming more common in the United Kingdom and occurs in 1 in 60–100 pregnancies. Mortality per case has reduced, but it accounts for 12% of maternal mortality in the United Kingdom [→ p.233]. It is more common with advanced maternal age and lower social class.

Pathology and sites of ectopic pregnancy

The most common site is in the fallopian tube (95%), although implantation can occur in the cornu, the cervix, the ovary and the abdominal cavity (Fig. 14.4). The thin-walled tube is unable to sustain trophoblastic invasion: it bleeds into its lumen or may rupture, when intraperitoneal blood loss can be catastrophic. The ectopic can also be naturally aborted.

Aetiology

No cause is evident with many, but any factor which damages the tube can cause the fertilized ovum to be caught. Commonly this is pelvic inflammatory disease, usually from sexually transmitted infection [→ p.61].

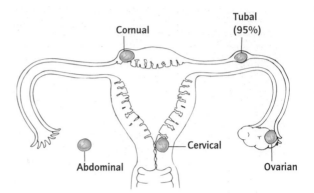

Fig. 14.4 Sites of ectopic pregnancy.

Assisted conception and pelvic, particularly tubal, surgery are additional risks.

Clinical features

The diagnosis is often missed. Abnormal vaginal bleeding, abdominal pain or collapse in any woman of reproductive age should all arouse suspicion. Increasing numbers of women are now diagnosed early and when asymptomatic, because of routine ultrasound.

History: Usually, lower abdominal pain is followed by scanty, dark vaginal bleeding. One may, however, be present without the other. The pain is variable in quality, often initially colicky as the tube tries to extrude the sac and then constant. Syncopal episodes and shoulder-tip pain suggest intraperitoneal blood loss. The 'classic' presentation of collapse with abdominal pain accounts for <25%. Amenorrhoea of 4–10 weeks is usual, but the patient may be unaware that she is pregnant.

Examination: Tachycardia suggests blood loss, and hypotension and collapse occur only *in extremis*. There is usually abdominal and often rebound tenderness. On pelvic examination, movement of the uterus may cause pain (cervical excitation) and either adnexum may be tender. The uterus is smaller than expected from the gestation and the cervical os is closed.

Investigations

A pregnancy test (urine HCG) *must* be performed on all women of reproductive age who present with pain, bleeding or collapse. It is almost invariably positive with an ectopic pregnancy.

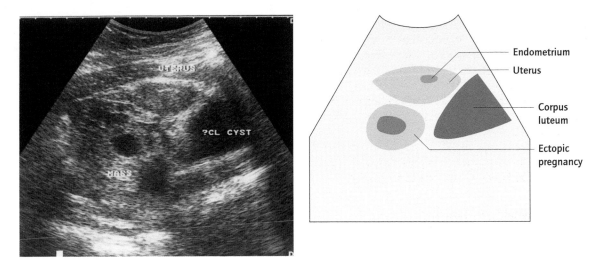

Fig. 14.5 Ultrasound of ectopic pregnancy. It is unusual to visualize the ectopic pregnancy with ultrasound.

Ultrasound (preferably transvaginal) does not always visualize an ectopic pregnancy (Fig. 14.5), but it should detect an intrauterine pregnancy. If the latter is not present, the gestation is either too early (<5 weeks) or there has been a complete miscarriage, or the pregnancy is elsewhere, i.e. ectopic.

Quantitative serum β-HCG is useful if the uterus is empty. If the maternal level is >1000 IU/mL then, if an intrauterine pregnancy is present, it will normally be visible on transvaginal ultrasound. If the level is lower than this, but rises by more than 66% in 48 h, an earlier but intrauterine pregnancy is likely. Declining or slower rising levels suggest an ectopic or non-viable intrauterine pregnancy. Caution is still required as, particularly with assisted conception, an intrauterine and an ectopic pregnancy can occasionally coexist.

Laparoscopy is the most sensitive investigation, but it is invasive. The combination of β-HCG and ultrasound allows for fewer 'negative' laparoscopies.

Management of the symptomatic suspected ectopic pregnancy
Nil by mouth
Full blood count (FBC) and cross-match blood
Pregnancy test
Ultrasound
Laparoscopy or consider medical management of criteria met

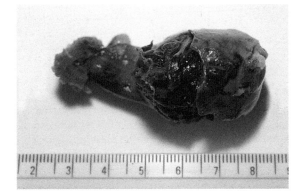

Fig. 14.6 The ectopic pregnancy (in Fig. 14.5) removed by salpingectomy.

Management

Where symptoms are present, the patient should be admitted. Intravenous access is inserted and blood is cross-matched. Anti-D is given if the patient is rhesus negative.

Acute presentations: If the patient is haemodynamically unstable, a laparotomy is performed. The affected tube is removed (salpingectomy) (Fig. 14.6).

Subacute presentations:

1 Classical management: At laparoscopy, the ectopic is usually removed from the tube (salpingostomy). This is preferable to laparotomy because recovery is faster and subsequent fertility rates are equivalent or better.

2 Non-surgical management: If the ectopic is unruptured with no cardiac activity, <35 mm in diameter, with a β-HCG level <5000 IU/mL, systemic single-dose methotrexate can also be used, without recourse to laparoscopy (*Int J Gynaecol Obstet* 1999; **65**: 97). Serial β-HCG levels are subsequently monitored to confirm that all trophoblastic tissue has gone: a second dose or surgery may still be required.

3 Conservative management: If the ectopic is small and unruptured and β-HCG levels are declining, observation may suffice as rupture is unlikely.

Complications

Particular support must be given to these patients, who have not only 'lost their baby' through a life-threatening condition but have also undergone surgery and had their fertility reduced. Only 70% of women will subsequently have a successful pregnancy and up to 10% will have another ectopic pregnancy.

Hyperemesis gravidarum

Definition and epidemiology

Hyperemesis gravidarum is when nausea and vomiting in early pregnancy are so severe as to cause severe dehydration, weight loss or electrolyte disturbance. This occurs in only 1 in 750 women. However, vomiting in pregnancy is a common cause of hospital admission, but most patients are only mildly dehydrated and therefore have 'moderate' nausea and vomiting of pregnancy (NVP). It seldom persists beyond 14 weeks and is more common in multiparous women.

Nausea and vomiting of pregnancy (NVP)	
Mild NVP	Nausea and occasional morning vomiting 50% of pregnant women No treatment required
Moderate NVP	More persistent vomiting 5% of pregnant women Often admitted to hospital
Severe NVP	Hyperemesis gravidarum

Management

Predisposing conditions, particularly urinary infection and multiple or molar pregnancy, are excluded. Intravenous rehydration is given, with thiamine and antiemetics. Steroids have been used in severe cases. Psychological support is essential, particularly as many of these women have social or emotional problems.

Gestational trophoblastic disease

Definitions and epidemiology

In this, trophoblastic tissue, which is the part of the blastocyst that normally invades the endometrium, proliferates in a more aggressive way than is normal. Human chorionic gonadotrophin is usually secreted in excess. Proliferation can be localized and non-invasive: this is called a *hydatidiform mole*. Alternatively, the proliferation may have characteristics of malignant tissue: if invasion is only present locally within the uterus, this is an '*invasive mole*'; if metastasis occurs, it is a *choriocarcinoma*. Molar pregnancy is rare, accounting for 1 in 500–1000 pregnancies, and is more common at the extremes of reproductive age.

Pathology

A complete mole is entirely paternal in origin, usually when one sperm fertilizes an empty ovum and undergoes mitosis. The result is diploid tissue, usually 46XX. There is no fetal tissue, merely a proliferation of swollen chorionic villi. Some 5–10% will turn malignant. *A partial mole* is usually triploid, derived from two sperms and one egg. There is variable evidence of a fetus and malignant change is rarer.

Clinical features

History: Vaginal bleeding is usual and may be heavy. Severe vomiting may occur. The condition may be detected on routine ultrasound.

Examination: The uterus is often large. Early pre-eclampsia and hyperthyroidism may occur.

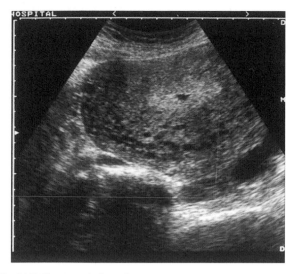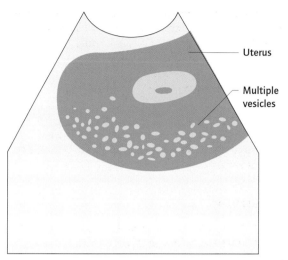

Fig. 14.7 Ultrasound of a molar pregnancy.

Investigations

Ultrasound characteristically shows a 'snowstorm' appearance of the swollen villi (Fig. 14.7), but the diagnosis can only be confirmed histologically.

Management and follow-up

The trophoblastic tissue is removed by suction curettage (ERPC) and the diagnosis confirmed histologically. Bleeding is often heavy. Thereafter, serial blood or urine HCG levels are taken: persistent or rising levels are suggestive of malignancy. This follow-up is normally done in a supra-regional centre. Pregnancy and the combined oral contraceptive are avoided until β-HCG levels are normal because they may increase the need for chemotherapy.

Complications

Recurrence of molar pregnancy occurs in about 1 in 60 subsequent pregnancies (*BJOG* 2003; **110**: 22).
Malignant trophoblastic disease, as an invasive mole or *choriocarcinoma*, follows 3% of complete moles. However, molar pregnancy precedes only 50% of malignancies, because malignancy can also follow miscarriages and normal pregnancies, usually presenting as persistent vaginal bleeding. The diagnosis of malignancy is made from persistently elevated or rising HCG levels, persistent vaginal bleeding or evidence of blood-borne metas-tasis, commonly to the lungs. The tumour is highly malignant, but is normally very sensitive to chemotherapy. Patients are scored into 'low-risk' and 'high-risk' categories according to prognostic variables. Low-risk patients receive methotrexate with folic acid, whereas higher-risk patients receive combination chemotherapy. Five-year survival rates approach 100%.

Further reading

Ballagh SA, Harris HA, Demasio K. Is curettage needed for uncomplicated incomplete spontaneous abortion? *American Journal of Obstetrics and Gynecology* 1998; **179**:1279–82.

Douchar N. Nausea and vomiting in pregnancy: a review. *British Journal of Obstetrics and Gynaecology* 1995; **102**: 6–8.

Hancock BW, Tidy JA. Current management of molar pregnancy. *The Journal of Reproductive Medicine* 2002; **47**: 347–54.

Li TC. Recurrent miscarriage: principles of management. *Human Reproduction (Oxford, England)* 1998; **13**: 478–82.

Royal College of Obstetricians and Gynaecologists. The investigation and treatment of couples with recurrent miscarriage. Guideline 17(B); 2003: www.rcog.org.uk.

Sau A, Hamilton-Fairley D. Nonsurgical diagnosis and management of ectopic pregnancy. *The Obstetrician and Gynaecologist* 2003; **5**: 29–33.

Spontaneous Miscarriage at a Glance

Definition	Expulsion or death of the fetus before 24 weeks
Epidemiology	15% of recognized pregnancies, up to 50% of all conceptions
Aetiology	>50% chromosomal abnormalities. Recurrent miscarriage also associated with autoimmune disorders, uterine abnormalities, polycystic ovary syndrome
Pathology	Products can be retained and cause haemorrhage and/or infection
Features	Heavy vaginal bleeding, often with pain. Little tenderness
Investigations	Ultrasound to confirm intrauterine site and fetal viability
Management	Depends on type. Anti-D if rhesus negative Evacuation of retained products of conception (ERPC) if heavy bleeding or definite missed miscarriage Conservative if threatened, diagnosis not certain, consider if inevitable/incomplete
Complications	Haemorrhage and infection, and of surgery

Ectopic Pregnancy at a Glance

Definition	Embryo implants outside the uterus	
Epidemiology	1%+ of pregnancies in United Kingdom	
Aetiology	Idiopathic, tubal damage from pelvic inflammatory disease, surgery, appendicitis	
Pathology	95% in fallopian tube. Occasionally cornu, cervix, ovary, abdomen Tubal implantation leads to tubal rupture and intraperitoneal bleeding	
Features	At 4–10 weeks of amenorrhoea	
	Acute:	Collapse with abdominal pain, patient shocked
	Subacute:	Abdominal pain, scanty dark per vaginum (PV) loss. Lower abdominal tenderness, cervical excitation, adnexal tenderness usual
	Incidental:	Detected at ultrasound
Investigations	Pregnancy test and transvaginal ultrasound, human chorionic gonadotrophin beta-subunit (β-HCG) Laparoscopy to confirm unless diagnosis certain and medical management proposed.	
Management	Surgical:	To stop/prevent bleeding: salpingectomy/salpingostomy
	Medical:	Methotrexate if criteria met
Complications	Haemorrhage can be fatal; repeat ectopic, subfertility	

15 Gynaecological Operations

There are three main routes to gain access to the pelvic organs:
1 The abdominal route involves opening the abdominal wall through a lower transverse or, occasionally, a vertical mid-line incision.
2 The vaginal route is used both to inspect and operate on the inside of the uterus and for vaginal and pelvic surgery.
3 Laparoscopic surgery, using closed-circuit television via a laparoscope with a camera attached; this and the instruments are inserted through small incisions in the abdominal wall.

Endoscopy and endoscopic surgery

Diagnostic hysteroscopy

The cavity is inspected using carbon dioxide insufflation or saline (Fig. 15.1). This can be performed without general anaesthesia. It is used as an adjunct to endometrial biopsy [→ p.12] or if menstrual problems [→ p.13] do not respond to medical treatment.

Hysteroscopic surgery

An operating hysteroscope is used. In the endometrial resection [→ p.13], the endometrium or intracavity fibroids and polyps are removed using cutting diathermy. The complications of uterine perforation and fluid overload are rare with experienced operators. Almost all patients have a significant reduction in blood loss. This technique is best used with dysfunctional bleeding that is heavy but regular and not painful, in women approaching the menopause. Sterility is not ensured. Endometrial diathermy, laser ablation or heating with a hot balloon produce similar effects but, because no specimen is produced, prior biopsies are essential.

Diagnostic laparoscopy

The peritoneal cavity is insufflated with carbon dioxide after carefully passing a small hollow needle through the abdominal wall. This enables a trocar to be inserted without damaging the pelvic organs. A laparoscope is then passed down the trocar to enable visualization of the pelvis (Fig. 15.1). Laparoscopy is used to assess macroscopic pelvic disease, in the management of pelvic pain and dysmenorrhoea, infertility (when dye is passed through the cervix to assess tubal patency), suspected ectopic pregnancy and pelvic masses.

Laparoscopic surgery

Instruments are inserted through separate 'ports' in the abdominal wall. Laparoscopic surgery is commonly performed to sterilize, to destroy areas of endometriosis or remove an ectopic pregnancy. Virtually every gynaecological operation has now been performed laparoscopically. The advantages are better visualization of tissues, less tissue handling, less infection, reduced hospital stay and faster postoperative recovery with less pain. However, serious visceral damage has occurred in less experienced hands.

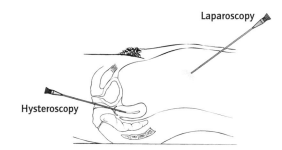

Fig. 15.1 Gynaecological endoscopy.

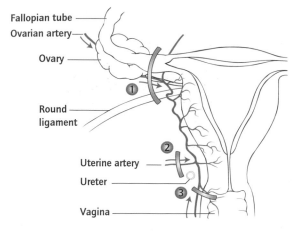

Fallopian tube
Ovarian artery
Ovary
Round ligament
Uterine artery
Ureter
Vagina

Fig. 15.2 Hysterectomy. (1) Blood: the anastomosis between uterine and ovarian arteries. If the ovaries are removed the ovarian artery and vein are ligated instead. Ligament: the round ligament. (2) Blood: the main uterine artery. Ligament: the cardinal ligament. The bladder is first dissected off the cervix and upper vagina, to prevent injury to it or to the ureters, which are close. (3) Blood: the cervico-vaginal branches of the uterine artery supplying the cervix and upper vagina. Ligament: the uterosacral ligament.

Hysterectomy

This is the commonest major gynaecological operation (Fig. 15.2). The ovaries can also be removed (bilateral salpingo-oöphorectomy, BSO). Because much of gynaecological management is based on symptoms rather than the disease itself, hysterectomy is most commonly performed for menstrual disorders, fibroids, endometriosis, chronic pelvic inflammatory disease and prolapse. The treatment of pelvic malignancies includes hysterectomy. Thromboprophylaxis is usual [→ p.105].

Types of hysterectomy

Total abdominal hysterectomy (TAH) is removal of the uterus and cervix through an abdominal incision. The above steps are performed from above, and therefore in the order 1, 2, 3 shown on Fig. 15.2. Specific indications include malignancy (ovarian and endometrial, in conjunction with a full laparotomy), a very large or immobile uterus and when abdominal inspection is required. In a subtotal hysterectomy, the cervix is retained and step 3 (Fig. 15.2) is omitted.

Vaginal hysterectomy (VH) is removal of the cervix and uterus after incising the vagina from below, and therefore in the order 3, 2, 1 (Fig. 15.2). The vaginal vault is closed after hysterectomy is complete. The specific indication is uterine prolapse, but absence of prolapse and moderate enlargement are not contraindications. Vaginal hysterectomy has a lower morbidity than abdominal hysterectomy.

Laparoscopic hysterectomy (LH) involves steps 1 and 2 (Fig. 15.2) from above with laparoscopic instruments, but step 3 is often completed vaginally. This is an alternative to TAH, not VH.

Wertheim's (radical) hysterectomy [→ p.32] involves removal of the parametrium, the upper third of the vagina and the pelvic lymph nodes. The usual indication is Stage 1a(ii)–2a *cervical carcinoma*. Occasionally, radical hysterectomy is performed vaginally (Schauta's radical hysterectomy).

Complications of hysterectomy	
Mortality:	1 in 10 000
Immediate:	Haemorrhage, bladder or ureteric injury
Postoperative:	Venous thromboembolism (use prophylactic low-molecular-weight heparin, LMWH), pain, retention and infection of urine, wound and chest infection (use prophylactic antibiotics), pelvic haematoma
Long term:	Prolapse, premature menopause, pain and psychosexual problems

Other common gynaecological operations

Dilatation and curettage (D&C)

The cervix is dilated with steel rods of increasing size; the endometrium is then curetted to biopsy it (Fig. 15.3). This is a diagnostic procedure and inferior to hysteroscopy because the cavity is not inspected.

Evacuation of retained products of conception (ERPC)

The cervix is dilated and a retained non-viable fetus or placental tissue is removed using suction. Surgical therapeutic abortion before 12 weeks uses a similar method.

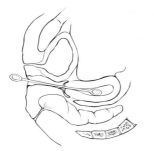

Fig. 15.3 Dilatation and curettage (D&C).

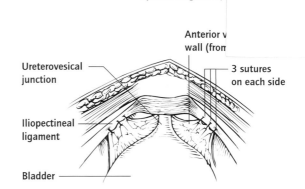

Fig. 15.4 The Burch colposuspension.

Cone biopsy [→p.31]

This removes the transformation zone and much of the endocervix by making a circular cut with a scalpel or laser in the cervix. It is used to stage apparently early cervical carcinoma and is sufficient treatment for Stage 1a(i) disease. The cervix can be left 'incompetent' and a cervical suture [→p.158] may be needed for future pregnancies.

Prolapse repair [→p.49]

An anterior repair (cystocoele) involves excision of prolapsed vaginal wall and plication of the bladder base and fascia. The vagina is then closed. A posterior repair (rectocoele) is similar, the levator ani muscle on either side being plicated between rectum and vagina. These operations are often performed together. Specific complications include retention of urine and overtightening of the vagina—it is important to ascertain if the patient is sexually active.

Operations for genuine stress incontinence

The principle is to elevate the bladder neck to allow it to be compressed when abdominal pressure rises [→p.54]. *Burch colposuspension* involves dissection through an abdominal incision in the extraperitoneal space over the bladder and anterior vaginal wall (Fig. 15.4). The vaginal wall on either side of the bladder neck is hitched up to the iliopectineal ligament on either side of the symphysis pubis with non-absorbable sutures.
Tension-free vaginal tape: The tape, made of polypropylene mesh, is approximately 2 cm wide and fixed to a trocar at each end. A small 3-cm vertical incision is made on the anterior vaginal wall over the mid-urethral section. After lateral dissection, the tape is introduced vaginally with the trocars entering the retropubic space. The tro-

cars are brought out through small transverse suprapubic incisions with the tape in position without tension and the vaginal skin is closed over.

Precautions in major gynaecological surgery

Thromboembolism

The combined oral contraceptive is usually stopped 4 weeks prior to major abdominal surgery. If hormone replacement therapy [→ p.90] is not stopped, low-molecular-weight heparin (LMWH) must be used. All women should be mobilized early, given thromboembolic disease stockings (TEDS) and kept hydrated; LMWH is given according to risk assessment (see box below).

Thromboprophylaxis in gynaecological surgery	
Low risk:	Minor surgery or major surgery <30 min, no risk factors
Moderate risk:	*Consider* anti-embolus stockings, low-molecular-weight heparin (LMWH), aspirin for: Surgery >30 min, obesity, gross varicose veins, current infection, prior immobility, major current illness
High risk:	*Use* LMWH prophylaxis for 5 days or until mobile for: Cancer surgery, prolonged surgery, history of deep vein thrombosis/thrombophilia, ≥3 of moderate risk factors above

Infection

Prophylactic antibiotics are used for major abdominal or vaginal surgery.

Urinary tract

Routine catheterization is only necessary after surgery for cancer or genuine stress incontinence, or when complications have arisen. Prophylactic antibiotics are used.

Further reading

Kadar N. *Atlas of Laparoscopic Pelvic Surgery.* Oxford: Blackwell Science, 1995.

Lee RA. *Atlas of Gynecologic Surgery.* The Mayo Foundation. Philadelphia: Saunders, 1992.

Obstetrics Section

16 The History and Examination in Obstetrics

The obstetric patient is usually a healthy woman undergoing a normal life event. The history and examination are to enable the doctor or midwife to safeguard both mother and fetus during this event, and are different from other specialities. Nevertheless, the student still needs to develop a consistent system of history-taking and examination to obtain the necessary information.

The obstetric history

Personal details

Ask her name, age, occupation, gestation and parity.

Presenting complaint/present circumstances

If she is an in-patient, why is she in hospital? Common reasons for admission are hypertension, pain, antepartum haemorrhage, unstable lie and possible ruptured membranes. If the pregnancy has hitherto been uncomplicated, say so.

History of present pregnancy

Dates: What was the first day of her last menstrual period (LMP)? What was the length of her menstrual cycle and was it regular? How many weeks gestation is she? (If a woman is at 38 weeks gestation, it is actually 36 weeks since conception.) To estimate the expected day of delivery (EDD), subtract 3 months from the date of the LMP, add 7 days and 1 year (Nägle's rule). In practice, this can be quickly calculated using an obstetric 'wheel' (Fig. 16.1). If a cycle is >28 days, the EDD will be later and needs to be adjusted: the number of days by which the cycle is longer than 28 is added to the date calculated using Nägle's rule. The reverse applies if the cycle is shorter than 28 days. If a woman has recently stopped the combined oral contraceptive, her cycles can be anovulatory and LMP is less useful.

Estimation of gestational age (Fig. 16.2)

From last menstrual period (LMP), allowing for cycle length

Ultrasound scan:
1 Measurement of crown–rump length between 7 and 14 weeks (if >1-week difference between LMP date and scan, use scan date)
2 Biparietal diameter or femur length between 14 and 20 weeks if no early scan and LMP unknown

Measurements to calculate gestational age are of little use beyond 20 weeks

---

Complications of pregnancy: Has there been any bleeding or hypertension, diabetes, anaemia, urine infections, concerns about fetal growth, or other problems? Ask if she has been admitted to hospital in the pregnancy?

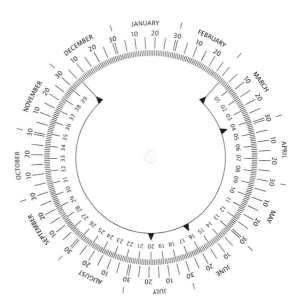

Fig. 16.1 The obstetric 'wheel'.

Tests: What tests have been performed (e.g. ultrasound scan, blood tests, prenatal diagnostic tests [→ p.124]).

Past obstetric history

Take details of past pregnancies in chronological order. Ask what was the mode and gestation of delivery and, if operative, why. Ask the birthweight and sex of the baby, and if the mother or the baby had any complications.

Parity. This is the number of times a woman has delivered potentially viable babies (in UK law this is defined as beyond 24 completed weeks). A woman who has had three term pregnancies is 'para 3', even if she is now in her fourth pregnancy. A suffix denotes the number of pregnancies that have miscarried (or been terminated) before 24 weeks; for example, if the same woman had had two prior miscarriages at 12 weeks, she would be described as 'para 3 + 2'. A nulliparous woman has never delivered a potentially live baby, although she may have had miscarriages or abortions; a multiparous woman has delivered at least one baby at 24 completed weeks or more.

Gravidity. This describes the number of times a woman has been pregnant: the woman above would be gravida 6, encompassing her three term deliveries, two miscarriages and the present pregnancy. The use of the term gravid is less descriptive and is best avoided.

Nulliparity and multiparity	
Nulliparous:	Has delivered no live/potentially live babies
Multiparous:	Has delivered live/potentially live (>24 week) babies

Symptoms of pregnancy
Amenorrhoea
Urinary frequency
Nausea ± vomiting
Breast tenderness

Other history

Past gynaecological history. This should be brief. Ask about intermenstrual and postcoital bleeding (IMB and PCB). Ask for the date of the last cervical smear and if one has ever been abnormal. Ask about prior contraception and any difficulty in conceiving.

Past medical history. Ask about operations, however distant. Ask about heart disease, hypertension, diabetes, anaemia, jaundice and epilepsy. If you elicit no history, ask 'have you ever been in hospital?'

Systems review. Ask the usual cardiovascular, respiratory, abdominal and neurological questions.

Drugs: Does she take any regular medication? Did she take preconceptual folic acid?

Family history. Is there a family history of twins, of diabetes, hypertension, pre-eclampsia, autoimmune disease or thrombophilia, or of any inherited disorder?

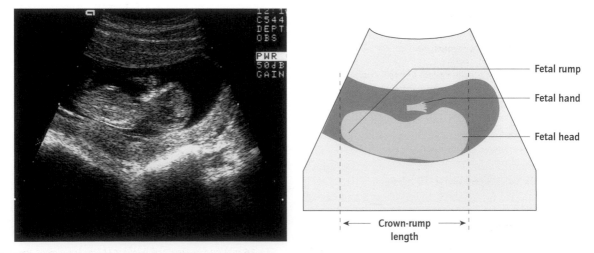

Fig. 16.2 Measurement of crown–rump length (12-week fetus).

Personal/social history: Does she smoke? Does she drink alcohol? If either, how much? Is she in a married or stable relationship and, if not, is there support at home? Where does she live, and what sort of accommodation is it?

Allergies: Ask specifically about penicillin and latex.

Other questions

Now ask: 'Is there anything else you think I ought to know'? The patient may be knowledgeable about her condition and this gives her the opportunity to help you if you have not discovered all the important facts.

Presenting the history

Start by summing up the important points, including important facts about any presenting complaint:
This is . . . aged . . ., who is . . . weeks into her . . . pregnancy and has been admitted to hospital because of . . . .

Example: This is Mrs X, aged 30 years, who is 38 weeks into her previously uncomplicated second pregnancy and has been admitted to hospital because of a painless antepartum haemorrhage.
N.B. You have demonstrated your understanding by mentioning the absence of pain, an important factor in the differential diagnosis of antepartum haemorrhage.

Now go through the history in some detail.

Then sum up again, in one sentence, including any important findings in the history.

Obstetric history: specific essential questions

Gestation and certainty
If in-patient, presenting complaint/reason for admission
Complications of the pregnancy
Parity and details of previous pregnancies
Gynaecological questions: intermenstrual bleeding (IMB), postcoital bleeding (PCB) and date of last cervical smear
Relevant past medical history
Relevant family history

The obstetric examination

General examination

General appearance, weight, height, temperature, oedema of the ankles and sacrum, and possible anaemia are assessed. At the booking visit, the chest, breasts, cardiovascular system and legs are also examined. The *blood pressure and urinalysis* tests should be performed together so that they are not forgotten (Fig. 16.3). The patient lies comfortably with her back semiprone at 45°. Diastolic blood pressure is recorded as Korotkoff V (when the sound disappears). If the blood pressure is raised or if there is proteinuria, examine elsewhere also [→ p.139] (e.g. for epigastric tenderness).

Abdominal examination

The patient should now lie as flat as is comfortable, discreetly exposed from just below the breasts to the symphysis pubis. In later pregnancy, the semiprone position or left lateral tilt will avoid aortocaval compression [→ p.205].

Why routinely palpate the abdomen?

<24 weeks:	To check dates, twins
>24 weeks:	To assess well-being by assessing size and liquor
>36 weeks:	To check lie, presentation and engagement

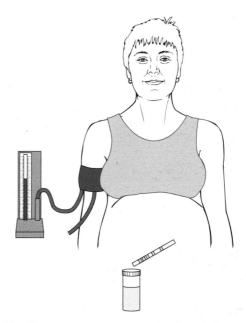

Fig. 16.3 Blood pressure measurement and urinalysis are essential.

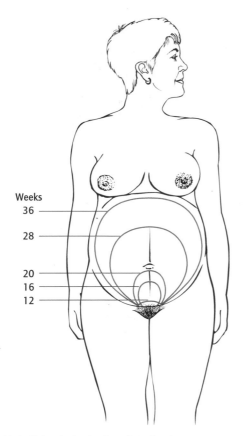

Fig. 16.4 Abdominal palpation of uterine size.

Weeks
36
28
20
16
12

The uterus is normally palpable abdominally at 12–14 weeks. By 20 weeks the fundus is usually at the level of the umbilicus. Before 20 weeks a uterus that is larger than expected is probably due to the gestation being incorrect, but could also be due to the presence of multiple pregnancy, uterine fibroids [→ p.20] or a pelvic mass.

Inspect
Look at the size of the pregnant uterus and look for striae, the linea nigra and scars, particularly in the suprapubic area (Fig. 16.4). Fetal movements are often visible in later pregnancy.

Palpation
This is purposeful and firm, but must be gentle. As you palpate ask yourself the reasons why you are doing it:
1 Is the fetus adequately grown?
2 Is the liquor volume normal?

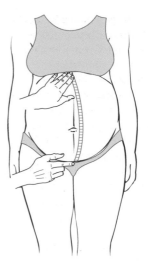

Fig. 16.5 Abdominal palpation. Step 1: Fundal palpation and measurement of symphysis–fundal height.

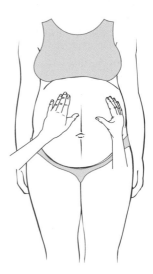

Fig. 16.6 Abdominal palpation. Step 2: Examination of fetal parts.

3 Is the lie longitudinal?
4 Is the presentation cephalic and, if so, is it engaged?
Palpation can be considered as consisting of three steps (Figs 16.5–16.7):
Step 1: Find the fundus using the fingers and ulnar border of the left hand. *Measure the distance to the symphysis pubis* with a tape measure (Fig. 16.5). After 24 weeks, the symphysis–fundal height in centimetres approximately

corresponds to the gestation ± 2 cm. This is the best clinical test for detecting the 'small for dates' fetus [→ p.169], but the sensitivity is only 70%. Also look for tenderness or uterine irritability.

Step 2: Next, facing the mother, use both hands to palpate down the fetus towards the pelvis (Fig. 16.6). Use 'dipping' movements to *palpate fetal parts* and *estimate the liquor volume*. Imagine an irregular potato in a small plastic bag containing water. Pressing on the outside of the bag will allow palpation of the potato, and the feel of the water is exactly how liquor feels. If none is present, the contents are easy to feel: if fluid volume is excessive (polyhydramnios), the bag will be tense and the fingers will need to dip in far to feel anything. Try to ascertain what you are feeling: the head is hard and, if free, can be gently 'bounced' or balloted between two hands, whereas the breech is softer, less easy to define and cannot be balloted.

The lie refers to the relationship between the fetus and the long axis of the uterus. If longitudinal, the head and buttocks are palpable at each end (Fig. 16.8). If transverse, the fetus is lying across the uterus and the pelvis will be empty (Fig. 16.9). If oblique, the head or buttocks are palpable in one of the iliac fossae.

Common causes of polyhydramnios
Diabetes/gestational diabetes
Fetal abnormality
Idiopathic

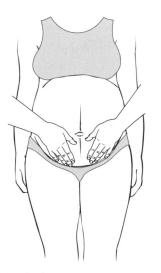

Fig. 16.7 Abdominal palpation. Step 3: Examination of presentation.

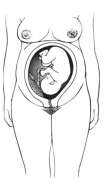

Fig. 16.8 Longitudinal lie (cephalic presentation in this instance).

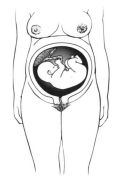

Fig. 16.9 Transverse lie.

Step 3: Turn to face the pelvis and press the fingers of both hands firmly down just above the symphysis pubis to assess the *presentation*: the fetal part that occupies the lower segment or pelvis (see Fig. 16.7). With a longitudinal lie (see Fig. 16.8), it is the head, or occasionally the buttocks. *Engagement of the head* (Fig. 16.10) occurs when the widest diameter descends into the pelvis: descent is described as 'fifths palpable'. If only two-fifths of the head is palpable abdominally, then more than half has entered the pelvis and so the head must be engaged. If more than two-fifths of the head is palpable, it is not engaged. If you are still unsure of the presentation, grasp the presenting fetal part between the thumb and index finger of the examining hand (Pawlik's grip). This can be uncomfortable for the patient and is seldom necessary.

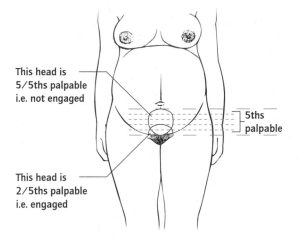

This head is 5/5ths palpable i.e. not engaged

5ths palpable

This head is 2/5ths palpable i.e. engaged

Fig. 16.10 Engagement of the fetal head.

Attempting to determine the *position* or *attitude* of the fetus is not a useful part of antenatal palpation of the abdomen. Where a woman has complained of pain or antepartum haemorrhage it is important to look for areas of tenderness and uterine irritability (it contracts when palpated).

Auscultate

Listening over the anterior shoulder (usually palpable between the head and the umbilicus), the fetal heart should be heard with a Pinard's stethoscope. Place this flat over the shoulder, press it on the abdomen with your ear, keeping both hands free and time the heart rate with your watch. It should be 110–160 beats per minute.

Vaginal examination is not a useful part of routine antenatal examination, unless labour is suspected or is to be induced and is therefore described in the chapters on labour.

Abdominal findings in pregnancy	
Uterine size:	Fundus palpable at 12–14 weeks
	At umbilicus at 20 weeks
	At xiphoid sternum at 36 weeks
	Fundal height increases approx. 1 cm/week after 24 weeks
Presentation:	Breech in 30% at 28 weeks
	Breech in 3% after 37 weeks
Engagement:	Usual in nulliparous after 37 weeks
	Multiparous often not engaged

Other features of relevance

Consider examination of fundi, reflexes, temperature, epigastrium, legs, chest, etc. if clinically indicated from history or other examination findings.

Presenting the examination

Present the examination findings, including relevant positive or negative findings:
Mrs X looks . . . (describe general appearance sensitively), her blood pressure is . . . and urinalysis shows . . . Her abdomen is distended compatible with pregnancy, the symphysis–fundal height is . . . , the lie is . . . and the presentation is . . . and is . . .(engagement). The fetal heart is audible and is . . . (rate). There is . . .(any important other positive or negative findings).

Example: Mrs X looks well, but has severe ankle and sacral oedema; her blood pressure is 150/110 and urinalysis shows 2+ of protein. Her abdomen is distended compatible with pregnancy and the symphysis–fundal height is 32 cm. The presentation is cephalic and the head is engaged. The fetal heart is 130 beats per minute. She has no epigastric tenderness.
N.B. You have shown understanding that this woman has pre-eclampsia by mentioning important negative findings (epigastric tenderness) pertinent to this diagnosis [→ p.139].

Management plan: You will now need to decide on a course of action. Plan what investigations (if any) are needed and what course of action (if any) is most appropriate.

The postnatal history and examination

History

Ascertain the name and age of the mother and the number of days since delivery.
Delivery: Ask about the gestation and mode of delivery, and if instrumental or Caesarean, ask why. Ask about the mode of onset (e.g. spontaneous or induced), length of labour, analgesia and any procedures in labour (e.g. fetal blood sampling). Was there excessive blood loss?
Infant: Ask about the infant's sex, birthweight and Apgar scores, cord pH if taken, and mode and success of feeding. Was vitamin K given?

History of puerperium so far: Ask about lochia (volume, any odour), have her bowels opened yet, is she passing urine normally, or is there difficulty, leaking or dysuria? Does she have pain, particularly in the perineum?

Plans for the puerperium: What contraception does she intend to use? (Progesterone-only contraception is suitable for breast-feeding mothers; the combined pill can be started at 4–6 weeks if bottle feeding.) What help is available at home?

History of pregnancy and obstetric history: This should be brief, but ask about her parity and major antenatal complications, for example pre-eclampsia, diabetes.

Social/personal history: Consider home conditions for the neonate.

Apgar scoring			
Sign	0	1	2
Heart rate	Absent	<100	>100
Respiratory effort	Absent	Weak, irregular	Strong cry
Muscle tone	Absent	Limb flexion	Active motion
Colour	All blue/pale	Extremities blue	All pink
Reflex irritability (stimulate foot)	No response	Grimace	Cry

Total score out of 10, at 1 and 5 min
1-min Apgar gives indication of need for resuscitation, but has little prognostic value
5-min Apgar correlates very vaguely with subsequent neurological outcome

Examination

General examination: Assess appearance, temperature, pulse, blood pressure, mood, possible anaemia. Also examine chest, breasts, any wound or intravenous site and legs if fever or tachycardia (Fig. 16.11).

Abdominal examination: Look for uterine involution and a palpable bladder. Examine the perineum if there is discomfort.

Presenting the postnatal history

Summarize her labour, delivery, and her and the neonate's current health:

Mrs X, aged . . . had a . . . delivery . . . (if not normal, state indication, i.e. for . . .) days ago and delivered a . . . (sex) infant, weighing . . . kilograms, with Apgar of . . . and . . . labour was . . . (mode of onset) at . . . weeks gestation and lasted . . . hours. This was her . . . pregnancy, which . . . (state any major complications). She is currently . . . (brief assessment of her health: blood pressure, anaemia, uterine involution), is . . . (bottle or breast) feeding and plans to use . . . as contraception.

Example: Mrs X, aged 32 years, had a ventouse delivery for prolonged second stage 2 days ago and delivered a girl weighing 3.7 kg. Labour was spontaneous at 40 weeks gestation and lasted 9 h. This was her first pregnancy and was uncomplicated. She is well, afebrile, her blood pressure is 120/80, her uterus is well contracted, she is breast-feeding and plans to use the progesterone-only pill.

Management/discharge plans. Mention anti-D and rubella vaccination if relevant.

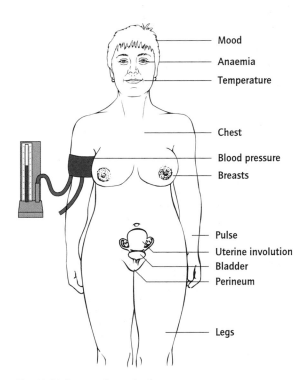

Fig. 16.11 Postnatal examination.

Basic neonatal assessment

History: Review the family history, antenatal course, labour course and delivery method and if resuscitation was required. Review birthweight, birthweight centile and weight gain/loss.

Examination: Examine the neonate in the presence of his/her mother. Undress the baby fully. Handle gently and wrap the neonate up after examination.

Neonatal examination	
General:	Colour (pallor/jaundice/cyanosis), features (dysmorphism/evidence of trauma/ birthmarks/any abnormalities) posture, behaviour and feeding movement (abnormal or restricted) respiration
Measure:	Heart rate, temperature, head measurements, weight
Examine:	Look for primitive reflexes (grasp, Moro, rooting) Inspect back and spine with baby prone Heart, check all pulses equal (e.g. radiofemoral delay) Abdomen, genitalia (undescended testes/ hernias/ambiguous genitalia), anus Look and examine for congenital dislocation of the hip and talipes

Investigations: SBR (serum bilirubin) if jaundiced. Day 7: Guthrie (phenylketonuria, thyroid)

Obstetric History at a Glance		
Personal details	Name, age, occupation, gestation, parity	
Presenting complaint or present circumstances		
History of present pregnancy	Dates:	Last menstrual period (LMP), cycle length, calculate expected day of delivery (EDD) and check present gestation
	Complications:	Specific complications, hospital admissions
	Tests done:	E.g. ultrasound scan, prenatal diagnosis, booking bloods [→ p.119]
Obstetric history	Past pregnancies: year, gestation, mode of delivery, complications, birthweight, ante/intra/postpartum complications	
Gynaecological history	Intermenstrual bleeding (IMB), postcoital bleeding (PCB), last cervical smear, contraception, subfertility	
Medical history	Operations; major illnesses, particularly diabetes, hypertension	
Systems review		
Drugs		
Personal	Smoking and alcohol	
Social	Stable relationship, finances, accommodation	
Allergies		
Is there anything else you think I should know?		

Obstetric Examination at a Glance

General	Appearance, weight, oedema (full examination at booking), blood pressure, urinalysis	
Abdomen	Inspect:	Size, scars, fetal movements
	Palpate:	Measure symphysis–fundal height, lie and presentation, liquor volume, engagement of presenting part
	Listen:	Fetal heart over anterior shoulder
Vaginal examination	Not usually indicated antenatally	
Other features	If relevant	

Antenatal Care

Pregnancy and childbirth are physiological events; most women are healthy and few need medical intervention. The main purpose of antenatal care is to identify mothers who do need medical attention. Some are identifiable at the booking visit, but most show no indication of the problems that can develop in pregnancy or labour.

The success of pregnancy care and the recognition that few pregnancies need intervention is now reflected in the United Kingdom by attempts to return to more natural labour and community-based care. The hospital-based, consultant-led system has been criticised as lacking in continuity of care and emphasizing the abnormal. Pressure from consumer groups has led to government support for more community-based care, and choice for women as to who is responsible for their care and where they deliver. These decisions are usually made early in the pregnancy but, because most problems are unpredictable at booking, they need to be constantly re-evaluated as the pregnancy proceeds.

The aims of antenatal care

1 Detect and manage pre-existing maternal disorders that may affect pregnancy outcome.
2 Prevent or detect and manage maternal complications of pregnancy.
3 Prevent or detect and manage fetal complications of pregnancy.
4 Detect congenital fetal problems, if requested by the patient.
5 Plan, with the mother, the circumstances of delivery to ensure maximum safety for the mother and baby, and maximum maternal satisfaction.
6 Provide education and advice regarding lifestyle and 'minor' conditions of pregnancy.

Preconceptual care and counselling

Many of the aims of antenatal care could be better fulfilled before conception. *Previous pregnancies* may have been traumatic and the implications of another can be discussed. The *health check* is better performed before conception and hitherto undetected problems such as cervical smear abnormalities can be treated. *Rubella status* can be checked so that immunization can occur before pregnancy. Health in women with chronic disease can be optimized; for instance, strict preconceptual *glucose control in diabetics* reduces the incidence of congenital abnormalities. Routine preconceptual administration of 0.4 mg of *folic acid* daily reduces the chance of neural tube defects (*Lancet* 1991; **338**: 132). Advice regarding *smoking* and *drugs* can be given. The woman should be encouraged to record *the dates of menstruation* so calculation of gestation is easier.

The booking visit

The first visit is usually made at about 12 weeks gestation. The most important purpose is to screen for possible complications that may arise in pregnancy, labour and the puerperium. 'Risk' is therefore assessed, using the history and examination and the investigations that are a standard feature of the booking visit. As discussed in Chapter 25, the benefits of this remain limited. Decisions about the type and frequency of antenatal care, as well as decisions about delivery, can be made in conjunction with the parents. These must be constantly re-evaluated as the pregnancy proceeds. At the same time, the gestation of the pregnancy is checked, appropriate prenatal screening is discussed and a general health check is accompanied by health advice.

History

Age. Women below the age of 17 years and above the age of 35 years have an increased risk of obstetric and medical complications in pregnancy. Chromosomal trisomies are more common with advancing maternal age.

History of present pregnancy. The accuracy of the last menstrual period is checked and the gestation adjusted for cycle length. The need for a dating ultrasound may be identified.

Past obstetric history. Many *obstetric disorders* have a small but significant recurrence rate. These include preterm labour, the small-for-dates and the 'growth-restricted' fetus [→ p.169], stillbirth, antepartum and postpartum haemorrhage, some congenital anomalies, rhesus disease, pre-eclampsia and gestational diabetes. Women with a history of preterm labour should be considered for cervical cerclage, or at least cervical ultrasound [→ p.159] and screening for bacterial vaginosis [→ p.158]. The *mode of delivery* of previous pregnancies will affect that of the current one: with one previous Caesarean section, vaginal delivery is usually attempted, but if more than one Caesarean has occurred, it is usual in the United Kingdom to perform an elective Caesarean.

Past gynaecological history. A history of subfertility increases perinatal risk; if fertility drugs or assisted conception have also been used, the likelihood of a multiple pregnancy is also increased. Women with previous uterine surgery (e.g. myomectomy) are often delivered by elective Caesarean section. A cervical smear history is taken.

Past medical history. Women with a history of hypertension, diabetes, autoimmune disease, haemoglobinopathy, thromboembolic disease, cardiac or renal disease, or other serious illnesses are at an increased risk of pregnancy problems and usually need input from the appropriate specialist.

Drugs. Drugs that are contraindicated in pregnancy should be changed to those considered to be safe. Ideally, this should have occurred at a preconceptual counselling visit.

Family history. Gestational diabetes is more common if a first-degree relative is diabetic. Hypertension, thromboembolic and autoimmune disease, and pre-eclampsia are also familial.

Personal/social history. Smoking, alcohol and drug abuse are sought.

Examination

General health and nutritional status are assessed: gestational diabetes is more common in women weighing >100 kg; dystocia in labour is more common in women <150 cm in height. A baseline blood pressure enables comparison if hypertension occurs in later pregnancy. If pre-existing hypertension is found, the risk of subsequent pre-eclampsia is increased. Incidental disease such as breast carcinoma may occasionally be detected.

Abdominal examination before the third trimester is limited. Once the uterus is palpable (12–14 weeks), the fetal heart can be auscultated with an electronic monitor. A uterus that is palpable before 12 weeks suggests multiple pregnancy. Routine vaginal examination and clinical assessment of pelvic capacity are inappropriate at this stage. If a smear has not been performed for 3 years it is usually done postnatally.

Booking visit investigations

Ultrasound scan

Ultrasound between 7 and 14 weeks will confirm gestation and viability, usually provide considerable maternal reassurance, and will diagnose multiple pregnancy (*Cochrane* 2000: CD000182). After 11 weeks it can also be used in screening for chromosomal abnormalities: nuchal translucency [→ p.125], preferably in conjunction with blood levels of human chorionic gonadotrophin beta-subunit (β-HCG) and pregnancy-associated plasma protein A (PAPPA). Early ultrasound is not routine in all hospitals.

Blood tests

A *full blood count* (FBC) check identifies pre-existing anaemia.

Serum antibodies (e.g. anti-D) identify those at risk of intrauterine isoimmunization [→ p.155]

Blood glucose levels, particularly if both fasting and postprandial, help identify pre-existing and gestational diabetics [→ p.145].

Blood tests for syphilis are still routine because of the serious implications for the fetus.

Rubella immunity [→ p.132] is checked: vaccination, if required, will be offered postnatally.

Human immunodeficiency virus (HIV) and *hepatitis B* counselling and screening is offered [→ p.134].

Haemoglobin electrophoresis is performed in women at risk of the *sickle-cell anaemias* or *thalassaemias* [→ p.153]. The former is common in Afro-Caribbean women, the latter in Mediterranean and Asian women. The partner can be tested if the woman is found to be a carrier, to identify women who should be offered prenatal diagnosis.

Other tests

Screening for infections implicated in preterm labour (e.g. *Chlamydia*, bacterial vaginosis [→ p.158]), could be performed at this stage.

Urine microscopy and culture are performed because asymptomatic bacteriuria in pregnancy commonly (20%) leads to pyelonephritis.

Urinalysis for *glucose*, *protein* and *nitrites* screen for underlying diabetes, renal disease and infection respectively.

Booking investigations
Urine culture
Full blood count (FBC)
Antibody screen
Glucose
Serological tests for syphilis
Rubella immunoglobulin G
Offer human immunodeficiency virus (HIV) and hepatitis B
Ultrasound scan
Screening for chromosomal abnormalities
Consider: Haemoglobin electrophoresis, cervix/vaginal swabs

Health promotion and advice

General

Medications are generally avoided in the first trimester, but teratogenicity is rare. *Diet* in pregnancy should be well balanced, with a daily energy intake of about 2500 calories. *Folic acid* supplementation, with 0.4 mg of folic acid daily, should continue until at least 12 weeks. *Vitamin D* supplementation is given to women who receive little exposure to sunlight (e.g. Asian women). Iron supplementation is no longer routine. A *dental check-up* is advised. *Exercise* in pregnancy is advised: swimming is ideal. Many women enquire about *travel* in pregnancy: most airlines will only carry women at <34–36 weeks. The risk of venous thromboembolism [→ p.151] is reduced by adequate hydration, but if additional risk factors are present, low-dose aspirin or heparin may be used. *Coitus* is not contraindicated in pregnancy, except when the placenta is known to be praevia or the membranes have ruptured. In the United Kingdom, *statutory maternity pay* is payable for 26 weeks: at 90% of average earnings for 6 weeks and then at a lower flat rate for 20 weeks.

Alcohol

A maximum of one drink per day is recommended. However, there is no known risk to consumption of <15 units of alcohol per week. Higher levels may decrease birthweight, and consumption of more than 20 units may affect the child's intelligence and may cause the fetal alcohol syndrome, characterized by growth restriction and neurological abnormalities.

Smoking

This reduces fertility and is associated with an increased risk of miscarriage, placental abruption, preterm labour, growth restriction and perinatal mortality.

Drug usage

Drug abuse is associated with preterm labour and increased perinatal mortality, and with drug dependence in the neonate.

Preparation for birth

Antenatal classes should educate women and their partners about pregnancy and labour. Knowledge and understanding help alleviate fear and pain, and allows women to have more control and make choices about their antepartum and intrapartum care. In addition, intrapartum techniques of posture, breathing and pushing are taught (Fig. 17.1).

Planning pregnancy care

At the end of the booking visit, the doctor or midwife can

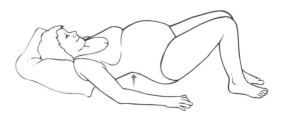

Fig. 17.1 Pelvic tilt at antenatal classes.

advise the woman of the most appropriate type of antenatal care, and a plan for visit frequency, extra surveillance or intervention is made. Women can choose between two care options:

Consultant-led care: Visits are shared by the general practitioner, or the midwife, and obstetricians. The latter may undertake all visits with some 'high-risk' women.

Community care: A core team of midwives is responsible for all antepartum and intrapartum care, usually with a general practitioner for the antepartum period. Delivery may be away from hospital.

Later pregnancy screening

Ultrasound for structural abnormalities

It is usual to arrange an ultrasound examination at 20 weeks. This 'anomaly scan' enables detection of most structural fetal abnormalities [→ p.127], although reported success rates vary widely.

Ultrasound screening for risk assessment

Doppler of the uterine arteries [→ p.171] at 23 weeks can be used as a screening test for intrauterine growth restriction and pre-eclampsia (*Ultrasound Obstet Gynecol* 2001 **18**: 441). Its use is imperfect, expensive and not routine. Nevertheless, it is far more effective at predicting major pregnancy complications than the medical or obstetric history. This could make the test cost effective in comparison to the current system, and, in the future, pregnancy risk assessment is likely to involve its routine use.

Continuing antenatal care

Frequency of antenatal visits

The woman is seen at decreasing intervals through the pregnancy because complications are more common later in the pregnancy. The frequency with which she is seen is dependent on the likelihood of complications and on the apparent fetal and maternal health as assessed in subsequent visits. NICE has recently recommended an antenatal appointment schedule (Fig. 17.2) (www.rcog.org.uk). This is the minimum in nulliparous women to detect pre-eclampsia, and more frequent visits are appropriate for many 'high-risk' pregnancies. Less intensive care is appropriate in multiparous patients with normal pregnancies, but is often less well accepted by women and health carers alike.

Conduct of antenatal visits

At each visit, the history is briefly reviewed. The woman is asked about her physical and mental state. Fetal movements are reviewed. She is normally weighed, though this is of little use unless gross oedema is found. The blood pressure is taken and the urine is checked for protein, glucose, leucocytes and nitrites. Urine culture is performed if the latter are detected. The abdomen is examined in the normal manner.

Before 26 weeks, the blood pressure, urinalysis and fundal height are checked. Serial measurements of fundal height can be plotted on a customized growth chart (*Obstet Gynecol* 1999; **94**: 591), to better identify the baby

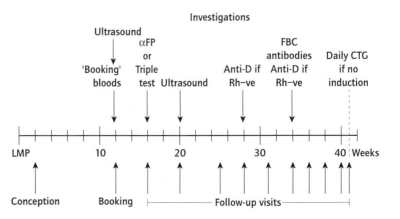

Fig. 17.2 Basic antenatal care in nulliparous women.

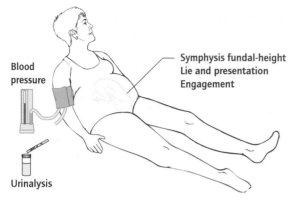

Fig. **17.3** Obstetric examination at antenatal visits in the late third trimester.

that is pathologically small and should be referred for ultrasound assessment [→ p.171].

At the 28–36-week visits, the blood pressure, urinalysis and fundal height are most important. Presentation is variable and less important. Anti-D is given to rhesus-negative women at 28 and 34 weeks (*Cochrane* 2000: CD000020).

At the 36–40-week visits, the lie, presentation and engagement of the presenting part are also established (Fig. 17.3). Pelvic examination is inappropriate unless induction is contemplated or there is suspicion of obstruction (and placenta praevia is excluded).

At 41 weeks, if induction of labour is not performed, particularly close surveillance is indicated. A cervical sweep [→ p.212] should be offered.

Conduct of antenatal visits	
History:	Physical and mental health Fetal movements
Examination:	Blood pressure and urinalysis Symphysis–fundal height Lie and presentation of fetus Engagement of presenting part Fetal heart auscultation

Further antenatal investigations

An FBC and antibody check is usually repeated at 34 weeks. The ultrasound examination is not routinely repeated (*Cochrane* 2000: CD001451) unless clinically indicated or obstetric risk factors are present [→ p.171]. Other tests are performed only if clinically indicated.

'Minor' conditions of pregnancy

Itching is common in pregnancy. The sclerae are checked for jaundice, and liver function tests and bile acids are assessed. Although rare, liver complications in pregnancy [→ p.149] often present with itching.

Symphisis pubis dysfunction is common (*Eur J Obstet Gynecol Reprod Biol* 2002; **105**: 143) and causes varying degrees of discomfort in the pubic and sacroiliac joints. Physiotherapy, corsets, analgesics and even crutches may be used. Care with leg abduction is required. It is usually but not invariably cured after delivery.

Abdominal pain is universal to some degree in pregnancy; it is usually benign and unexplained. However, medical and surgical problems are no less common in pregnancy, and may have a worse prognosis, particularly appendicitis and pancreatitis. Urinary tract infections and fibroids [→ p.20] can cause pain in pregnancy.

Heartburn affects 70% and is most marked in the supine position. Extra pillows are helpful; antacids are not contraindicated. Pre-eclampsia can present with epigastric pain.

Backache is almost universal and may cause sciatica. Most cases resolve after delivery. Physiotherapy, advice on posture and lifting, a firm mattress and a corset may all help.

Constipation is common and often exacerbated by oral iron. A high fibre intake is needed. Bulking agents or stool softeners are used if this fails.

Ankle oedema is common, worsens towards the end of pregnancy and is an unreliable sign of pre-eclampsia. However, a sudden increase in oedema warrants careful assessment and follow-up of blood pressure and urinalysis: if associated with pre-eclampsia, the sacrum, fingers and even the face are often affected. Benign oedema is helped by raising the foot of the bed at night; diuretics should not be given.

Leg cramps affect 30% of women. Treatments are generally unproven, but sodium chloride tablets, calcium salts or quinine may be safely tried.

Carpal tunnel syndrome is due to fluid retention compressing the median nerve. It is seldom severe and is usually temporary. Splints on the wrists may help.

Vaginitis due to candidiasis is common in pregnancy and more difficult to treat. There is an itchy, non-offensive white–grey discharge associated with excoriation.

Imidazole vaginal pessaries (e.g. clotrimazole) are used for symptomatic infection.

Tiredness is almost universal and is often incorrectly attributed to anaemia.

Further reading

Carroli G, Villar J, Piaggio G *et al.* WHO Antenatal Care Trial Research Group. WHO systematic review of randomised controlled trials of routine antenatal care. *Lancet* 2001; **357**: 1565–70.

Villar J, Carroli G, Khan-Neelofur D, Piaggio G, Gulmezoglu M. Patterns of routine antenatal care for low-risk pregnancy. *Cochrane Database System Review (Online: Update Software)* 2001; **4**: CD000934.

www.rcog.org.uk/resources/Public/Antenatal_Care.pdf

Appendix: Physiological changes in pregnancy	
Weight gain	10–15 kg
Genital tract	Uterus weight increase from 50 to 1000 g Muscle hypertrophy, increased blood flow and contractility Cervix softens, may start to efface in late third trimester
Blood	Blood volume: 50% increase Red cell mass: increase Haemoglobin: decrease (normal lower limit 10.5 g/dL) White blood cell count (WBC) increase
Cardiovascular system	Cardiac output: 40% increase Peripheral resistance: 50% reduction Blood pressure: small mid-pregnancy fall
Lungs	Tidal volume: 40% increase Respiratory rate: no change
Others	Renal blood flow: glomerular filtration rate 40% increase, so creatinine/urea decrease Reduced gut motility: delayed gastric emptying/constipation Thyroid enlargement

18 Congenital Abnormalities and their Identification

Congenital abnormalities affect 2% of pregnancies (1% major). They can be *structural deformities* (e.g. diaphragmatic hernia) or *chromosomal abnormalities* (most commonly trisomies, e.g. Down's syndrome) or *inherited diseases* (e.g. cystic fibrosis), or are the result of *intrauterine infection* (e.g. rubella) or *drug exposure* (e.g. antiepileptics).

They account for about 25% of perinatal deaths and are a major cause of disability in later life. Prenatal identification of such abnormalities is important to prepare the parents, to allow delivery to be at an appropriate time and place, to prepare neonatal services and, in the case of untreatable severe disabilities, to enable the parents to terminate the pregnancy if they wish. Parental attitudes vary with age, religion and social background: counselling must be non-directive and allow the parents to make an informed choice about screening or diagnostic testing. This is an essential part of the booking visit.

The difference between screening and diagnostic tests

A screening test is available for all (women) and gives a measure of the risk of (the fetus) being affected by a particular disorder. The 'higher-risk' patient can then be offered a diagnostic test. A result might be: 'the risk of Down's syndrome in this pregnancy is 1 in 50'

A diagnostic test is performed on women with a 'high risk' to confirm or refute the possibility, e.g. 'this fetus does not have Down's syndrome'

Criteria for screening and diagnostic tests

A screening test should be widely available and cheap; it must have a high sensitivity (i.e. not miss affected individuals) and specificity (i.e. not many false positives), and it must be non-invasive and safe. There must also be

an acceptable diagnostic test for the disorder for which it is screening.

A diagnostic test must be highly sensitive and safe. Further, the implications of being affected by the disorder should be serious enough to warrant the often-invasive test.

Methods of prenatal testing

Maternal blood testing

As a screening test: Alpha fetoprotein (AFP) is a product of the fetal liver. When the fetus has an open neural tube defect (NTD), maternal levels are raised: this can be confirmed or refuted by ultrasound after 16 weeks. Raised levels in the absence of NTDs indicate a higher risk of third trimester complications, so allowing high-risk care (see Chapter 25).

The levels of several blood markers are altered in maternal blood where a fetus is affected by Down's syndrome. These include human chorionic gonadotrophin beta-subunit (β-HCG), pregnancy-associated plasma protein A (PAPP-A), AFP, oestriol and inhibin A. The triple test, a blood test at 15 weeks, uses AFP, HCG and oestriol; many different tests using a combination of markers now exist, and some can be performed around 10 weeks. The best screening test uses a combination of blood markers and ultrasound [→ p.126].

As a diagnostic test: Prenatal diagnosis from the few fetal cells in the maternal circulation is likely to revolutionize prenatal diagnosis in the future.

Ultrasound

To confirm dates: Ultrasound scan is used to confirm the gestation and exclude multiple pregnancy.

As a diagnostic test: Some structural abnormalities are

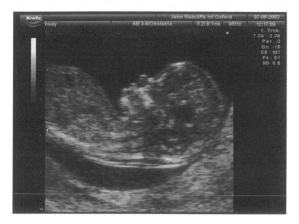

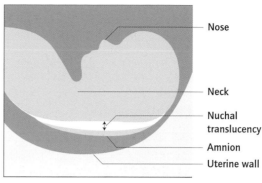

Nose

Neck

Nuchal translucency

Amnion

Uterine wall

Fig. 18.1 Normal nuchal translucency.

clear on ultrasound before 14 weeks (e.g. anencephaly; see Fig. 18.4), but most are best seen at 20 weeks. A prenatal diagnosis of many abnormalities such as club foot, cleft lip or cardiac defects can often be made, although in practice many are missed. Polyhydramnios [→ p.131] may be due to fetal abnormality, particularly of the upper gastrointestinal tract and warrants repeat ultrasound in later pregnancy.

As a screening test for abnormalities: Measurement of nuchal translucency (the space between skin and soft tissue overlying the cervical spine) between 11 and 14 weeks is a screening test for trisomies (Fig. 18.1). The presence or length of the nasal bone can also be used at this gestation (*Lancet* 2001; **358**: 1655) and later. In addition, 50% of fetuses with trisomies have structural abnormalities that are visible at a 20-week ultrasound. The identification of structural abnormalities increases the risk of trisomies and may prompt the use of amniocentesis.

To aid other diagnostic tests: Amniocentesis and chorionic villus sampling (CVS) are performed under ultrasound guidance.

Amniocentesis

This is a diagnostic test, involving removal of amniotic fluid using a fine gauge needle under ultrasound guidance (Fig. 18.2). It is performed after 15 weeks gestation, but it may be done later. This enables prenatal diagnosis of chromosomal abnormalities and inherited disorders such as sickle-cell anaemia, thalassaemia and cystic

fibrosis. The chance of miscarriage is increased by 1% (*Lancet* 1986; **1**: 1287).

Chorionic villus sampling (CVS)

This diagnostic test involves biopsy of the trophoblast, by passing a small needle through the abdominal wall or cervix and into the placenta, after 11 weeks (*Cochrane* 2000: CD000077). The test result is obtained faster than with amniocentesis and allows an abnormal fetus to be identified at a time when abortion, if requested, could be performed under general anaesthesia. The miscarriage rate is slightly higher than after amniocentesis, but this is because it is performed earlier, when spontaneous miscarriage is more common. It is used to diagnose chromosomal problems and autosomal dominant and recessive conditions.

With both amniocentesis and CVS, fluorescence *in situ* hybridization (FISH) and polymerase chain reaction (PCR) can both be used to diagnose the most common abnormalities in less than 48 h.

Preimplantation genetic diagnosis (PGD)

In vitro fertilization (IVF) [→ p.76] allows cell(s) from a developing embryo to be removed for genetic analysis before the embryo is transferred to the uterus (*Hum Reprod* 2003; **18**: 465). This allows selection, and therefore implantation, only of embryos that will not be affected by the disorder for which it is being tested. The technique is expensive and presents ethical dilemmas, but has been used in prenatal diagnosis of sex-linked disorders, trisomies, and both autosomal dominant and recessive conditions. It does require IVF, even in couples who are fertile.

Chromosomal abnormalities

These affect 6 per 1000 live births, but they are also the main cause (60%) of isolated spontaneous miscarriage. Most are trisomies.

Down's syndrome

Trisomy 21 is the commonest chromosomal abnormality among live births. It is usually the result of random non-dysjunction at meiosis, although occasionally (6%) it arises as a result of a balanced chromosomal translocation in the parents. It is more common with advancing maternal age (Fig. 18.3). The affected infant has mental retardation, characteristic facies and often (50%) congenital cardiac disease. Other structural abnormalities may also be present.

Other chromosomal abnormalities

Trisomy 18 and *trisomy 13* are associated with major structural defects, and therefore usually diagnosed after ultrasound has identified the characteristic abnormalities. They are more common with advanced maternal age. Affected fetuses die *in utero* or shortly after birth. Sex chromosome abnormalities include *Klinefelter's syndrome* (47 XXY). These males have normal intellect, small testes and are infertile. In *Turner's syndrome* (a single X chromosome only: X0), affected individuals are female, infertile but with normal intellect [→ p.15].

Risk factors for Down's syndrome	
History:	High maternal age
	Previous affected baby (risk increased 1%)
	Balanced parental translocation (rare)
Ultrasound:	Thickened nuchal translucency
	Some structural abnormalities
	Absent or shortened nasal bone
Blood tests:	See text

Screening and diagnosis of chromosomal abnormalities

Amniocentesis and *CVS* are diagnostic tests for chromosomal abnormalities. Traditionally they have been offered to women over the age of about 35 years. However, younger women have more babies and therefore, despite a lower individual risk, account for about 70% of all Down's syndrome pregnancies. These would go unde-

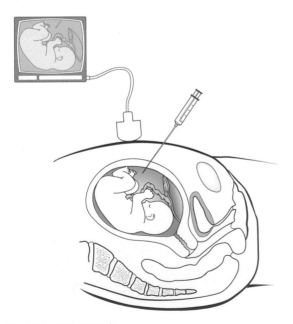

Fig. 18.2 Amniocentesis.

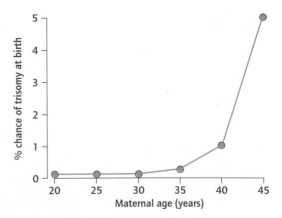

Fig. 18.3 Maternal age and risk of trisomies.

tected without a screening programme for all consenting women.

Both blood tests and ultrasound can be used as screening tests. The most effective, however, involves a combination. Where risk factors are independent of each other, they can be 'integrated', taking into account the results of several screening tests to reach a single risk figure. The most effective in common usage is a combination of maternal age with blood tests and a nuchal translucency scan at 11–14 weeks. This will detect approximately 90% of Down's syndrome babies for a false positive rate of 5% (*Ultrasound Obstet Gynecol* 2002; **20**: 219).

Theoretical projections suggest that incorporating also the presence or absence of the nasal bone, blood tests at 15 weeks, and even markers on the 20 week scan, will improve both the sensitivity and false positive rate considerably.

Structural abnormalities

Open neural tube defects (NTDs)

These are the result of failure of closure of the neural tube. Neural tissue is exposed, to varying degrees, and may degenerate. Less than 1 in 200 pregnancies are affected, and the incidence is declining. The type and severity of defect depends on its site and degree. The best known examples are *spina bifida* and *anencephaly* (Fig. 18.4): in the former, severe disability is usual; the latter is incompatible with life. Preconceptual daily folic acid supplementation (0.4 mg) reduces the incidence of NTDs and should be taken by all women considering pregnancy. Neural tube defects recur in 1 in 10 pregnancies, but this risk is greatly reduced by higher dose folic acid (4 mg).

Screening and diagnosis of NTDs

Alpha fetoprotein levels are elevated in pregnancies affected by open NTDs and this has been used as a screening test. The now almost routine use of *ultrasound* at 20 weeks, which may diagnose NTDs with a sensitivity of >95%, has rendered screening almost redundant.

Cardiac anomalies

These occur in 0.8% of pregnancies. They are more common in women with cardiac disease, diabetes and when previous offspring have been affected (overall recurrence risk 3%). Most are non-lethal; others may be correctable with surgery after birth. The most common are ventricular septal defects. Ultrasound can be used to detect and diagnose prenatal cardiac disease very accurately, but, in practice, less than a third of cases are diagnosed prenatally (Fig. 18.5). Particularly where other abnormalities coexist, and with certain abnormalities, the risk of chromosomal abnormalities is increased.

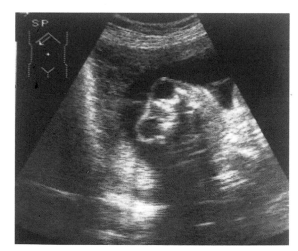

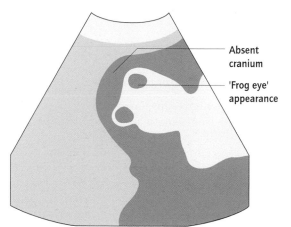

Absent cranium

'Frog eye' appearance

Fig. 18.4 Neural tube defect (NTD): anencephaly.

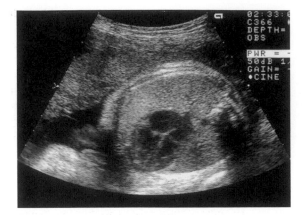
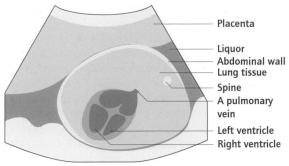

Placenta
Liquor
Abdominal wall
Lung tissue
Spine
A pulmonary
vein
Left ventricle
Right ventricle

Fig. 18.5 Normal heart: transverse view of chest.

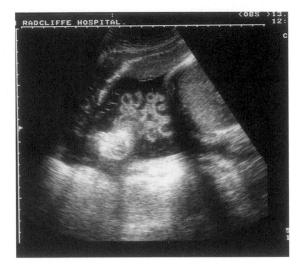
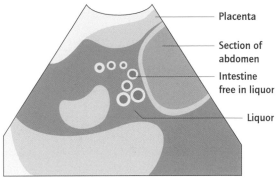

Placenta

Section of
abdomen

Intestine
free in liquor

Liquor

Fig. 18.6 Gastroschisis.

Other structural abnormalities

Polyhydramnios (excessive amniotic fluid) [→ p.131] is common with many abnormalities. *Exomphalos* is characterized by partial extrusion of abdominal contents in a peritoneal sac. Fifty per cent of affected infants have a chromosomal problem and amniocentesis is offered. *Gastroschisis* (Fig. 18.6) is characterized by free loops of bowel in the amniotic cavity and is rarely associated with chromosomal defects. *Diaphragmatic hernias* occur when the abdominal contents herniate into the chest. Many neonates die because of associated anomalies or pulmonary hypoplasia. These disorders are all visible on ultrasound at 20 weeks and can be seen as early as 12 weeks.

Fetal hydrops

This occurs when extra fluid accumulates in 2+ areas in the fetus. It occurs in 1 in 500 pregnancies and, because of its high mortality, is rarer in late pregnancy. It can be 'immune', in association with anaemia and haemolysis as a result of antibodies including Rhesus disease [→ p.155]. Or it can be 'non-immune', secondary to another cause. There are five main categories of non-immune hydrops. *Chromosomal abnormalities* such as trisomy 21 are most common in early pregnancy. Many *structural abnormalities* (e.g. diaphragmatic hernia) can cause hydrops, the presence of which usually worsens the fetal prognosis. Congenital *cardiac abnormalities* or arrhythmias may be present. Cardiac failure due to *anaemia* (e.g. parvovirus infection [→ p.133], feto–maternal haemorrhage or fetal alpha thalassaemia major may also be responsible. Hydrops occurs in monochorionic twins in association with severe *twin–twin transfusion syndrome* [→ p.183].

Investigation involves careful ultrasound assessment, including a specialist cardiac scan and assessment of the middle cerebral artery [→ p.156]. Maternal blood is taken for Kleihauer and parvovirus immunoglobulin M testing. Fetal blood sampling may also assess anaemia; it or amniocentesis are performed for karyotyping. The management and prognosis depends on the cause.

Single gene disorders

Autosomal dominant conditions (e.g. neurofibromatosis) affect 1 in 150 live births. One affected parent has a 50% chance of passing on the condition.

Autosomal recessive genes (e.g. cystic fibrosis or sickle-cell disease) have different prevalences in different populations. If both parents are carriers, the neonate has a one in four chance of being affected by the disease, whilst half will be carriers. Detection of carrier status for most cystic fibrosis genes and for haemoglobinopathies is possible. Partners of women who have or are carriers of recessively inherited disease may be tested to see if they too are carriers. Prenatal diagnosis, usually with CVS, may then be offered.

Further reading

Bui TH, Blennow E, Nordenskjold M. Prenatal diagnosis: molecular genetics and cytogenetics. *Best Practice & Research. Clinical Obstetrics & Gynaecology* 2002; **16**(5): 629–43.

Gilbert RE, Augood C, Gupta R *et al*. Screening for Down's syndrome: effects, safety, and cost effectiveness of first and second trimester strategies. *BMJ* 2001; **323**: 423–5.

Snijders R, Smith E. The role of fetal nuchal translucency in prenatal screening. *Current Opinion in Obstetrics & Gynecology* 2002; **14**(6): 577–85.

www.fetalmedicine.com

Ultrasound at a Glance

Definition		3.5–7.0 MHz sound waves are passed into the body; the intensity of deflection from different tissues depends on their densities: this can be represented in two-dimensional form
Gynaecology		Assessment of pelvic mass [→ p.37] and normal pelvic anatomy. 'Follicle tracking' in ovulation induction [→ p.73]. Endometrial cavity assessment in abnormal menstrual bleeding [→ p.14]
Obstetric	First trimester:	In exclusion of ectopic pregnancy [→ p.98], assessment of pregnancy viability, detection of retained products of conception after miscarriage Estimation of gestational age (e.g. crown–rump length at 7–14 weeks) [→ p.119] Detection of multiple pregnancy and determination of chorionicity [→ p.182] Screening for chromosomal abnormalities (nuchal translucency) [→ p.127]
	Second trimester:	Diagnosis of structural abnormalities [→ p.127] Screening for chromosomal abnormalities Help other diagnostic (e.g. amniocentesis) or therapeutic (e.g. transfusion [→ p.157]) techniques Doppler for fetal assessment [→ p.171] or of uterine arteries [→ p.171]
	Third trimester:	Assessment of fetal growth [→ p.171] As part of biophysical profile for fetal well being [→ p.172] Diagnosis of placenta praevia [→ p.162] Determining presentation in difficult cases Doppler for fetal assessment [→ p.171]
	Benefits:	Aids diagnosis in gynaecology and first trimester Maternal reassurance, screening for abnormalities Reduction of perinatal mortality in high risk pregnancy Benefit in low risk pregnancy mainly better diagnosis of abnormalities
	Safety:	Extremely safe. Possible small increase in left-handedness and lower birthweight

Prenatal Screening and Diagnosis of Congenital Abnormalities at a Glance

Booking	Counsel all regarding prenatal diagnosis options Check rubella immunity to identify need for postnatal immunization Check hepatitis B to allow immunoglobulin administration to neonate Check for syphilis infection and HIV status Arrange genetic counselling ± later chorionic villus sampling (CVS) or amniocentesis if risk of inherited disorder
7–14 weeks	Ultrasound scan to date pregnancy and identify twins: Advise regarding screening for chromosomal trisomies: with nuchal translucency, OR
15 weeks	Maternal serum tests to screen for chromosomal trisomies Counsel and offer amniocentesis if the risk is high
20 weeks	Routine anomaly ultrasound to detect structural abnormalities Counsel and consider amniocentesis if abnormalities found Offer cardiac scan if high risk
Later	Some abnormalities only visible in later pregnancy: ultrasound if polyhydramnios, breech, suspected intrauterine growth restriction (IUGR)

Polyhydramnios at a Glance

Definition	Liquor volume increased. Normal volume varies with gestation, but deepest liquor pool >10 cm considered abnormal
Epidemiology	1% of pregnancies
Aetiology	Idiopathic; maternal disorders (established and gestational diabetes, renal failure); twins (particularly twin–twin transfusion syndrome [→ p.183]); fetal anomaly (20%) (particularly upper gastrointestinal obstructions or inability to swallow, chest abnormalities, myotonic dystrophy)
Clinical features	Maternal discomfort. Large for dates, taut uterus, fetal parts difficult to palpate
Complications	Preterm labour; maternal discomfort, abnormal lie and malpresentation

Management

To diagnose fetal anomaly:	Detailed ultrasound screening
To diagnose diabetes:	Maternal blood glucose testing [→ p.146]
To reduce liquor:	If <34 weeks and severe, amnioreduction [→ p.146], or use of non-steroidal anti-inflammatory drugs (NSAIDS) to reduce fetal urine output Consider steroids if <34 weeks
Delivery:	Vaginal unless persistent unstable lie or other obstetric indication

19 Infections in Pregnancy

Cytomegalovirus (CMV)

In the adult, this virus usually causes subclinical infection; about 35% of women are immune. Infection at any stage in pregnancy (1%) causes neonatal infection in 40%: of these, most remain asymptomatic and are unlikely to develop long-term sequelae. Such sequelae, including hearing, visual and mental impairment, often follow symptomatic neonatal infection, but occasionally occur in infants who were asymptomatic and undiagnosed at birth. About 250 neonates have clinical evidence of CMV infection every year in the United Kingdom. *Screening* is impractical in pregnancy since vaccination is not available, the disease is usually subclinical, and most maternal infections do not result in neonatal sequelae.

Herpes simplex [→p.63]

The type 2 deoxyribonucleic acid (DNA) virus is responsible for most genital herpes (Fig. 19.1 and Fig. 9.2). Less than 5% of pregnant women have a history of prior infection, but many more have antibodies. Neonatal herpes is rare, but has a mortality of 50%. Infection is transmitted at vaginal delivery particularly if vesicles are present. This is most likely to follow primary maternal infection, because the fetus will not have passive immunity from maternal antibodies. Caesarean section is therefore recommended (*BJOG* 1998; **105**: 255) for those developing symptoms within 6 weeks of a primary attack, or in women with recurrent herpes who have vesicles are present at the time of labour. Aciclovir in pregnancy may reduce the frequency of attacks. Swabs are of little use in pregnancy, and *screening* for asymptomatic herpes is of little benefit.

Rubella

This virus usually affects children and causes a mild febrile illness with a macular rash, which is often called 'German measles'. Immunity is lifelong; however, maternal infection in early pregnancy frequently causes multiple fetal abnormalities, including deafness, cardiac disease, eye problems and mental retardation. The probability and severity of malformation decreases with advancing gestation: after 16 weeks, the risk is very low (Fig. 19.3). Widespread immunization of girls means that <10 affected neonates are born each year (*BMJ* 1999; **7186**: 769). *Screening* for rubella immunity at booking remains routine to identify those in need of vaccination after the end of pregnancy. If a non-immune woman develops rubella before 16 weeks gestation, termination of pregnancy is offered. Rubella vaccine is live and contraindicated in pregnancy, although harm has not been recorded.

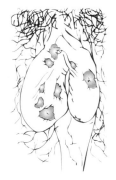

Fig. 19.1 Herpes simplex.

Herpes simplex virus (HSV)	Cold sores (type 1) Genital herpes (type 2)
Cytomegalovirus (CMV)	Cytomegalic inclusion disease in neonates

Fig. 19.2 Herpesvirus.

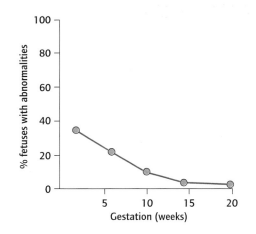

% fetuses with abnormalities

Fig. 19.3 Infection with rubella in early pregnancy.

Toxoplasmosis

Infection with protozoan parasite *Toxoplasma gondii* often causes no symptoms and follows contact with cat faeces and eating infected meat. In the United Kingdom, 20% of adults have antibodies, but it is far more common in mainland Europe. Infection in pregnancy occurs in 0.2% of women: fetal infection follows in under half, and very few have the sequelae of mental retardation, convulsions, spasticities and visual impairment (<10 per year in the United Kingdom). Diagnosis can be difficult: subsequently proven cases may have no detectable antibodies. *Screening* is controversial but is not currently routine in the United Kingdom, as most maternal infections do not result in neonatal sequelae and confirmation of infection is difficult. Proven cases of infection are treated with spiramycin.

Syphilis [→ p.63]

This sexually transmitted disease due to *Treponema pallidum* is rare in the United Kingdom, although endemic in developing countries. Active disease in pregnancy usually causes miscarriage, severe congenital disease or stillbirth. Prompt treatment with benzylpenicillin is safe and will prevent, but not reverse, fetal damage. Therefore *screening tests*, such as the Venereal Disease Research Laboratories (VDRL) test, which are cheap and accurate, are still in routine use.

Herpes zoster

Primary infection with this virus causes chickenpox, a common childhood illness. Reactivation of latent infection is shingles, which usually affects adults in one or two dermatomes. A woman who is not immune to zoster can develop chickenpox after exposure to chickenpox or shingles. Chickenpox in pregnancy is rare (0.05%), but can cause severe maternal illness and is immediately treated with oral aciclovir. Infection before 20 weeks is teratogenic, but only to 1–2% of fetuses. Maternal infection in the week preceding delivery causes neonatal infection in up to 50%, with a high mortality. Neonates delivered at this time, or if the mother develops vesicles within 2 days of delivery, are given zoster immunoglobulin. *Screening* for zoster is of no use.

Infections suitable for screening
Syphilis
Hepatitis B
Rubella
Probably: *Chlamydia*
Bacterial vaginosis
β-haemolytic streptococcus

Teratogenic infections
Cytomegalovirus (CMV)
Rubella
Toxoplasmosis
Syphilis
Chickenpox

Parvovirus

The B19 virus infects 0.25% of women, and more during epidemics. A 'slapped cheek' appearance (erythema infectiosum) is classic but many have arthralgia or are asymptomatic. Infection is usually from children and 50% of adults are immune. The virus suppresses fetal erythropoesis causing anaemia and fetal death in 9% of infected fetuses (*BJOG* 1998; **105**: 174), usually with infection before 20 weeks gestation. Anaemia is detectable on ultrasound, initially as increased blood flow velocity in the fetal middle cerebral artery [→ p.156] and subsequently as oedema (hydrops [→ p.128]) from cardiac failure. *In utero* blood transfusion of hydropic fetuses may prevent demise, although spontaneous resolution may also occur. There are no long-term sequelae among survivors.

Prevention of vertical transmission of Group B streptococcus	
Strategy 1: Risk factors alone	Strategy 2: Risk factors + screening
No screening	High vaginal swab (HVS) and rectal swab at 34–36 weeks

Treat with intravenous penicillin in labour if:
  Previous history
  Intrapartum fever >38°C
  Current preterm labour
  Rupture of the membranes (>18 h)
	Treat with intravenous penicillin in labour if: swabs positive, OR any risk factor presents (except prolonged rupture of membranes)

Group B streptococcus (GBS)

The bacterium *Streptococcus agalactiae* is present in the genital tract of about 20% of pregnant women; 75% of their babies are colonized, and 1% of these develop streptococcal sepsis. This is the most common cause of severe sepsis in neonates and has a mortality of 6% in term infants and 18% in preterm infants. Intravenous penicillin in carriers at the onset of labour reduces early neonatal infection (*Cochrane* 2000: CD000115) to about 0.04%.

Preventative strategies are based on risk factors either alone or in conjunction with *screening* (see box below) (RCOG Guideline 36, 2003: www.rcog.org.uk), but are under-used in the United Kingdom. Indeed the sensitivity of many available tests for the bacterium is poor: special culture media are required.

Group A streptococcus remains an important cause of puerperal sepsis [→ p.227], particularly in developing countries.

Hepatitis C

In the United Kingdom, infection is mostly limited to high-risk groups, particularly human immunodeficiency virus (HIV) -infected women (30%). Most are asymptomatic. Vertical transmission occurs in 6%, is increased by concomitant HIV infection and a high viral load. Infected neonates are prone to chronic hepatitis. Most data suggest that elective Caesarean section does not reduce vertical transmission rates. *Screening* is restricted to high-risk groups.

Hepatitis B

Hepatitis B is rare in the West but not in the developing world. Its infectivity depends on antibody status: indi-viduals with the 'surface' antibody (HBsAb positive) are immunologically cured and of low infectivity to others and their fetus. Those with the surface antigen but not the antibody (HBsAg positive) and those with the E antigen (HBeAg positive) are more infectious.

Vertical transmission occurs at delivery. Importantly, 90% of infected neonates become chronic carriers, compared with only 10% of infected adults. This can be reduced by over 90% by immunization of the neonate. *Screening*, therefore, has important benefits and is now routine: screening of women at high risk because of origin (developing world) or behaviour (intravenous drug abusers and their partners; prostitutes) identifies only 50% of chronic carriers. Known carriers should be handled with sensitive precautions for fear of infecting staff.

Mycobacterium tuberculosis (TB)

Worldwide, TB is very common, and its incidence in the United Kingdom is increasing because of immigration, HIV infection and travel. Tuberculin testing is safe; Bacille bilié de Calmette-Guérin (BCG) vaccination is live and contraindicated. Diagnosis in late pregnancy is associated with worse neonatal outcomes, and TB is a significant cause of maternal mortality in the developing world. Treatment with first-line drugs and additional vitamin B_6 is safe in pregnancy, but streptomycin is contraindicated. Congenital TB is very rare, but the neonate is at risk of infection.

Human immunodeficiency virus (HIV)

The retroviruses that cause acquired immune deficiency syndrome (AIDS) have infected 0.6% of women in some inner city areas in the United Kingdom, and most women are unaware of their infection. Stillbirth, intrauterine growth restriction (IUGR) [→ p.169] and prematurity are more common in HIV-positive women. However, pregnancy does not hasten progression to AIDS. Vertical transmission to the fetus occurs mostly intrapartum or during breastfeeding and occurs in 15%, although passively acquired antibodies in the neonate are universal because of transplacental transfer. Transmission is greater with low CD4 counts and high viral load (early- and late-stage disease), membrane rupture for more than 4 h and low birthweight. Twenty-five per cent of HIV-infected neonates develop AIDS by 1 year and 40% will develop AIDS by 5 years.

Strategies to reduce vertical transmission are expensive and therefore depend upon local resources. The most effective is combination therapy, currently including zidovudine and lamuvidine, aimed at reducing maternal disease progression. This is continued throughout pregnancy and labour, and the neonate is also treated. Caesarean section and the avoidance of breastfeeding are usual, although it is uncertain if elective Caesarean section is beneficial in those on treatment with an undetectable viral load. This 'best' strategy reduces vertical transmission to <2%. In the developing world, however, expensive drugs may be unavailable and elective Caesarean section and failure to breastfeed may have serious adverse effects. There, nevirapine, as single doses in labour and to the neonate, greatly reduces vertical transmission in women delivering vaginally and breastfeeding.

Screening in pregnancy is routinely available in antenatal clinics. Human immunodeficiency virus outside the inner city areas in the United Kingdom is rare, and the benefits of treatment and Caesarean section must be weighed against the cost and the social and behavioural implications of knowledge of HIV status.

Malaria

Although rare in the United Kingdom, malaria infection is very common in developing countries. Maternal complications are more frequent in pregnancy, and IUGR [→ p.169] and stillbirth are more common. Treatment with either chloroquine or mefloquine according to the area reduces these risks.

Listeriosis

Infection with the bacterium *Listeria monocytogenes* can occur from consumption of pâtés, soft cheeses and pre-packed meals, and causes a non-specific febrile illness. It is common in human faeces, but if bacteraemia occurs in pregnancy (0.01% of women) potentially fatal infection of the fetus may follow. The diagnosis is established from blood cultures. *Screening* is impractical. Prevention involves the avoidance of high-risk foods in pregnancy.

Chlamydia and gonorrhoea [→p.62]

Chlamydia trachomatis infection in pregnancy occurs in about 5% of women and *Neisseria gonorrhoeae* in 0.1%. Most women are asymptomatic. Although best known as causes of pelvic inflammatory disease and subfertility, both have been associated with preterm labour and with neonatal conjunctivitis. *Chlamydia* is treated with azithromycin or erythromycin; tetracyclines cause fetal tooth discoloration. Gonorrhoea is treated with cephalosporins as resistance to penicillin is common. *Screening* to identify neonates at risk is worthwhile in developing countries. Furthermore, treatment of asymptomatic *Chlamydia* infection may reduce the incidence of preterm birth. Screening is currently not routine in the United Kingdom, but at least for *Chlamydia* may be of benefit.

Bacterial vaginosis [→p.61]

This overgrowth of normal vaginal lactobacilli by anaerobes, *Gardnerella vaginalis* and *Mycoplasma hominis* can be asymptomatic or cause an offensive vaginal discharge in women. Preterm labour [→ p.158] is more common, and antibiotic treatment with clindamycin or metronidazole may reduce this risk (*Lancet* 2003; **361**: 983). *Screening*, therefore, is essential for woman with a previous history of preterm labour, and may even become routine for all. Screening involves a 'whiff test' with vaginal pH assessment.

Other obstetric infections

- Urinary tract infections and pyelonephritis [→ p.150]
- Endometritis [→ p.227]
- Chorioamnionitis [→ p.160]

Further reading

Brocklehurst P, Volmink J. Antiretrovirals for reducing the risk of mother-to-child transmission of HIV infection. *Cochrane Database System Review (Online: Update Software)* 2002; **2**: CD003510.

Gaytant MA, Steegers EA, Semmekrot BA, Merkus HM, Galama JM. Congenital cytomegalovirus infection: review of the epidemiology and outcome. *Obstetrical & Gynecological Survey* 2002; **57**: 245–56.

Herbert M, Impey L. Infections in pregnancy. In: Warrell D, Cox T, Firth J, Benz E, eds. *Oxford Textbook of Medicine*, Vol. 2, 4th edn. Oxford: Oxford University Press, 2003: 449–55.

Ormerod P. Tuberculosis in pregnancy and the puerperium. *Thorax* 2001; **56**: 494–9.

Platt JS, O'Brien WF. Group B streptococcus: prevention of early-onset neonatal sepsis. *Obstetrical & Gynecological Survey* 2003; **58**: 191–6.

Infections in Pregnancy at a Glance

Cytomegalovirus (CMV)	1% maternal infection rate but low percentage of fetuses affected. No treatment, screening or vaccination
Rubella	Most women immune, so low infection rate. High percentage of fetuses affected, most if early gestation. Termination of pregnancy (TOP) offered if infection <16 weeks. Screening identifies those in need of postnatal immunization
Toxoplasmosis	Low percentage of fetuses permanently affected. Screening not routine in the United Kingdom. Proven fetal toxoplasmosis treated with spiramycin
Syphilis	Rare. Screening routine because treatment prevents congenital syphilis
Herpes simplex virus (HSV)	Common. Neonatal infection is rare but very serious. High risk of neonatal herpes (therefore Caesarean is indicated) if primary infection within 6 weeks of delivery, or active vesicles at time of labour
Group B streptococcus	High maternal carrier rate; major cause of neonatal sepsis. Treatment with intrapartum penicillin of high-risk groups ± positive third trimester screen reduces neonatal infection
Herpes zoster	Many immune. Severe maternal illness in pregnancy. Infection <20 weeks is occasionally teratogenic. Infection just before delivery can cause severe neonatal infection, so immunoglobulin given to neonate
Hepatitis B	Carriage common in high-risk women. High transmission rate, high mortality in neonate. Universal screening identifies neonates in need of immunoglobulin
Hepatitis C	Mostly in high-risk (e.g. human immunodeficiency virus, HIV) women: 6% vertical transmission
HIV	Disease unaffected by pregnancy. Adverse fetal outcome more common. Vertical transmission increased by early and late disease, prolonged membrane rupture. Vertical transmission reduced (from 15% to 2%) by combination antiretrovirals, avoidance of breastfeeding and Caesarean section (strategy recommended in the West). Nevirapine recommended if resources scarce
Chlamydia	5% in pregnancy. Neonatal conjunctivitis and preterm labour. Antibiotics may prevent latter, so screening probably worthwhile
Bacterial vaginosis	Common. Associated with preterm labour. Screening and treatment if previous preterm labour

20 Hypertensive Disorders in Pregnancy

Normal blood pressure changes in pregnancy

Blood pressure is dependent on systemic vascular resistance and cardiac output. It normally falls to a minimum level in the second trimester, by about 30/15 mmHg, because of reduced vascular resistance. This occurs in both normotensive and chronically hypertensive women. By term, the blood pressure again rises to pre-pregnant levels (Fig. 20.1). Hypertension due to pre-eclampsia is largely due to an increase in systemic vascular resistance. Protein excretion in normal pregnancy is increased, but is less than 0.5 g/24 h.

Classification of hypertensive disorders in pregnancy

The classification of these is diverse and often inconsistent. The definitions below are used because they are simple and best represent the pathological processes involved.

Pregnancy-induced hypertension
This is when the blood pressure rises above 140/90. It can be due to either pre-eclampsia or transient hypertension. *Pre-eclampsia* is a disorder in which hypertension and proteinuria appear in the second half of pregnancy, usually with oedema. Eclampsia, or the occurrence of epileptiform seizures, is the most dramatic complication. Proteinuria is occasionally absent, e.g. in early disease, when it is not always distinguishable from *transient hypertension*. These patients without significant (<0.5 g/24 h) proteinuria are 'latent' hypertensives who commonly develop hypertension in later life.

Pre-existing or chronic hypertension
This is present when the diastolic blood pressure is more than 140/90 mmHg before pregnancy or before 20 weeks gestation. This may be *essential hypertension*, or it may be *secondary* to renal or other disease. There may be pre-existing proteinuria because of renal disease. Patients with underlying hypertension are at an increased risk (sixfold) of developing 'superimposed' pre-eclampsia.

Classification of hypertension	
Pregnancy induced:	Pre-eclampsia Transient
Pre-existing:	Essential Secondary

Pre-eclampsia

Definitions and terminology

Pre-eclampsia is a multisystem disease, which usually manifests as hypertension and proteinuria. It is peculiar to pregnancy, of placental origin, and cured only by delivery. Blood vessel endothelial cell damage, in

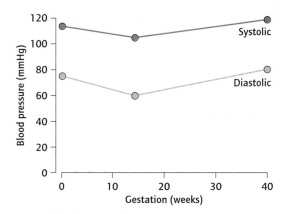

Fig. 20.1 Blood pressure changes in pregnancy.

association with an exaggerated maternal inflammatory response (*AmJOG* 1999; **180**: 499) leads to vasospasm, increased capillary permeability and clotting dysfunction (Fig. 20.2). These can affect all the maternal organs *to varying degrees* and account for all manifestations and complications. Increased vascular resistance accounts for the hypertension, increased vascular permeability for proteinuria, reduced placental blood flow for intrauterine growth restriction (IUGR) and reduced cerebral perfusion for eclampsia.

The multisystem nature of the disease explains why the clinical features are variable. Hypertension is just a sign rather than the disease itself, and is even occasionally absent until late stages; proteinuria is often absent in early disease. Although traditionally central to *establishing* the diagnosis, one or other of these features may nevertheless be absent in a woman who has pre-eclampsia (*BMJ* 1994; **309**: 1395). Furthermore, eclampsia, the most dramatic complication, is just one of many. Differing definitions confuse the issue: 'pregnancy-induced hypertension' encompasses 'transient hypertension', which, although often indistinguishable from mild pre-eclampsia on clinical grounds, is a different disease entity.

Establishing the diagnosis of pre-eclampsia

Blood pressure rises above 140/90 WITH
Proteinuria >0.5 g/24 h

Course and degrees of the disease

The disease is progressive, but variable and unpredictable. Hypertension usually precedes proteinuria, a relatively late sign. Some women develop life-threatening disease at 24 weeks; others merely develop mild hypertension at term. Although only partly reflecting the severity of disease, the degree of hypertension can be used to help assess it (see box below).

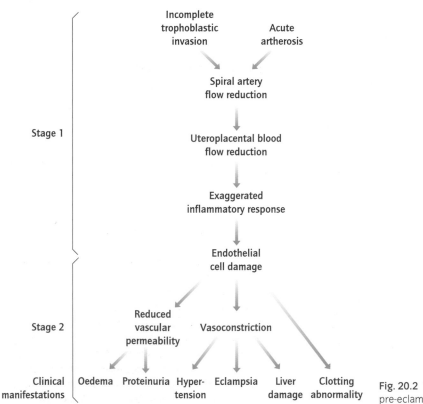

Fig. 20.2 The possible pathogenesis of pre-eclampsia.

Degrees of pre-eclampsia	
Classifications vary: the one below encompasses the principles and diversity of the disease	
Mild:	Proteinuria and hypertension <170/110
Moderate:	Proteinuria and hypertension ≥170/110
Severe:	Proteinuria and hypertension <32 weeks or with maternal complications

Principal risk factors for pre-eclampsia
Nulliparity
Previous history, family history
Extremes of maternal age
Chronic hypertension
Diabetes
Twin pregnancies
Autoimmune disease
Renal disease
Obesity

Epidemiology

Pre-eclampsia affects 6% of nulliparous women to varying degrees. It is unusual in multiparous women unless the first pregnancy was affected (12% recurrence risk), or the current pregnancy is the first with a new partner.

Pathophysiology

The mechanism is incompletely understood but it appears to be a two-stage process (see Fig. 20.2).

Stage 1 accounts for the development of the disease, occurs before 20 weeks and causes no symptoms. In normal pregnancy, trophoblastic invasion of spiral arterioles leads to vasodilatation of vessel walls. In pre-eclampsia this invasion is incomplete. This impaired materno–fetal trophoblast interaction may be caused by altered immune responses. In addition, spiral arterioles may contain atheromatous lesions. The result is decreased uteroplacental blood flow.

Stage 2 is the manifestation of the disease: The ischaemic placenta, probably via an exaggerated maternal inflammatory response, induces widespread endothelial cell damage, causing vasoconstriction, increased vascular permeability and clotting dysfunction. These cause the clinical manifestations of disease.

Aetiology

Predisposing factors include nulliparity, a previous or family history of pre-eclampsia, a new partner, the extremes of maternal age, disorders characterized by microvascular disease (chronic hypertension, chronic renal disease, sickle-cell disease [→ p.153], diabetes, autoimmune disease) and pregnancies with a large placenta (twins, molar pregnancy).

Clinical features

History: Pre-eclampsia is usually asymptomatic, but a headache, drowsiness, visual disturbances, nausea/vomiting or epigastric pain may occur at a late stage.

Examination: Hypertension is usually the first sign, but it is occasionally absent until the late stages. Oedema is found in most pregnancies but in pre-eclampsia may be massive, not postural or of sudden onset. The presence of ankle clonus or epigastric tenderness is suggestive of impending complications. Urine testing for protein with dipsticks should be regarded as part of the clinical examination (Fig. 20.3).

Significance of dipstick urinalysis	
Trace:	Seldom significant
1+:	Possible significant proteinuria: quantify with 24-h collection
2+ or more:	Significant proteinuria likely: quantify
N.B. Mild proteinuria may also be due to urinary infection, so do urine culture	

Complications of pre-eclampsia (Fig. 20.4)
Maternal

Early-onset disease tends to be more severe. The occurrence of any of the following complications, which may occur together, is an indication for delivery whatever the gestation. They may also occur postpartum as it takes at least 24 h for delivery to 'cure' the disease.

Eclampsia is grand mal seizures (0.2% of all pregnancies), probably resulting from cerebrovascular vasospasm. Mortality can result from hypoxia and concomitant complications of severe disease. Treatment is with magnesium sulphate (*Lancet* 1995; **345**: 1455).

Timing of delivery

Pre-eclampsia is progressive, unpredictable and cured only by delivery. As a general rule, one or more fetal or maternal complications are likely to occur within 2 weeks of the onset of proteinuria (*Lancet* 1993; **341**: 1451).

Mild hypertension without fetal compromise is monitored for deterioration. Induction of labour at term is wise.

Moderate or severe pre-eclampsia requires delivery if gestation exceeds 34–36 weeks, after which time complications of prematurity are seldom a problem. Hypertension reaching 170/110 mmHg must be controlled first. Before 34 weeks, conservative management may be appropriate, in a specialist unit with full neonatal care facilities, but the possible benefits of increasing fetal maturity must be weighed against the risks of disease complications. Steroids are given prophylactically, hypertension is treated and there is intensive maternal and fetal surveillance involving daily clinical assessment, CTG and fluid balance, and frequent blood testing. Clinical deterioration will prompt delivery.

Severe pre-eclampsia with complications or fetal distress requires delivery whatever the gestation.

Conduct of delivery

Before 34 weeks, Caesarean section is usual. After 34 weeks, labour can usually be induced with prostaglandins. Epidural analgesia helps reduce the blood pressure. The fetus is monitored with CTG and the blood pressure closely observed. Antihypertensives can be used in labour. If the pressure reaches 170/110 mmHg in second stage, an elective forceps delivery is performed, as maternal pushing raises intracranial pressure and increases the risk of cerebral haemorrhage. Oxytocin rather than ergometrine is used in the third stage as the latter can increase the blood pressure.

Potential pitfalls in managing pre-eclampsia

Pre-eclampsia is unpredictable

Admit patients with proteinuria only: hypertension may be absent

Epigastric pain is ominous and liver function testing is mandatory

Treatment of hypertension may disguise pre-eclampsia

Excessive fluid administration causes pulmonary oedema

Complications may still arise after delivery

Postnatal care of the pre-eclamptic patient

Whilst delivery is the only cure for pre-eclampsia it often takes at least 24 h for severe disease to improve, and the maternal complications may need to be managed in an intensive care unit. *Liver enzymes*, platelets and *renal function* are still monitored closely. Low platelet levels usually return to normal within a few days. *Fluid balance* is essential: pulmonary oedema and respiratory failure may follow uncontrolled administration of intravenous fluid. If the urine output is low, central venous pressure (CVP) monitoring will guide management. If the CVP is high (suggesting overload), frusemide is given. If it is low, fluid but not albumin is given. If it is normal and oliguria persists, renal failure is likely. The *blood pressure* is maintained at 90–100 mmHg diastolic, usually with a beta-blocker, which may be needed for several weeks. Second-line drugs in the postnatal period include nifedipine and angiotensin-converting enzyme (ACE) inhibitors.

Pre-exisiting hypertension in pregnancy

Definitions and epidemiology

This is diagnosed when the diastolic blood pressure exceeds 140/90 before 20 weeks. Patients with pregnancy-induced hypertension that is 'transient' also have an underlying predisposition to hypertension and may need treatment later in life. Underlying hypertension is present in about 5% of pregnancies, and is more common in older and obese women, and in women with a positive family history or who developed hypertension taking the combined oral contraceptive.

Aetiology

Essential or 'idiopathic' hypertension is the most common cause. Secondary hypertension is commonly associated with diabetes or renal disease such as polycystic disease, renal artery stenosis or chronic pyelonephritis. Other rarer causes are phaeochromocytoma, Cushing's syndrome, cardiac disease and coarctation of the aorta.

Clinical features

Hypertension often increases in late pregnancy. Symptoms are often absent, although fundal changes, renal bruits and radiofemoral delay should be excluded in all hypertensives. Proteinuria in patients with renal disease may be present from booking.

Investigations

To identify secondary hypertension: Phaeochromocytoma is excluded by performing at least two 24 h urine collections for vanillylmandelic acid (VMA). This is worthwhile because the maternal mortality of this condition is very high. Renal function is assessed and a renal ultrasound is performed.

Management

The principal dangers are worsening hypertension and superimposed pre-eclampsia; in the absence of these, perinatal mortality is only marginally increased. Methyldopa is used to control hypertension, with nifedpine as a second-line agent. Angiotensin-converting enzyme inhibitors affect fetal urine production and are contraindicated. The pregnancy is treated as 'high risk' and fortnightly ultrasound examinations in the third trimester are usual. Pre-eclampsia is six times more common, and confirmed by the finding of significant proteinuria for the first time after 20 weeks.

Further reading

Myers JE, Baker PN. Hypertensive diseases and eclampsia. *Current Opinion in Obstetrics & Gynecology* 2002; **14**: 119–25

Redman CWG, Roberts JM. Management of pre-eclampsia. *Lancet* 1993; **341**: 1451–4.

Roberts JM, Redman CWG. Pre-eclampsia: more than pregnancy induced hypertension. *Lancet* 1993; **341**: 1447–51.

www.doorbar.co.uk/apec.html for information on pre-eclampsia.

Pre-eclampsia at a Glance

Definition	Multisystem disease unique to pregnancy that usually manifests as hypertension (blood pressure, BP, >140/90) after 20 weeks and proteinuria that is due to:	
Pathology	Endothelial cell damage and vasospasm, which can affect the fetus and almost all maternal organs. It is of placental origin and cured only by delivery	
Degrees	Mild:	Proteinuria and BP <170/110
	Moderate:	Proteinuria and BP ≥170/110
	Severe:	Proteinuria and hypertension before 32 weeks or with maternal complications
Epidemiology	6%	
Aetiology	Nulliparity, previous history, maternal age, twins, molar pregnancy, pre-existing hypertension, diabetes or autoimmune disease	
Features	None until late stage, then headache, epigastric pain, visual disturbances	
Complications	Maternal:	Eclampsia, cerebrovascular accidents (CVAs), liver/renal failure, haemolysis, elevated liver enzymes and low platelet count (HELLP), disseminated intravascular coagulation (DIC), pulmonary oedema
	Fetal:	Intrauterine growth restriction (IUGR), fetal morbidity and mortality
Investigations	To confirm diagnosis:	Mid-stream urine (MSU) and urine protein measurement
	To monitor:	Watch BP, serial full blood count (FBC), urea and electrolytes (U&E), liver function tests (LFTs) and fetal surveillance
Screening	Observation of high-risk pregnancies. Uterine artery Doppler	
Prevention	Aspirin and vitamins C and E have limited role	
Management	Investigate if BP > 140/90; admit if proteinuria or moderate/severe disease Antihypertensives if BP reaches 170/110; steroids if moderate/severe at < 34 weeks	
	Delivery:	Deliver mild by term Deliver moderate/severe after 34–36 weeks if possible Deliver if maternal complications whatever the gestation
	Magnesium sulphate if eclamspia; consider prophylactic use in severe disease Postnatally, watch BP, urine output, blood tests: FBC, U&E, LFTs	

21 Other Medical Disorders in Pregnancy

Diabetes and gestational diabetes

Physiology

Glucose tolerance decreases in pregnancy due to altered carbohydrate metabolism and the antagonistic effects of human placental lactogen, progesterone and cortisol. Glucose tolerance is not bimodally distributed in the general population (Fig. 21.1), and there is a spectrum of glucose intolerance. Pregnancy is 'diabetogenic': women without diabetes but with impaired or potentially impaired glucose tolerance often 'deteriorate' enough to be classified as diabetic in pregnancy. They are called 'gestational diabetics' and have a high chance of developing subsequent overt diabetes. The absence of a bimodal distribution also means that definitions are artificial and even variable, and that the incidence of gestational diabetes varies accordingly.

The kidneys of non-pregnant women start to excrete glucose at a threshold level of 11 mmol/L. In pregnancy this varies more but often decreases, so glycosuria may occur at physiological blood glucose concentrations. Raised fetal blood glucose levels induce fetal hyperinsulinaemia, causing fetal fat deposition and excessive growth (macrosomia).

Definition and epidemiology

Pre-existing insulin-dependent diabetes affects 0.1–0.3% of pregnant women. Increasing amounts of insulin will be required in these pregnancies to maintain normoglycaemia.

Gestational diabetes describes the development of significant glucose intolerance in pregnancy that disappears after the end of pregnancy. Definitions vary, but the most practical definition is when a glucose level in pregnancy is >9.0 mmol 2h after a 75-g glucose load. This definition encompasses 2% of pregnant women.

Risk factors are a previous history of gestational diabetes, a fetus >4 kg, a previous unexplained stillbirth, a family history of diabetes, weight >100 kg or polycystic ovary syndrome (PCOS) [→ p.70]. In pregnancy, the presence of polyhydramnios or persistent glycosuria also indicate increased risk. In women with PCOS, antenatal metformin reduces the risk of gestational diabetes (*Hum Reprod* 2002; **17**: 2858).

Diabetes in pregnancy	
Pre-existing diabetes (<0.3%):	Insulin requirements increase in pregnancy
Gestational diabetes (2%):	Glucose levels rise temporarily to diabetic level

Fetal complications (Fig. 21.2)

Complications are related to glucose levels, so gestational diabetics are usually less affected than established diabetics. *Congenital abnormalities*, e.g. cardiac abnormalities, are three to five times more common in established diabetics, and are related to periconceptual glucose control. *Preterm labour*, natural or

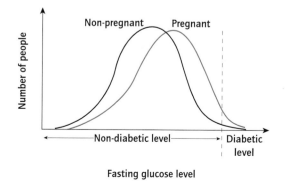

Fig. 21.1 Distribution of glucose tolerance in the non-pregnant and pregnant population.

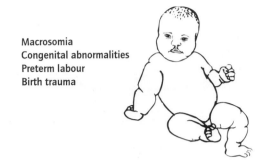

Macrosomia
Congenital abnormalities
Preterm labour
Birth trauma

Fig. 21.2 Fetal complications of diabetes.

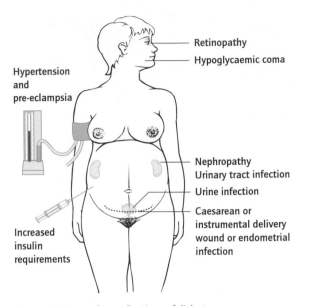

Retinopathy
Hypoglycaemic coma

Hypertension and pre-eclampsia

Increased insulin requirements

Nephropathy
Urinary tract infection

Urine infection

Caesarean or instrumental delivery wound or endometrial infection

Fig. 21.3 Maternal complications of diabetes.

induced, occurs in 10% of established diabetics, and *fetal lung maturity* at any given gestation is less than with non-diabetic pregnancies. *Polyhydramnios* (increased liquor) [→ p.131] is common. As the fetus tends to be larger, *dystocia* and *birth trauma* (particularly shoulder dystocia) are more common. *Fetal compromise*, *fetal distress* in labour and *sudden fetal death* are more common, and related particularly to poor third-trimester glucose control.

Maternal complications (Fig. 21.3)

Insulin requirements normally increase considerably by the end of pregnancy. *Ketoacidosis* is rare, but *hypoglycaemia* may result from attempts to achieve optimum glucose control. *Urinary tract infection* and *wound or endometrial infection* after delivery are more common. Pre-existing *hypertension* is detected in up to 25% of overt diabetics and *pre-eclampsia* is more common. *Caesarean* or *instrumental delivery* is more likely because of fetal compromise and increased fetal size. Diabetic *nephropathy* is associated with poorer fetal outcomes but does not usually deteriorate. Diabetic *retinopathy* often deteriorates and may need to be treated in pregnancy.

Detection of and screening for gestational diabetes

Screening is widely practised, but is of limited proven benefit, as complications are less than with pre-existing diabetics. Regimes are variable and that outlined in the box below is one example. The aim is to detect a level of glucose intolerance that is potentially harmful to the fetus.

Detection and screening for gestational diabetes

Step 1: Screening the general population
Screen for glycosuria. If detected on 2+ occasions, undergo Step 2
   If at high risk of gestational diabetes (history), undergo Step 2 at 28 and 34 weeks routinely

Step 2: More intensive screening of the higher risk groups
Perform 'timed' glucose level. If >6 mmol/L when preprandial or >2 h after a meal, or >7 mmol/L <2 h after a meal, go to Step 3

Step 3: Diagnostic testing
Perform glucose tolerance test with a 75-g oral glucose load. If abnormal (2-h level >9.0 mmol/L), gestational diabetes is diagnosed. Start on a high-fibre, low-carbohydrate diet, and after a few days proceed to Step 4

Step 4: Assessing need for insulin
Perform 'glucose series' measuring several levels in a day. If preprandial glucose levels are consistently >6 mmol/L, insulin therapy is started. If not, diet may be adequate

Risk factors for gestational diabetes

Previous history of gestational diabetes
Previous fetus >4 kg
Previous unexplained stillbirth
First-degree relative with diabetes
Polyhydramnios
Persistent glycosuria
Weight >100 kg
Polycystic ovary syndrome (PCOS)

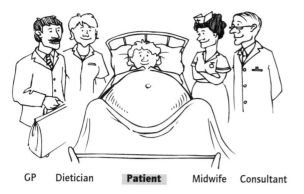

GP   Dietician   **Patient**   Midwife   Consultant

Fig. 21.4 The multidisciplinary approach to diabetes in pregnancy.

Management of diabetes in pregnancy

Precise glucose control and fetal monitoring for evidence of compromise are the cornerstones of management. Antenatal care is consultant-based, with delivery in a unit with neonatal intensive care facilities. A multidisciplinary approach is necessary (Fig. 21.4).

Preconceptual care and early pregnancy assessment. Insulin-dependent diabetic women wishing to undergo pregnancy should have their renal function and retinae assessed. Glucose control is optimized, and folic acid is prescribed.

Organization and patient education. Care is based on a 'team approach', consisting of an obstetrician, midwife, general practitioner, dietician and often a physician. The key member, however, is the woman, who has day-to-day control of her diabetes and needs to be educated about optimizing control. If she is not motivated, normoglycaemia will not be achieved.

Monitoring the diabetes. Glucose levels are checked by the patient several times daily with a home 'glucometer'. The ideal is levels consistently between 4 and 6 mmol/L: this is usually achieved by a combination of one nighttime-long/intermediate-acting and three preprandial short-acting insulin injections. Doses will usually need to be progressively increased as the pregnancy advances. Oral hypoglycaemic agents are not used in women with established diabetes, although metformin reduces the incidence of gestational diabetes in women with PCOS. High concentrations of glycosylated haemoglobin (HbA1c) reflect poor prior control.

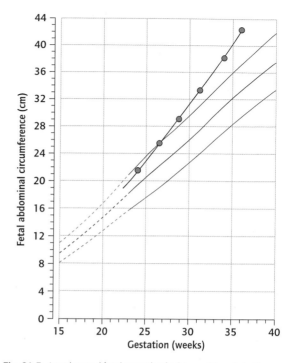

Fig. 21.5 Accelerated fetal growth of a fetus with a diabetic mother.

Visits occur fortnightly up to 34 weeks and weekly thereafter.

Monitoring the fetus. A 20-week ultrasound scan is used to check the gestation and detect abnormalities, and a specialist cardiac scan is arranged. Serial ultrasound examinations monitor fetal growth and liquor volume. Even where glucose control has been good, macrosomia and polyhydramnios can occur (Fig. 21.5).

Timing and mode of delivery. Evidence is limited (*Cochrane* 2001: CD001997). The *gestational diabetic* with good glucose control can be managed in the normal manner. The *pre-existing diabetic* normally undergoes induction of labour at 39 weeks. Delivery is earlier if glucose control has been poor. Birth trauma is more likely and, although prediction is imprecise, elective Caesarean section is often used where the abdominal circumference exceeds the head circumference, as this pattern is associated with an increased risk of shoulder dystocia [→ p.221]. During labour, glucose levels are maintained with a 'sliding scale' of insulin and a 10% dextrose infusion.

The neonate commonly develops hypoglycaemia because it has become 'accustomed to' hyperglycaemia and its insulin levels are high. Respiratory distress syndrome occasionally occurs, even after 38 weeks. A careful examination is made to reveal hitherto undetected congenital abnormalities.

The puerperium and postnatal period. In the pre-existing diabetic, insulin can be rapidly changed to pre-pregnant doses. In the gestational diabetic, insulin is discontinued. A glucose tolerance test should be performed on gestational diabetics at 3 months: 50% will be diagnosed as diabetic within the next 10 years.

Management of diabetes

Preconceptual glucose control
Assessment of maternal diabetic complications
Patient education and team involvement
Glucose monitoring and insulin adjustment
Anomaly and cardiac ultrasound and fetal surveillance
Delivery by 39 weeks

Cardiac disease

In pregnancy there is a 40% increase in cardiac output, due to both an increase in stroke volume and heart rate, and a 40% increase in blood volume. There is also a 50% reduction in systemic vascular resistance: blood pressure often drops in the second trimester, but is usually normal by term. The increased blood flow produces a flow (ejection systolic) murmur in 90% of pregnant women.

Epidemiology

Cardiac disease affects 0.3% of pregnant women. The maternal risk is dependent on the cardiac status and most encounter no problems. However, acquired and uncorrected congenital disease mean that it remains a major cause of maternal mortality, usually as a result of cardiac failure.

Risks of pregnancy

Increased cardiac output acts as an 'exercise test' with which the heart may be unable to cope. This usually manifests before 24 weeks or in labour, but decompensa-

tion may also occur with blood loss or fluid overload. The latter can occur in the early puerperium, as uterine involution 'squeezes' a large 'fluid load' into the circulation.

Types of cardiac disease

Congenital heart disease has usually been corrected, or is relatively benign if the woman has reached reproductive age. However, uncorrected cyanotic disease and primary pulmonary hypertension (50% maternal mortality) are particular risks and avoidance or even termination of pregnancy is advised. *Rheumatic heart disease* is now rare, but usually manifests as mitral stenosis. This usually causes few problems. *Myocardial infarction* is unusual in women of reproductive age; mortality is greater at later gestations.

Management principles

Patients are seen in conjunction with a *cardiologist.* Those with severe decompensated disease are advised against pregnancy. Regular *cardiac assessment,* particularly echocardiography, is needed. Fetal cardiac anomalies are more common (3%) and are best detected on *ultrasound* at 20 weeks gestation. *Hypertension* should be treated. Regular checks for anaemia are made. *Labour* is usually more appropriate than elective Caesarean. Unless the lesion is mild, delivery is in a unit with *intensive care facilities;* cardiac monitoring is continued postnatally for at least 24 h. *Epidural analgesia* is safe unless there is severe outflow obstruction. The *left lateral position* is encouraged to avoid the supine hypotension syndrome [→ p.205] and attention is paid to *fluid balance.* *Elective forceps* delivery helps avoid the additional stress of pushing in severe cases. Operative delivery and prolonged labour are covered by *antibiotic prophylaxis.*

Respiratory disease

Tidal volume increases by 40% in pregnancy, although there is no change in respiratory rate. Asthma is common in pregnancy. Pregnancy has a variable effect on the disease: drugs should not be withheld, because they are generally safe and because a severe asthma attack is potentially lethal to mother and fetus. Well-controlled asthma has little detrimental effect on perinatal outcome. Women on long-term steroids require an increased dose in labour because the chronically suppressed adrenal cortex is unable to produce adequate steroids for the stress of labour.

Epilepsy

Epilepsy affects 0.5% of pregnant women. Seizure control can deteriorate in pregnancy, and epilepsy is a significant cause of maternal death. The risk of congenital abnormalities (e.g. neural tube defects, NTDs) is increased (4% overall): this is largely due to drug therapy and is increased with polypharmacy. The fetus has a 3% risk of developing epilepsy.

Optimum management involves preconceptual seizure control on the minimum number of drugs and folic acid supplementation. Ideally, sodium valproate should not be used because it is associated with lower intelligence in children. Carbamazepine or preferably lamotrigine (*Epilepsia* 2002; **43**: 1161) are used. Because of the maternal risks of seizures, drug therapy is continued; ultrasound is used to exclude fetal abnormalities. In women without complete seizure control, drug levels should be checked 4-weekly and the doses may need to be increased. Folic acid 5 mg is continued throughout pregnancy and vitamin K 10 mg is given orally, to the woman from 36 weeks and to the neonate. If a seizure occurs, it is important to exclude eclampsia.

Thyroid disease in pregnancy

Thyroid status does not alter in pregnancy, although iodine clearance is increased. Goitre is more common. Fetal thyroxine production starts at 12 weeks; before, it is dependent on maternal thyroxine. Maternal thyroid-stimulating hormone (TSH) is increased in early pregnancy.

Hypothyroidism
This affects 1% of pregnant women. In the United Kingdom, most cases of hypothyroidism are due to Hashimoto's thyroiditis or thyroid surgery, but hypothyroidism is common where dietary iodine is deficient.

Untreated disease is rare as anovulation is usual but is associated with a high perinatal mortality. Inadequate replacement may affect childhood development. Thyroxine replacement is maintained and may need to be increased: monthly thyroid function tests are performed. Thyroxine hardly crosses the placenta.

Hyperthyroidism
This affects 0.2% of pregnant women and is usually due to Graves' disease. Untreated disease is rare as anovulation is usual. In untreated women, perinatal mortality is high and crises can occur at delivery. Symptoms may be confused with those of pregnancy. Hyperthyroidism is treated with propylthiouracil. This crosses the placenta and can cause neonatal hypothyroidism: the lowest possible dose is used and thyroid function is tested monthly. Antithyroid antibodies also cross the placenta: rarely, this causes neonatal thyrotoxicosis and goitre. Graves' disease often worsens postpartum.

Postpartum thyroiditis
This is common (5–10%) and can cause postnatal depression. In affected patients, there is a transient and usually subclinical hyperthyroidism, followed after about 4 months by hypothyroidism. This is permanent in 20%.

Liver disease

Acute fatty liver
This is a very rare (1 in 9000) condition that may be part of the spectrum of pre-eclampsia. Acute hepatorenal failure, disseminated intravascular coagulation (DIC) and hypoglycaemia lead to a high maternal and fetal mortality. There is extensive fatty change in the liver. Malaise, vomiting, jaundice and vague epigastric pain are early features, while thirst may occur weeks earlier. Early diagnosis and prompt delivery are essential, although correction of clotting defects and hypoglycaemia are needed first. Treatment is then supportive, with further dextrose, blood products, careful fluid balance and, occasionally, dialysis. The recurrence rate is very low.

Intrahepatic cholestasis of pregnancy
This is due to abnormal sensitivity to the cholestatic effects of oestrogens. It occurs in 1% of pregnant women

in the West, is familial and tends to recur. It is associated with an increased perinatal mortality and morbidity. This is difficult to predict, but is due to the toxic effects of bile salts on the fetus, possibly by precipitating fetal arrhythmia. Pruritus of the hands and feet is usual; serum bile acids and, usually, liver enzymes are raised. Ursodeoxycholic acid helps relieve itching and may reduce the obstetric risks. Close fetal surveillance and induction of labour at 38 weeks are advised. Because there is an increased maternal and fetal tendency to haemorrhage, vitamin K 10 mg is given daily from 36 weeks.

Thrombophilias and the antiphospholipid syndrome

Antiphospholipid syndrome
This is when the lupus anticoagulant and/or anticardiolipin antibodies occur (measured on two occasions at least 3 months apart) in association with adverse pregnancy complications, but in the absence of the other clinical manifestations of lupus. Recurrent miscarriage [→ p.96], intrauterine growth restriction (IUGR) and early pre-eclampsia are common, and the fetal loss rate is high. Placental thrombosis appears to be responsible. Low levels of these antibodies are also present in nearly 2% of all pregnant women and therefore treatment, normally with aspirin and low-molecular-weight heparin (LMWH) (*BMJ* 1997; **314**: 253) is restricted to those with the *syndrome*. The pregnancy is managed as 'high risk', with serial ultrasound and elective induction of labour at least by term. Postnatal anticoagulation is also recommended to prevent venous thromboembolism.

Other prothrombotic disorders
In addition to the risk of venous thromboembolism, activated protein C resistance, the prothrombin gene variant, the Factor V Leyden gene, protein S deficiency or antithrombin III deficiency are all more common in women with recurrent pregnancy loss (*Lancet* 2003; **361**: 901), early pre-eclampsia, placental abruption and IUGR. A family or personal history of venous thrombosis is also common (*BJOG* 2003; **110**: 462). Indeed many thrombophilias have been associated with an increased risk of cerebral palsy (*Ann Neurol* 1998; **44**: 665). Women with prothrombotic tendencies and an adverse pregnancy history are usually treated as for antiphospholipid syndrome, although the effectiveness of this is currently unproven.

Systemic lupus erythematosus (SLE)
This affects 0.1–0.2% of pregnant women. In absence of the lupus anticoagulant or anticardiolipin antibodies (see above), the risks to the pregnancy are largely confined to those of associated hypertension or renal disease. Maternal symptoms often relapse after delivery.

Renal disease

In pregnancy, the glomerular filtration rate increases 40%, causing urea and creatinine levels to decrease.

Chronic renal disease
This affects 0.2% of pregnant women. Fetal and maternal complications are dependent on the degree of renal impairment, and pregnancy is inadvisable if the creatinine level is >200 μmol/L. Renal function can deteriorate in pregnancy. Rejection of renal transplants is not more common; immunosuppressive therapy is continued. Proteinuria can cause diagnostic confusion with pre-eclampsia, which is more common, but will usually have been present before 20 weeks. Fetal complications include pre-eclampsia, IUGR and preterm delivery. Management involves serial ultrasounds to assess fetal growth, measurement of renal function, screening for urinary infection (which may exacerbate renal disease) and control of hypertension. Vaginal delivery is usually appropriate.

Urinary infection
Urine infection is associated with preterm labour, anaemia and increased perinatal morbidity and mortality. Asymptomatic bacteriuria affects 5% of women, but in pregnancy is more likely (20%) to lead to pyelonephritis (Fig. 21.6). The urine should be cultured at the booking visit, and asymptomatic bacteriuria is treated. Subsequently, culture is performed if leucocytes, nitrites or protein are detected on routine urinalysis. Pyelonephritis affects 1–2% of women, causing loin pain, rigors, vomiting and a fever. *Escherichia coli* accounts for 75%. Intravenous antibiotics are needed.

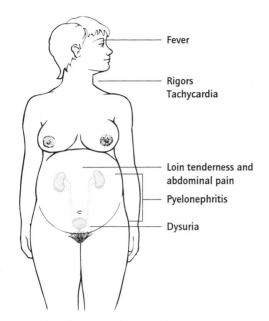

Fig. 21.6 Clinical features of pyelonephritis.

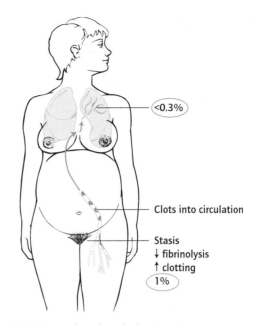

Fig. 21.7 Venous thromboembolism in pregnancy.

Venous thromboembolic disease

Pregnancy is prothrombotic and the incidence of venous thrombosis increases sixfold. Blood clotting factors are increased, fibrinolytic activity is reduced and blood flow is altered by mechanical obstruction and immobility. Women with inherited prothrombotic conditions, such as carriers of the Factor V Leyden mutation (*Lancet* 1996; **347**: 1346), and those with a family or personal history, are particularly prone to thromboses.

Pulmonary embolus
This is an important cause of maternal death [→ p.232] in developed countries. Embolism occurs in <0.3%, with a mortality of 1–3% (Fig. 21.7).

Deep vein thrombosis (DVT)
This occurs in about 1% of pregnant women. Doppler examination of the leg and/or a venogram are used.

With both conditions, clinical signs may be absent, and many women with a pulmonary embolus are not diagnosed before death. Diagnosis is as in the non-pregnant woman, although D-dimers are often raised in preg-nancy. A thrombophilia screen is performed before treatment. Venous thromboembolism is treated initially with a bolus and then an infusion of unfractionated intravenous heparin. This is followed by subcutaneous LMWH as maintenance therapy because this may be safer (*Ann Intern Med* 1999: **130**: 800), and treatment is continued into the puerperium. Low-molecular-weight heparin doses are adjusted according to the anti-Factor Xa level. Warfarin is teratogenic, may cause fetal bleeding and is seldom used antenatally.

Thromboprophylaxis
General measures include maintenance of hydration and mobilization. *Antenatal prophylaxis* with LMWH is restricted to women at very high risk. *Postpartum prophylaxis* with LMWH or warfarin is usually con-tinued for 6 weeks and is used more often: 50% of the mortality occurs at this time. Low-molecular-weight heparin is given to women with a previous or strong family history, a known prothrombotic tendency, and those who have had a Caesarean section and have three or more moderate risk factors (age >35 years, high parity, obesity, gross varicose veins, infection, pre-eclampsia, immobility or major current illness). Current thrombo-prophylactic practice is unfortunately less extensive than this.

Drug abuse in pregnancy

About 1 in 400 births occur to narcotic abusers; more use cocaine or 'crack'. Abuse is associated with infections including human immunodeficiency virus (HIV) and other sexually transmitted infections (STIs), preterm labour, IUGR and placental abruption ('crack' usage). Fetal narcotic dependence is usual. Many women use methadone, but 'top-ups' of heroin are still common. Acute opiate withdrawal in pregnancy can cause *in utero* death and methadone-only maintenance is appropriate. The patient is screened for STIs and monitored for signs of fetal compromise [→ p.199], particularly in labour, when meconium is common. Neonatal abstinence causes irritability and convulsions and is treated with phenobarbital. Subsequently the infant will need increased social care and is at increased risk of sudden infant death syndrome (SIDS).

Anaemias

The 40% increase in blood volume in pregnancy is relatively greater than the increase in red cell mass. The result is a net fall in haemoglobin concentration, such that 10.4 g/dL should be considered the lower limit of normal. More iron and folic acid are required in pregnancy because of the increase in red cell mass, uterine growth and fetal requirements and iron absorption increases (Fig. 21.8).

Iron deficiency anaemia

This affects 10% of pregnant women. Symptoms are usually absent unless the haemoglobin is <8 g/dL, and the fetus is unaffected unless severe anaemia is present. Folic acid deficiency may coexist. The blood film shows reduced mean cell volume and mean cell haemoglobin (Fig. 21.9). Ferritin levels are reduced. Treatment (*Cochrane* 2001: CD003094) is with oral iron, but this can cause gastrointestinal upset, when intramuscular iron can be used. Both methods can achieve an increase of 0.8 g/dL per week.

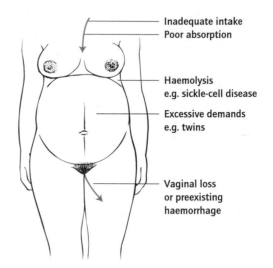

Fig. 21.8 Anaemia in pregnancy.

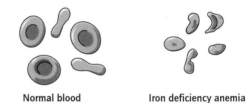

Fig. 21.9 Picture of blood film of iron deficiency anaemia.

Folic acid deficiency anaemia

This is rarer but often is missed. The mean cell volume is usually increased, neutrophils are hypersegmented and red cell folic acid is low. Folic acid deficiency should always be considered (measure red cell folic acid) if anaemia is present without marked microcytosis. Treatment is with oral folic acid.

Prophylaxis against anaemia

Routine iron supplements reduce the incidence of anaemia without affecting perinatal outcome (*Cochrane* 2000: CD001135). Postnatal blood transfusion may be required less frequently. However, iron is often poorly tolerated, particularly during the first trimester. Routine supplementation is not necessary: all women are given dietary advice, and the haemoglobin is checked at booking and again at 28 weeks. Iron is then given if the haemoglobin drops below 10.4 g/dL. Because routine preconceptual folic acid supplements (0.4 mg) reduce the incidence of NTDs, these are recommended to all women. In those with epilepsy or a previous history of a NTD, a higher dose (5 mg) is used.

Dietary advice to avoid anaemia	
Food rich in iron:	Meat, particularly kidney and liver, eggs, green vegetables
Food rich in folic acid:	Lightly cooked or raw green vegetables, fish

Haemoglobinopathies

The adult haemoglobin molecule (HbA) is made of two α chains and two β chains, bound together in a tetramer. Fetal haemoglobin (HbF), which is normally gradually replaced by the adult type after birth, is made of two α chains and two γ chains.

Sickle-cell disease

This recessive disorder is due to abnormal β-chain formation (called an S chain) in the haemoglobin molecule. The result is an abnormal haemoglobin molecule made of two α chains bound to two S chains. Sickle S is found in people of Afro-Caribbean origin, and of those in the United Kingdom, 10% are heterozygotes or 'carriers'. Haemoglobin electrophoresis is routinely performed in all pregnant women who are not of northern European origin. The partners of heterozygotes are also tested: if positive, prenatal diagnosis is offered [→ p.126].
Homozygotes have only HbS, and many have been affected with 'crises' and chronic haemolytic anaemia all their life. In pregnancy, maternal complications include more frequent crises (35%), pre-eclampsia, thrombosis and infections. Fetal complications are miscarriage, IUGR [→ p.169], preterm labour and death. Regular exchange blood transfusions, screening for infection and maintenance of hydration are needed. Folic acid supplements are given; iron is avoided because of overload.
Heterozygotes have 35% HbS and usually have no problems, but may develop 'crises' under extreme conditions.

Thalassaemias

Alpha thalassaemia results from impaired synthesis of the α chain in the haemoglobin molecule. It occurs largely in people of south-east Asian origin. Four genes are responsible for α chain synthesis. Individuals with four gene deletions die *in utero*. Heterozygous individuals have one or two gene deletions, are usually anaemic, and require folic acid and iron supplementation.
Beta thalassaemia results from impaired β-chain synthesis. It occurs largely in people of south-east Asian and Mediterranean origin. Homozygous individuals are usually affected by iron overload and pregnancy is unusual, but folic acid *without* oral iron is needed. Heterozygous women have a chronic anaemia, which can worsen during pregnancy.

Prenatal diagnosis using chorionic villus sampling (CVS) [→ p.126] by mutation analysis from polymerase chain reaction (PCR) -amplified deoxyribonucleic acid (DNA) must be offered if the partner is heterozygous for either the β or α form.

Further reading

Burrows RF. Haematological problems in pregnancy. *Current Opinion in Obstetrics & Gynecology* 2003; **15**: 85–90.

Cao A, Galanello R, Rosatelli MC. Prenatal diagnosis and screening of the haemoglobinopathies. *Bailliere's Clinical Haematology* 1998; **11**: 215–38.

Girling J. Thyroid disease in pregnancy. *Hospital Medicine (London, England: 1998)* 2000; **61**: 834–40.

Greer IA. Prevention of venous thromboembolism in pregnancy. *Best Practice & Research. Clinical Haematology* 2003; **16**: 261–78.

Holmes LB. The teratogenicity of anticonvulsant drugs: a progress report. *Journal of Medical Genetics* 2002; **39**: 251–9.

Kelly A, Nelson-Piercy C. Obstetric cholestasis. *The Obstetrician and Gynaecologist* 2000; **2**: 29–31.

Lupton M, Oteng-Ntim E, Ayida G, Steer PJ. Cardiac disease in pregnancy. *Current Opinion in Obstetrics & Gynecology* 2002; **14**: 137–43.

Regan L, Rai R. Thrombophilia and pregnancy loss. *Journal of Reproductive Immunology* 2002; **55**: 163–80.

Royal College of Obstetricians and Gynaecologists. Thromboembolic disease in pregnancy and the puerperium: acute management. Guideline 28: www.rcog.org.uk.

Sanders CL, Lucas MJ. Renal disease in pregnancy. *Obstetrics and Gynecology Clinics of North America* 2001; **28**: 593–600.

Tamas G, Kerenyi Z. Current controversies in the mechanisms and treatment of gestational diabetes. *Current Diabetes Reports* 2002; **2**: 337–46.

Woods J. Adverse consequences of prenatal illicit drug exposure. *Current Opinion in Obstetrics & Gynaecology* 1996; **8**: 403–11.

Diabetes in Pregnancy and Gestational Diabetes at a Glance

Definitions/ Epidemiology	Pre-existing diabetes: 0.1–0.3% Gestational diabetes: impaired glucose tolerance in pregnancy 2% of women
Aetiology	Gestational diabetes: worsening glucose tolerance in pregnancy in susceptible women Risk factors: family or previous history, polycystic ovary syndrome (PCOS), previous large baby/unexplained stillbirth, weight >100 kg, persistent glycosuria, polyhydramnios
Complications	Related to glucose control; rarer in gestational diabetes
	Fetal: Congenital abnormalities, preterm labour, birth trauma, fetal compromise, distress and sudden death
	Maternal: Increased insulin requirements, ketoacidosis/hypoglycaemia, worsening retinopathy, preeclampsia, infections, operative delivery
Management	Preconceptual glucose stabilization; patient education/involvement Increase insulin to achieve 'tight' control; reduce post-delivery Anomaly ultrasound, then close fetal surveillance Induction/lower segment Caesarean section (LSCS) by 39 weeks unless well-controlled gestational diabetes

Thrombophilia in Pregnancy at a Glance

Main types	Antiphospholipid syndrome, protein S deficiency, activated protein C resistance and Factor V Leyden, prothrombin gene variant, antithrombin III deficiency
Complications	Venous thromboembolism, miscarriage, preterm delivery, pre-eclampsia, placental abruption, intrauterine growth restriction (IUGR), fetal death
Management	Individualized: high-risk pregnancy care. Aspirin and low-molecular-weight heparin (LMWH) usually only if adverse previous obstetric history. Postnatal LMWH

Anaemia in Pregnancy at a Glance

Iron deficiency	10% of women. Mean cell volume (MCV), mean cell haemoglobin concentration (MCHC) and ferritin reduced Prophylaxis: disputed. Treat if haemoglobin (Hb) <10.4
Folic acid deficiency	Rarer, MCV often raised. Red cell folate reduced Prophylaxis: routine in early pregnancy and preconceptually High dose if epileptic or previous neural tube defect (NTD)
Sickle-cell disease	10% of Afro-Caribbeans in the United Kingdom carry gene Increased perinatal mortality, thrombosis, sickle crises Management: exchange transfusions, folic acid, avoid precipitating factors for crises. Avoid iron Test partner and offer prenatal diagnosis if carrier
Thalassaemias	Alpha: south-east Asian origin. Beta: Mediterranean origin as well Management: Give folic acid, avoid iron (Beta thalassaemia). May need transfusions Test partner and offer prenatal diagnosis if carrier

22 Red Blood Cell Isoimmunization

Definition

Red blood cell isoimmunization occurs when the mother mounts an immune response against antigens on fetal red cells that enter her circulation. The resulting antibodies then cross the placenta and cause fetal red blood cell destruction.

Pathophysiology

Blood is classified according to its ABO and rhesus genotype. The rhesus system consists of three linked gene pairs; one allele of each pair is dominant to the other: *C*/*c*, *D*/*d* and *E*/*e*. An individual inherits one allele of each pair from each parent in a mendelian fashion. The most significant in isoimmunization is the *D* gene. As *D* is dominant to *d*, only individuals who are *DD* or *Dd* (i.e. homozygous or heterozygous) express the D antigen and are 'D rhesus positive' (Fig. 22.1). Individuals homozygous for the recessive *d* (*dd*) are 'D rhesus negative', and their immune system will recognize the D antigen as foreign if they are exposed to it.

Small amounts of fetal blood cross the placenta and enter the maternal circulation during uncomplicated pregnancies and particularly at sensitizing events such as delivery, placental abruption and amniocentesis [→ p.125]. If the fetus is 'D rhesus positive' and the mother is 'D rhesus negative', the mother will mount an immune response (sensitization), creating anti-D antibodies. Immunity is permanent, and if the mother's immune system is again exposed to the antigen, large numbers of antibodies are rapidly created. They can cross the placenta and bind to fetal red blood cells, which are then destroyed in the fetal reticuloendothelial system (Fig. 22.2). This can cause haemolytic anaemia and ultimately death, and is called rhesus haemolytic disease. A similar immune response can be mounted against other red blood cell antigens (e.g. after blood transfusion): the most important antibodies are anti-c and anti-Kell (a non-rhesus antibody).

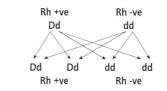

Fig. 22.1 Mendelian inheritance of *D*/*d* gene pair.

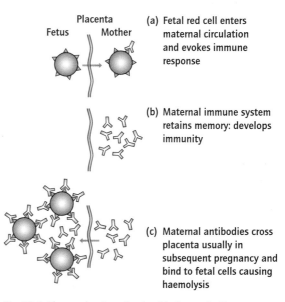

Fig. 22.2 The mechanism of red cell isoimmunization.

Prevention: using anti-D

Production of maternal anti-D can be prevented by the administration of exogenous anti-D to the mother. This 'mops up' fetal red cells that have crossed the placenta, by binding to their antigens, thereby preventing recognition by the mother's immune system. Anti-D (500 iµ) should be given to all women who are rhesus negative at 28 and 34 weeks (*Cochrane* 2000: CD000020): this alone will reduce the rate of isoimmunization in a first pregnancy from 1.5% to 0.2%. Anti-D is also given within 72 h of any sensitizing event, although some benefit is gained within 9 days, and if the neonate is found to be rhesus positive after delivery. It is unnecessary if the neonate is rhesus negative; its status is therefore routinely checked at birth. It is also pointless if maternal anti-D is already present, as sensitization has already occurred.

Prevention of rhesus disease	
Booking and 34 weeks:	Check all women for antibodies
Rhesus-negative women:	Give anti-D at 28 and 34 weeks, after any bleeding or potentially sensitizing event, and after delivery if neonate is rhesus positive

Epidemiology

Fifteen per cent of Caucasian women, but fewer African or Asian women, are D rhesus negative. In the absence of prophylaxis, many will develop anti-D antibodies. The use of anti-D, smaller family size, and good management of isoimmunization has resulted in perinatal deaths attributable to rhesus disease being extremely rare. Currently only 1.7% of D rhesus-negative women have been sensitized.

Aetiology of isoimmunization

Anti-D: Although now rare, D rhesus isoimmunization still occurs because of omitted and inadequate doses of prophylactic anti-D. If both parents are known to be D rhesus negative, the fetus must be rhesus negative also and therefore will be unaffected.

Other antibodies: Anti-c, anti-E and anti-Kell have assumed greater relative importance, largely because of the decline in anti-D rhesus disease. Many other rare antibodies can cause mild fetal anaemia and postnatal jaundice.

Manifestations of rhesus disease

As antibody levels rise in a sensitized woman, the antibodies will cross the placenta and cause haemolysis, but only if the fetus is rhesus positive. In mild disease, this may lead to *neonatal jaundice* only. Or there may be sufficient haemolysis to cause neonatal anaemia (haemolytic disease of the newborn). More severe disease causes *in utero* anaemia and, as this worsens, cardiac failure, ascites and oedema (hydrops) and fetal death follow. Rhesus disease generally worsens with successive pregnancies as maternal antibody production increases.

Management of isoimmunization

The management of rhesus isoimmunization varies widely but comprises: (i) identification of women at risk of fetal haemolysis and anaemia; (ii) assessing if/how severely the fetus is anaemic; and (iii) blood transfusion *in utero* or delivery for affected fetuses.

Identification

Unsensitized women are screened for antibodies at booking and again at 34 weeks gestation. If anti-D levels are <10 IU/mL, a significant fetal problem is very unlikely and levels are subsequently checked every 2 weeks. Higher levels warrant further investigation. Amniocentesis, and more recently maternal blood sampling for fetal cells (*Prenat Diagn* 2001; **21**: 321), is sometimes used where the father is a heterozygote. Anti-Kell antibody levels are less predictive of disease severity.

Assessing severity of fetal anaemia

Pregnancies at risk of fetal anaemia are assessed using ultrasound. Only severe anemia (e.g. <5 g/dL) is detectable as fetal hydrops or excessive fetal fluid. Doppler ultrasound of the peak velocity in systole (PSV) of the fetal middle cerebral artery (MCA) (Fig. 22.3) has a high sensitivity for significant anaemia (*NEJM* 2000; **342**: 9), at least before 36 weeks. It is therefore used at least fortnightly in at-risk pregnancies.

If anaemia is suspected from this, fetal blood sampling is performed under ultrasound guidance, using a needle

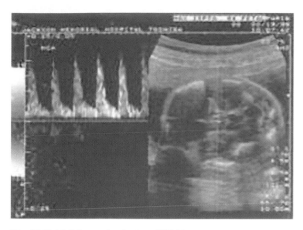

Fig. 22.3 Middle cerebral artery (MCA).

in the umbilical vein. The risk of fetal loss is 1%, and after 28 weeks it should be performed with facilities for immediate delivery if complications arise.

Blood transfusion

Fetal blood sampling is performed with rhesus negative high-haematocrit blood ready, which can be injected down the needle into the umbilical vein if anaemia is found. This process of quantification of anaemia and transfusion will need to be repeated at increasing intervals until about 36 weeks, after which time delivery is undertaken. Blood is more easily administered to the neonate: both top-up (for anaemia) and exchange (for hyperbilirubinaemia) transfusions may be required.

Postnatally, all neonates born to rhesus-negative women should have a full blood count (FBC), blood film, bilirubin and indirect Coombs' test: these detect lesser degrees of isoimmunization.

Further reading

Crowther CA, Keirse MJ. Anti-D administration in pregnancy for preventing rhesus alloimmunisation. *Cochrane Database System Review (Online: Update Software)* 2000; **2**: CD000020.

Moise K. Management of rhesus alloimmunisation in pregnancy. *Obstetrics and Gynecology* 2002; **100**: 600–11

Rhesus Isoimmunization at a Glance		
Definition	Maternal antibody response against fetal red cell antigen entering her circulation; passage of antibodies into fetus leads to haemolysis	
Aetiology	Anti-D still prevalent because of inadequate/failed prophylaxis Other major antibodies: anti-c and anti-Kell	
Epidemiology	15% of Caucasian women are rhesus negative; anti-D responses in 1.7%	
Pathology	Haemolysis causes anaemia. Neonatal jaundice ± anaemia if less severe; hydrops and fetal death if severe	
Prevention	Administer anti-D to rhesus-negative women at 28 and 34 weeks, and after potentially sensitizing events	
Management	Identification:	Antibody testing and past obstetric history
	Assess severity:	Doppler of fetal middle cerebral artery (MCA); fetal blood sampling to confirm
	Treat:	Transfuse if fetus anaemic, deliver if >36 weeks
	Postnatally:	Check full blood count (FBC), bilirubin, rhesus group, Coombs' test

23 Preterm Delivery and its Management

Definition

A preterm delivery is when preterm labour results in delivery between 24 and 37 weeks gestation. Before 24 weeks, labour is tantamount to a miscarriage, although exceptionally fetal survival occurs at 23 weeks.

Epidemiology

Some 8% of deliveries are preterm. A further 6% of deliveries present preterm with contractions but deliver at term. Prematurity accounts for 80% of neonatal intensive care occupancy and 20% of perinatal mortality. Long-term morbidity, including cerebral palsy, lung disease and blindness is common (Fig. 23.1). Fetuses delivered before 28 weeks are most affected. Preterm labour is more common in intravenous drug abusers, in women from poorer backgrounds, in Afro-Caribbean women, and in those with a previous preterm birth, medical disorders or sexually transmitted infections (STIs) [→p.135].

Aetiology (Fig. 23.2)

Genital tract infection, usually subclinical, is implicated in about 60%. The organisms are seldom isolated, but bacterial vaginosis [→ p.135] and urinary tract infections (UTIs) are associated. The mechanism is poorly understood. *Cervical incompetence* presents with painless cervical dilatation or preterm rupture of the membranes. It is often associated with previous cervical trauma but may coexist with infection because the latter causes softening and shortening of the cervix, and may cross intact membranes. *Fetal compromise* and severe pre-eclampsia can also lead to preterm delivery, either spontaneous, as a 'fetal survival response', or *iatrogenic*. *Multiple pregnancy* is increasing, due to assisted conception, and 40% deliver preterm. *Other causes* include diabetes, antepartum haemorrhage, polyhydramnios [→ p.131] and uterine anomalies such as congenital defects or fibroids. Many cases, however, remain *idiopathic*.

Prediction of preterm labour

Besides the above risk factors, investigations may predict preterm delivery. The *cervical length* on transvaginal sonography (TVS) (Fig 23.3) is sensitive and specific: at 23 weeks, a cervical length of <15 mm on TVS at 23

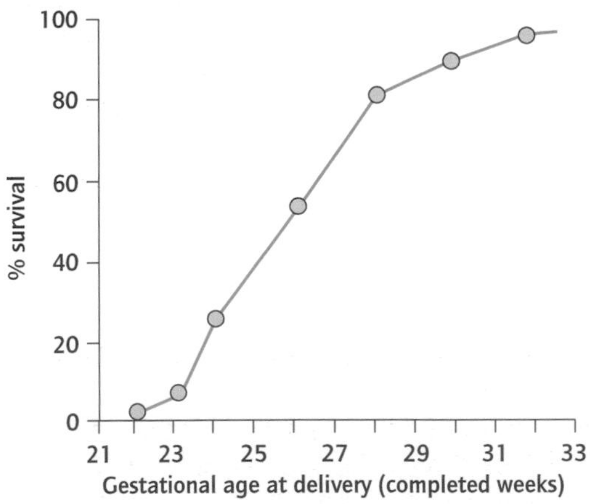

Fig. 23.1 Survival of preterm infants.

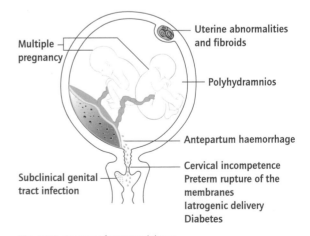

Fig. 23.2 Causes of preterm labour.

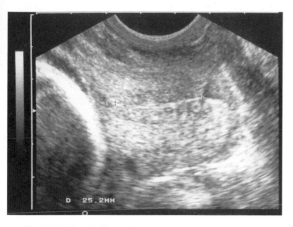

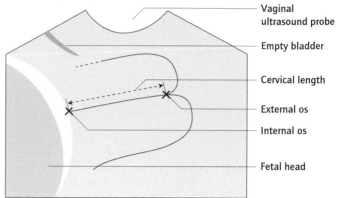

Vaginal
ultrasound probe

Empty bladder

Cervical length

External os

Internal os

Fetal head

Fig. 23.3 Cervical length.

weeks predicts 85% of spontaneous deliveries before 28 weeks (*Ultrasound Obstet Gynecol* 1998; **12**: 312), with a false positive rate of 1.5%. Cervical length may also be used to determine which women with preterm contractions are likely to labour. The latter may also be determined by *fetal fibronectin assay* (collected vaginally and assayed at the bedside), although with a poor specificity (*BMJ* 2002; **325**: 301).

Prevention of preterm labour

Screening and treatment of *UTIs* and *bacterial vaginosis* (*Lancet* 2003; **361**: 983) reduces the incidence of preterm labour. Bedrest and prolonged oral tocolysis do not prevent preterm delivery. The role of cervical cerclage is unclear (*Cochrane* 2003: CD003253). Cerclage, with a non-absorbable suture (Fig. 23.4), is often inserted at 12–14 weeks in women have had painless preterm deliveries; regular cervical scanning and use of the suture in women with a shortening cervix is an acceptable alternative (*Ultrasound Obstet Gynecol* 2002; **19**: 475). Although sutures are normally inserted vaginally, the abdominal route can be used if the cervix is very short or scarred. Although cervical length is predictive of preterm delivery, it is unclear if the universal use of cervical length ultrasound could help prevent preterm birth.

Risk factors for preterm labour
Previous history
Urinary and subclinical genital tract infection
Multiple pregnancy
Diabetes, polyhydramnios
Uterine abnormalities
Short cervix on transvaginal sonography (TVS)

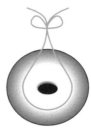

Fig. 23.4 Cervical suture. Transverse section of the cervix.

Clinical features

History: Women without cervical incompetence usually present with painful contractions. Antepartum haemorrhage or a dull suprapubic pain may also occur. The passage of fluid suggests ruptured membranes.

Examination: Fever is uncommon. The lie and presentation of the fetus are checked with abdominal palpation (Fig. 23.5). Digital vaginal examination is performed unless the membranes have ruptured. An effaced or dilating cervix confirms that labour is ensuing, but an uneffaced cervix does not mean that the patient will not labour preterm: the course of preterm labour is unpredictable and may be extremely rapid or very slow.

Investigations

To assess fetal state, cardiotocography (CTG) and ultrasound are used.

To assess the likelihood of delivery if the cervix is uneffaced, fetal fibronectin assay is helpful (*BMJ* 2002; **325**: 301), in that a negative result means preterm delivery is unlikely. Assessment of cervical length using ultrasound is also predictive.

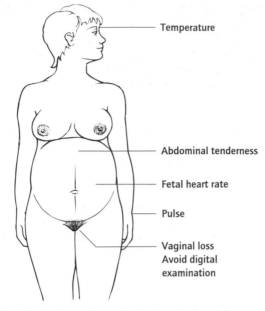

Temperature

Abdominal tenderness

Fetal heart rate

Pulse

Vaginal loss
Avoid digital
examination

Fig. 23.5 Monitoring the patient with preterm prelabour rupture of the membranes.

To look for bacteria, vaginal swabs should be taken, using a sterile speculum if the membranes have ruptured. The C-reactive protein (CRP) usually rises with chorioamnionitis; white cell count estimation is often unhelpful because steroids may cause it to rise.

Management
Promoting pulmonary maturity
Steroids are given between 24 and 34 weeks. These reduce perinatal morbidity and mortality by promoting pulmonary maturity (*Cochrane* 2000: CD000065) They do not increase the risk of infection, but careful glucose control is needed in diabetic patients. As they take 24 h to act, delivery is often artificially delayed using tocolysis.
Tocolysis: Nifedipine or atosiban, an oxytocin-receptor antagonist, can be given to allow steroids time to act or to allow *in utero* transfer to a unit with neonatal intensive care facilities. These delay rather than stop preterm labour and should not be used for more than 24 h. Ritodrine or salbutamol and non-steroidal anti-inflammatory drugs (NSAIDs) also delay delivery but are seldom used because of side effects.

Detection and prevention of infection
The presence of infection risks maternal health and con-

siderably worsens the outlook for the neonate (*Lancet* 1995; **346**: 1449). This may occur even where the membranes have not ruptured: chorioamnionitis warrants intravenous antibiotics and immediate delivery, whatever the gestation.

Delivery
Mode of delivery: Vaginal delivery reduces the incidence of respiratory distress syndrome in the neonate and Caesarean section is undertaken only for the usual obstetric indications. Breech presentation [→ p.177] is more common in preterm labour: at term, elective Caesarean section is safer for breech babies. This has meant a loss of operator skills, and although the evidence in preterm labour is lacking, most preterm breeches in labour now undergo Caesarean section.

Conduct of delivery: Paediatric facilities are mobilized. The membranes are not ruptured in labour, at least up to 32 weeks: labour may be slow, allowing steroids more time to act, and the membranes might cushion the delicate preterm fetus against trauma. Forceps are used only for the usual obstetric indications, and the ventouse is contraindicated.

Antibiotics for delivery are recommended, because of the increased risk and morbidity of Group B streptococcus [→ p.134].

Preterm prelabour rupture of the membranes

Definition

The membranes rupture before labour at <37 weeks. Often the cause is unknown, but all the causes of preterm labour may be implicated. It occurs in one-third of preterm deliveries.

Complications

Preterm delivery is the principal complication and follows within 48 h in >50% of cases. *Infection* is also common, resulting in chorioamnionitis. This may occur before, and therefore be the cause of the membranes rupture, or it may be ascending. *Prolapse of the umbilical cord* may occur rarely. Absence of liquor (usually before

24 weeks) can result in *pulmonary hypoplasia* and postural deformities.

Clinical features

History: A gush of clear fluid is normal, followed by further leaking.

Examination: The lie and presentation are checked. A pool of fluid is visible in the posterior fornix on speculum examination. Digital examination is best avoided, although it is performed to exclude cord prolapse if the presentation is not cephalic. Chorioamnionitis is characterized by a fever, tachycardia, uterine tenderness and coloured or offensive liquor, although clinical signs appear late.

Investigations

To confirm the diagnosis in doubtful cases, commercially available tests are available. Ultrasound may reveal reduced liquor, but the volume can also be normal as fetal urine production continues.

To look for infection, a high vaginal swab (HVS), full blood count (FBC) and CRP are taken. In doubtful cases, amniocentesis [→ p.125] with Gram staining and culture is occasionally used.

Fetal well being is assessed by CTG. A persistent fetal tachycardia is suggestive of infection.

Management
Principles
The risk of preterm delivery must be balanced against the risk of infection, which, if present, greatly increases neonatal mortality and long-term morbidity. Prevention, identification and treatment of this are therefore essential. The woman is admitted and given steroids. Close maternal (signs of infection) and fetal surveillance is performed, and if the gestation reaches 36 weeks, induction is normally performed.

Prevention of infection
The prophylactic use of erythromycin in women even without clinical evidence of infection is recommended (*Cochrane* 2003: CD001058). Co-amoxiclav is contraindicated.

Identification and management of infection
Early chorioamnionitis produces few signs. If signs of infection appear, intravenous antibiotics are given immediately and the fetus is delivered whatever the gestation.

Further reading

Odibo AO, Elkousy M, Ural SH, Macones GA. Prevention of preterm birth by cervical cerclage compared with expectant management: a systematic review. *Obstetrical & Gynecological Survey* 2003; **58**: 130–6.

Slattery MM, Morrison JJ. Preterm delivery. *Lancet* 2002; **360**: 1489–97.

Spong CY. Recent developments in preventing recurrent preterm birth. *Obstetrics and Gynecology* 2003; **101**: 1153–4.

Welsh A, Nicolaides K. Cervical screening for preterm delivery. *Current Opinion in Obstetrics & Gynecology* 2002; **14**: 195–202.

Preterm Delivery at a Glance

Epidemiology	8% of deliveries, 20% of perinatal mortality
Aetiology	Subclinical infection, cervical incompetence, iatrogenic, multiple pregnancy, antepartum haemorrhage, diabetes, polyhydramnios, fetal compromise, uterine abnormalities, idiopathic
Prediction	Ultrasound (transvaginal ultrasound, TVS) of cervical length at 23 weeks
Prevention	Antibiotics if bacterial vaginosis or urinary tract infection (UTI); cervical suture if cervical incompetence likely: either at 12 weeks or if cervix shortens
Features	Abdominal pains, antepartum haemorrhage, ruptured membranes
Investigations	High vaginal swab (HVS), cardiotocography (CTG), ultrasound
Management	Steroids if <34 weeks, tocolysis for max. 24 h Antibiotics in labour Caesarean for normal indications Inform neonatologists

24 Antepartum Haemorrhage

Definition

Antepartum haemorrhage (APH) is bleeding from the genital tract after 24 weeks gestation. This is the time at which neonatal survival is better than anecdotal.

Causes of antepartum haemorrhage (APH)	
Common:	Undetermined origin
	Placental abruption
	Placenta praevia
Rarer:	Incidental genital tract pathology
	Uterine rupture
	Vasa praevia
	Placenta praevia

Placenta praevia

Definitions and epidemiology

Placenta praevia occurs when the placenta is implanted in the lower segment of the uterus. It complicates 0.4% of pregnancies at term. At early ultrasound scan the placenta is 'low-lying' in many more pregnancies, but appears to 'move' upwards as the pregnancy continues. This is because of the formation of the lower segment of the uterus in the third trimester: it is the myometrium where the placenta implants that moves away from the internal cervical os. Therefore, only 1 in 10 apparently low-lying placentas will be praevia at term.

Classification

Placenta praevia is classified according to the proximity

Classification of placenta praevia	
Marginal (previously types I–II):	Placenta in lower segment, not over os (Fig. 24.1a)
Major (previously types III–IV):	Placenta completely or partially covering os (Fig. 24.1b)

of the placenta to the internal os of the cervix. It may be predominantly on the anterior or posterior uterine wall.

Aetiology

This is unknown, but placenta praevia is slightly more common with twins, in women of high parity and age, and if the uterus is scarred (e.g. previous Caesarean) (*J Matern Fetal Neonatal Med* 2003; **13**: 175).

Complications

The placenta in the lower segment obstructs engagement of the head: except for some marginal praevias, this necessitates *Caesarean section* and may also cause the lie to be *transverse*. *Haemorrhage* can be severe and may continue after delivery as the lower segment is less able to contract and constrict the maternal blood supply. If a placenta implants in a previous Caesarean section scar, it may be so deep as to prevent separation (placenta accreta). This is often only adequately treated by *hysterectomy*.

Clinical features

History: Typically, there are intermittent painless APHs, which increase in frequency and intensity over several weeks. Such bleeding may be catastrophic. One third

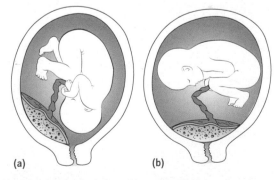

Fig. 24.1 (a) Marginal placenta praevia. (b) Major placenta praevia (abnormal lie and malpresentation are common).

of women, however, have not experienced bleeding before the diagnosis is made.

Examination: Breech presentation and transverse lie are common. An engaged head excludes the possibility of major placenta praevia. Vaginal examination can provoke massive bleeding and is *never* performed in a woman who is bleeding vaginally unless placenta praevia has been excluded.

Presentation of placenta praevia
Incidental finding on ultrasound scan
Vaginal bleeding
Abnormal lie, breech presentation

Investigations

To make the diagnosis, ultrasound is used (Fig. 24.2). If a low-lying placenta has been diagnosed at a second trimester ultrasound, this is usually repeated at 32 weeks to exclude placenta praevia. Lower segment growth is such that the marginal placenta praevia may still 'move' up until 36 weeks: the ultrasound should be repeated at this time in such women.

To assess fetal and maternal well being, cardiotocography (CTG), a full blood count (FBC), clotting studies and cross-match are needed. Fetal distress [→ p.169] is uncommon.

Management
Admission
This is necessary for all women with APH. If placenta praevia is then found on ultrasound, such women normally stay in hospital until delivery because of the danger of massive haemorrhage. Blood is kept available; anti-D is administered to rhesus-negative women; intravenous access is maintained; steroids [→ p.160] are administered if the gestation is <34 weeks. In women with asymptomatic placenta praevia, admission can be delayed until 37 weeks, provided they can get to hospital easily.

Delivery
This is by elective Caesarean section at 39 weeks by the most senior person available. Blood loss may be great during delivery; postpartum haemorrhage is also common because the lower segment does not contract well after delivery. Earlier, emergency delivery is needed if bleeding is severe before this time. However, pregnancy can often be prolonged with observation and, if necessary, blood transfusion. Only if the degree of praevia is marginal and the fetal head is past the lower edge (on ultrasound), can vaginal delivery be contemplated. In exceptional, doubtful cases, vaginal examination is performed in theatre with full facilities for an immediate Caesarean.

Massive haemorrhage
This requires maternal resuscitation and immediate delivery.

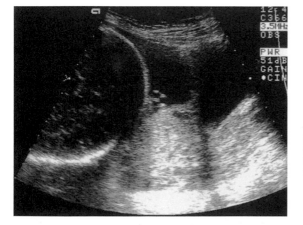 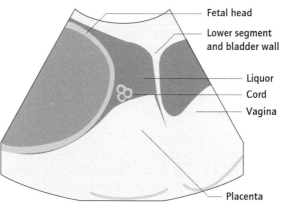

Fig. 24.2 Ultrasound of placenta praevia and labelled drawing.

Differentiation between placental abruption and placenta praevia		
	Abruption	Placenta praevia
Shock	Inconsistent with external loss	Consistent with external loss
Pain	Common, often severe Constant with exacerbations	No. Contractions occasionally
Bleeding	May be absent Often dark	Red and often profuse Often smaller previous antepartum haemorrhage (APHs)
Tenderness	Usual, often severe Uterus may be hard	Rare
Fetus	Lie normal, often engaged May be dead or distressed	Lie often abnormal/head high Heart rate usually normal
Ultrasound	Often normal, placenta not low	Placenta low

Placental abruption

Definition

Placenta abruption is when part (or all) of the placenta separates before delivery of the fetus. It occurs in 1% of pregnancies. However, it is likely that many APHs of undetermined origin are in fact small placental abruptions and that this figure is therefore higher.

Pathology

When part of the placenta separates, considerable maternal bleeding may occur behind it. This can have several consequences. Further placental separation and acute fetal distress may follow. Blood usually also tracks down between the membranes and the myometrium to be revealed as APH. It may also enter the liquor. Or it may simply enter the myometrium: visible haemorrhage is absent in 20% (Fig. 24.3).

Complications

Fetal death is common (30% of proven abruptions). Haemorrhage often necessitates blood transfusion; disseminated intravascular coagulation (DIC) and renal failure may rarely lead to maternal death.

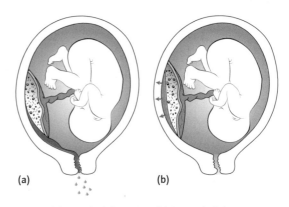

(a)   (b)

Fig. 24.3 (a) Revealed abruption. (b) Concealed abruption.

Aetiology

Many affected women have no risk factors. However, intrauterine growth restriction (IUGR), pre-eclampsia, autoimmune disease, maternal smoking, cocaine usage, a previous history of placental abruption (risk 6%), multiple pregnancy and high maternal parity all predispose to abruption. It has also been occasionally associated with trauma or a sudden reduction in uterine volume (e.g. rupture of the membranes in a woman with polyhydramnios).

Major risk factors for placental abruption
Intrauterine growth restriction (IUGR) Pre-eclampsia Pre-existing hypertension Maternal smoking Previous abruption

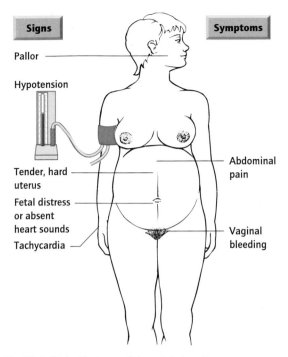

Signs | Symptoms

Pallor

Hypotension

Tender, hard uterus

Fetal distress or absent heart sounds

Tachycardia

Abdominal pain

Vaginal bleeding

Fig. 24.4 Clinical features of placental abruption.

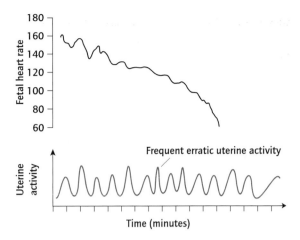

Fig. 24.5 Terminal fetal heart bradycardia with placental abruption.

Clinical features (Fig. 24.4)

History: Classically, there is painful APH. The pain is due to blood behind the placenta and in the myometrium, and is usually constant with exacerbations; the blood is often dark. The degree of vaginal bleeding does not reflect the severity of the abruption because some may not escape from the uterus. Indeed, pain or bleeding may occur alone. If pain occurs alone, the abruption is 'concealed'. If vaginal bleeding is evident, it is 're-vealed'.

Examination: Tachycardia suggests profound blood loss, which may be out of proportion to the vaginal loss because of 'concealed' loss. Hypotension only occurs after massive blood loss. The uterus is tender and often contracting: labour usually ensues. In severe cases, the uterus is 'woody' hard and the fetus is very difficult to feel. Fetal heart tones are often abnormal or even absent. If coagulation failure has occurred, widespread bleeding is evident.

Investigations

The diagnosis is usually made on clinical grounds. Investigations help to establish the severity of the abruption, to plan appropriate resuscitation, and whether and how to deliver the fetus.

To establish fetal well being, CTG [→ p.173] is performed. In addition to fetal distress, frequent uterine activity may be evident on the tocograph (Fig. 24.5).

To establish maternal well being, full blood count (FBC), coagulation screen and cross-match are performed. Catheterization with hourly urine output, central venous pressure (CVP) monitoring, regular FBC, coagulation, and urea and creatinine estimations are required in severe cases. Ultrasound has little place in the diagnosis of placental abruption, except to exclude placenta praevia.

Features of major placental abruption
Maternal collapse
Coagulopathy
Fetal distress or demise
'Woody' hard uterus
Poor urine output or renal failure
N.B. Degree of vaginal loss is often unhelpful

Management
Assessment and resuscitation
Admission is required, even without vaginal bleeding if there is pain and uterine tenderness. Intravenous fluid is

given, with steroids if the gestation is <34 weeks. Blood transfusion must not be delayed. Opiate analgesia is used; anti-D is given to rhesus-negative women.

Delivery

This depends on the fetal state and gestation. The mother must be stabilized first.

If there is fetal distress, urgent delivery by Caesarean section is required.

If there is no fetal distress, but the gestation is 37 weeks or more, induction of labour with amniotomy is performed. The fetal heart is monitored continuously, maternal condition is closely observed and Caesarean section is performed if fetal distress ensues.

If the fetus is dead, coagulopathy is also likely. Blood products are given and labour is induced.

Conservative management

If there is no fetal distress, the pregnancy is preterm and the degree of abruption appears to be minor, steroids are given (if <34 weeks) and the patient is closely monitored on the antenatal ward. If all symptoms settle, she may be discharged after 3–5 days, but the pregnancy is now 'high risk': ultrasound scans for fetal growth are arranged.

Postpartum management

Whatever the mode of delivery, postpartum haemorrhage [→ p.225] is a major risk.

Principles of management of major placental abruption
Fetal condition: cardiotocography (CTG)
Maternal condition: fluid balance, renal function, full blood count (FBC) and clotting. Central venous pressure (CVP) if appropriate
Early delivery
Blood ± blood-products transfusion

Other causes of antepartum haemorrhage (APH)

Bleeding of undetermined origin

When APH is small and painless but the placenta is not praevia, it may be difficult to find a cause. Ultrasound is of little diagnostic use. Many episodes are likely to be minor degrees of placental abruption: there is no such thing as a 'heavy show' (a show is the occasionally slightly blood-stained mucus plug that usually drops from the cervix around the time that labour begins). This, and indeed the 'recurrent show', are likely to be minor abruptions, and patients should be managed as such.

Ruptured vasa praevia

This is rupture of a blood vessel from a velamentous cord insertion (running in the membranes) in front of the presenting part (Fig. 24.6a). When the membranes rupture, fetal bleeding and rapid exsanguination occurs. It occurs in about 1 in 5000 pregnancies. The typical presentation is painless, moderate vaginal bleeding at amniotomy or spontaneous rupture of the membranes, which is accompanied by severe fetal distress. Caesarean section is seldom fast enough to save the fetus.

Uterine rupture [→ p.222]

This condition (Fig. 24.6b) very occasionally occurs before labour in women with a scarred or congenitally abnormal uterus.

Bleeding of gynaecological origin

Cervical carcinoma can present in pregnancy (Fig. 24.6c). If a cervical smear is overdue, the woman with small recurrent or postcoital haemorrhage should undergo speculum examination and colposcopy. Cervical

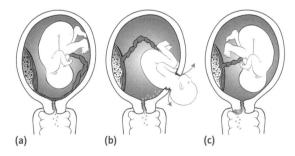

Fig. 24.6 Other causes of antepartum haemorrhage (APH). (a) Vasa praevia. (b) Ruptured uterus (intra-abdominal loss usually predominates). (c) Cervical carcinoma.

polyps, ectropions and vaginal lacerations may also be evident.

Further reading

Hladky K, Yankowitz J, Hansen WF. Placental abruption. *Obstetrical & Gynecological Survey* 2002; **57**: 299–305.

Kayani SI, Walkinshaw SA, Preston C. Pregnancy out-come in severe placental abruption. *BJOG: an International Journal of Obstetrics and Gynaecology* 2003; **110**: 679–83.

Neilson JP. Interventions for suspected placenta praevia. *Cochrane Database System Review (Online: Update Software)* 2003; **2**: CD001998.

Placenta Praevia at a Glance		
Definition	Placenta implanted in uterine lower segment 'Low-lying' refers to placental site before lower segment formation	
Types	Marginal praevia:	Near/adjacent to cervical os
	Major praevia:	Over/partly covering cervical os
Epidemiology	0.4% of pregnancies. Low-lying placenta in early pregnancy 5%	
Aetiology	Usually idiopathic. Large placenta, scarred uterus, high parity/age	
Complications	Haemorrhage. Need for preterm or Caesarean delivery	
Features	Painless antepartum haemorrhage (APH), often multiple and increasing in frequency and severity Also abnormal lie, incidental ultrasound finding	
Investigations	Ultrasound to locate the placenta. Full blood count (FBC) and cross-match if bleeding	
Management	If low-lying placenta on early ultrasound, repeat at 32 weeks	
	Asymptomatic:	Admission at 37 weeks
	Bleeding:	Admit whatever gestation. Have blood ready. Steroids if <34 weeks. Blood transfusion if necessary
	Delivery:	Caesarean at 39 weeks; before if bleeding heavy

Placental Abruption at a Glance

Definition	Separation of part/all of placenta before delivery; after 24 weeks
Epidemiology	1% of pregnancies
Aetiology	Idiopathic; common associations: intrauterine growth restriction (IUGR), pre-eclampsia, autoimmune disease, smoking, previous abruption
Complications	Fetal death, massive haemorrhage causing disseminated intravascular coagulation (DIC), renal failure, maternal death. Postpartum haemorrhage
Features	Painful antepartum haemorrhage (APH), but pain or bleeding can be in isolation. Uterine tenderness and contractions: if major, absent fetal heart, 'woody' uterus, maternal collapse, coagulopathy
Investigations	Cardiotocography (CTG) to assess fetus. Full blood count (FBC), clotting to assess maternal state Ultrasound scan excludes placenta praevia if diagnosis in doubt If severe, intensive maternal monitoring (central venous pressure, CVP, urine output, etc.)

Management		
	Admit:	If severe, resuscitate with blood
	Fetal distress present:	Deliver by Caesarean section
	Fetal distress absent:	>37 weeks, induce labour
	Fetus dead:	Induce labour. Coagulopathy likely
	Minor preterm abruption:	Wait. Serial ultrasound scans

25 Fetal Growth, Compromise and Surveillance

The aim of pregnancy care of the fetus is to prevent bad outcomes: particularly death or poor health. Pursuit of this aim must take account maternal health, of resources, and the fact that most pregnancies are normal. Poor health encompasses cerebral palsy particularly, but also the need for neonatal care or resuscitation. Furthermore, there is growing evidence that *in utero* health and growth influences health, particularly cardiac disease, in later life. The principal causes of perinatal mortality and cerebral palsy are outlined in in the boxes below.

Principal causes of perinatal mortality

Unexplained
Intrauterine growth restriction (IUGR)
Prematurity
Congenital abnormalities
Intrapartum fetal distress
Placental abruption

Principal associations of cerebral palsy

Major:	Prematurity (see Chapter 23)
	Intrauterine growth restriction (IUGR)
	Infection
	Pre-eclampsia (see Chapter 20)
	Congenital abnormalities (see Chapter 18)
	Intrapartum 'fetal distress' (see Chapter 29)
	Postnatal events
Other:	Autoimmune disease (see Chapter 21)
	Multiple pregnancy (see Chapter 27)
	Placental abruption (see Chapter 24)

Terminology

Because there are so many associations of adverse neonatal outcomes, and because their mechanisms of action are poorly understood, our use of terms such as compromise and fetal distress is simplistic.

Fetal compromise is a chronic situation and should be defined as when conditions for the normal growth and neurological development are not optimal. Most identifiable causes involve poor nutrient transfer through the placenta, often called 'placental dysfunction'. Commonly there is intra-uterine growth restriction, but this may also be absent (e.g. maternal diabetes or prolonged pregnancy).

Small for dates (gestational age) means that the weight of the fetus is less than the tenth centile for its gestation (if at term: 2.7 kg). Other cut-off points (e.g. third centile) can also be used. Traditionally, small size was felt to reflect chronic compromise due to placental dysfunction. However, most fetuses are simply constitutionally small, have grown consistently (Fig. 25.1) and are not compromised. Assessment of fetal weight is better at identifying IUGR if customized (www.preg.info) according to that would be expected for the individual [→ p.170] rather than the overall population.

Intrauterine growth restriction (IUGR) describes fetuses that have failed to reach their own 'growth potential'. Their growth *in utero* is slowed: many end up 'small for dates' (SFD), but some do not: many stillbirths or fetuses distressed in labour are of apparently 'normal' weight. If a fetus was genetically determined to be 4 kg at term and delivers at term weighing 3 kg, its growth has been restricted, and it may have placental dysfunction (Fig. 25.2). Similarly, an ill, malnourished tall adult may weigh more than a healthy shorter one.

Fetal distress refers to an acute situation, as hypoxia that may result in fetal damage or death if it is not reversed, or if the fetus delivered urgently. As such it is usually used in labour (see Chapter 29). Nevertheless, most babies that subsequently develop cerebral palsy were not born hypoxic.

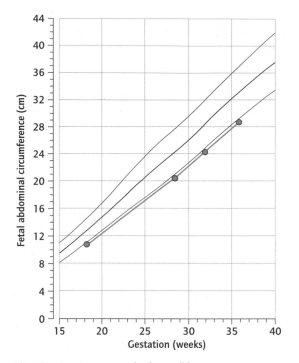

Fig. 25.1 Consistent growth of a small fetus.

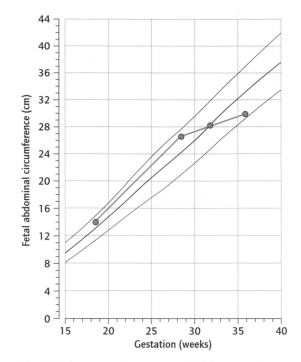

Fig. 25.2 Slowed growth suggestive of fetal compromise.

Fetal growth

Constitutional determinants: Low maternal height, weight, parity, non-Caucasian ethnic group and female fetal gender can lead to small for dates but do not themselves cause IUGR.

Pathological determinants of fetal growth include pre-existing maternal disease (e.g. renal disease and autoimmune disease), maternal pregnancy complications (e.g. pre-eclampsia) [→ p.137], smoking, drug usage and congenital abnormalities. These may cause IUGR.

If adjustment is made for constitutional determinants, a large proportion (up to 70%) of so-called unexplained antepartum stillbirths are growth restricted. Fetal growth assessment is therefore a key element of fetal surveillance.

Fetal surveillance

Aims of fetal surveillance

1 Identify the 'high-risk' pregnancy using history or events during pregnancy, or using specific investigations.
2 Monitor the high-risk fetus for growth and well being.
3 Intervene (usually expedite delivery) at an appropriate time, balancing the risks of *in utero* compromise against those of intervention and prematurity. The latter is itself a major cause of mortality and morbidity.

Problems with fetal surveillance

All methods of surveillance have a false positive rate: that is, they can be over-interpreted. Whilst they may identify problems, they do not necessarily solve them and prevent adverse outcomes. In addition, they 'medicalize' pregnancy by concentrating on the abnormal, and they are expensive. For these reasons, 'risk assessment' has become important. This is done by using past obstetric or medical history (see below box) and the standard pregnancy monitoring outlined in Chapter 17. The principal difficulty is that in most pregnancies with adverse outcomes no visible risk factors are present. For this reason, screening tests for all women are under evaluation. Currently they are not universally employed.

Identification of the high-risk pregnancy	
Pre-pregnancy:	Poor past obstetric history or very small baby
	Maternal disease
	Assisted conception
	Extremes of reproductive age
	Heavy smoking or drug abuse
During pregnancy:	Hypertension/proteinuria
	Vaginal bleeding
	Small-for-dates (SFD) baby
	Prolonged pregnancy
	Multiple pregnancy
	Recurrent urinary tract infections (UTIs)
Investigations:	Cervical scan at 23 weeks [→ p.158]
	Uterine artery Doppler at 23 weeks

Investigations to identify a high-risk pregnancy

Maternal uterine artery Doppler at 23 weeks: The uterine circulation normally develops a very low resistance in normal pregnancy. Abnormal waveforms, indicating failure of development of a low resistance circulation, identify 75% of pregnancies at risk of adverse neonatal outcomes in the early third trimester, particularly early pre-eclampsia, IUGR or placental abruption (*Ultrasound Obstet Gynecol* 2001; **18**: 441). This test is less predictive of later problems. Nevertheless, it is far superior to the current risk assessment based on history alone.

Blood tests: Whilst human chorionic gonadotrophin (HCG) and alpha fetoprotein (AFP) can be used to screen for chromosomal abnormalities [→ p.124]), elevated AFP levels in normally formed fetuses are associated with increased risk. As such, however, they are less effective than uterine artery Doppler.

Methods to assess fetal growth and well being

These tests are not routine in low-risk pregnancy, and must be used in conjunction with urinalysis and measurement of symphysis–fundal height and blood pressure as part of routine antenatal care.

Ultrasound assessment of fetal growth

What it is: Ultrasound scan is used to measure fetal size after the first trimester, using the abdominal and head circumferences, or (biparietal) diameter. These changes are recorded on centile charts (Fig. 25.3). Three factors help to differentiate between the healthy small fetus and the 'growth-restricted' fetus:
1 The rate of growth can be determined by previous scans, or a later examination, at least 2 weeks apart.
2 The pattern of 'smallness' may help: the fetal abdomen will often stop enlarging before the head, which is 'spared'. The result is a 'thin' fetus or asymmetrical growth restriction.
3 Allowance for constitutional non-pathological determinants of fetal growth enables 'customization' of individual fetal growth (*BJOG* 2001; **108**: 830), assessing actual growth according to expected growth.
Benefits: Serial ultrasound is safe and useful in confirming consistent growth in high-risk and multiple pregnancies. The use of ultrasound in dating and identification of abnormalities is discussed elsewhere [→ p.124].
Limitations: 'One-off' ultrasound scans in later pregnancy are of limited benefit in 'low-risk' pregnancies (*Cochrane* 2000: CD001451). Inaccurate measurements are common, misleading and potentially harmful.

Doppler umbilical artery waveforms

What it is: Doppler is used to measure velocity waveforms in the umbilical arteries (Fig. 25.4). Evidence of a high resistance circulation, i.e. reduced flow in fetal diastole compared to systole, suggests placental dysfunction.
Benefits: Umbilical artery waveforms help identify which SFD fetuses are actually growth restricted and therefore compromised (*Cochrane* 2000: CD000073). Its usage improves perinatal outcome in high-risk pregnancy whilst reducing intervention in those not compromised.

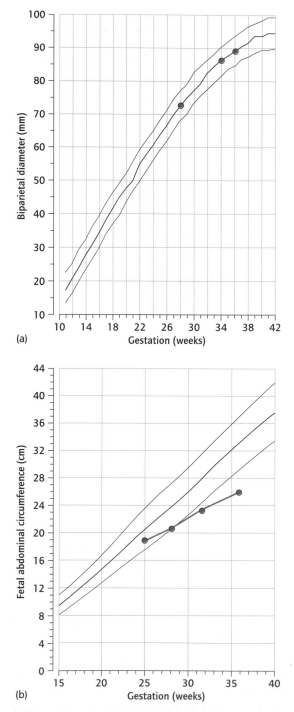

(a)

(b)

Fig. 25.3 (a) Normal growth of the head; (b) slowed growth of the abdomen.

In addition, the absence of flow in diastole usually predates cardiotocograph (CTG) abnormalities and correlates well with severe compromise.

Limitations: Doppler is not a useful screening tool in low-risk pregnancies (*Cochrane* 2000: CD001450) and is less effective at identifying the normal-weight compromised fetus.

Doppler waveforms of the fetal circulation

What it is: All major fetal vessels can be seen, but the most commonly measured are the middle cerebral arteries and the ductus venosus. With fetal compromise, the middle cerebral artery often develops a low resistance pattern in comparison to the thoracic aorta or renal vessels. This reflects a head-sparing effect. The velocity of flow also increases with fetal anaemia [→ p.156]. The ductus venosus waveform has been used as an alternative to antepartum CTG.

Benefits: The use of these is restricted to high-risk pregnancy and generally contributes to, rather than dictates, decisions regarding intervention.

Limitations: there is currently little evidence that their use reduces perinatal mortality or morbidity.

Ultrasound assessment of biophysical profile/amniotic fluid volume

What it is: Four variables (limb movements, tone, breathing movements and liquor volume) are 'scored' zero or two each, to a total out of eight. In the traditional biophysical profile, CTG is also included and the total score is out of 10. It takes up to 30 mins. A low score suggests severe compromise. Reduced liquor volume is associated with a higher risk of fetal distress in labour.

Benefits: It is useful in high-risk pregnancy where CTG or Doppler give equivocal results.

Limitations: It is time consuming and is of little use in the low-risk pregnancy.

Kick chart

What it is: The mother records the number of individual movements that she experiences every day. Ten is considered normal, but it is a change in number rather than the actual number of movements that is important.

Benefits: Most compromised fetuses have reduced movements in the days or hours before demise. A reduction in

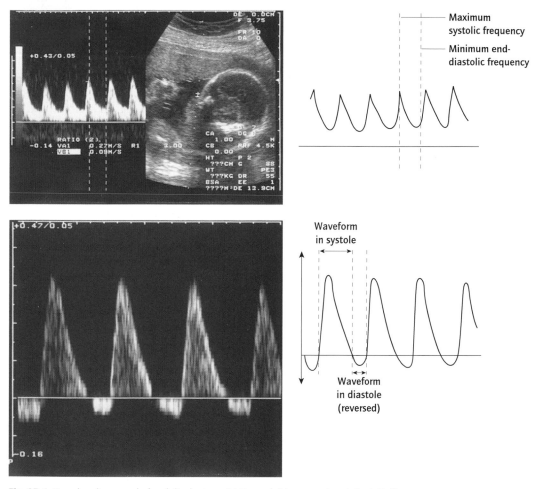

Maximum
systolic frequency

Minimum end-
diastolic frequency

Waveform
in systole

Waveform
in diastole
(reversed)

Fig. 25.4 Doppler ultrasound of umbilical artery: (a) Normal; (b) reversed end-diastolic flow.

fetal movements is an indication for more sophisticated testing. Kick charts are simple and cheap.

Limitations: Compromised fetuses stop moving only shortly before death. Routine counting is of limited benefit in reducing perinatal mortality. The high false positive rate can lead to unnecessary intervention, and maternal anxiety is common.

Cardiotocography (CTG) or non-stress test

What it is: The fetal heart is recorded electronically for up to an hour (this can be combined with ultrasound as a biophysical profile). Accelerations and variability >5 beats per min should be present, decelera-tions absent and the rate in the range of 110–60 (Fig. 25.5).

Benefits: Antenatal abnormalities represent a late stage in fetal compromise and delivery is indicated. Computerized interpretation of variability is of benefit in 'buying time': delaying delivery of chronically compromised premature fetuses.

Limitations: CTGs alone are of no use as an antenatal screening test. Indeed, reliance on occasional CTGs as tests of well being leads to increased perinatal mortality. The best a normal antenatal CTG means is that, barring an acute event, the fetus will not die in the next 24 h. Therefore, to be useful in high-risk pregnancy it needs to be performed daily.

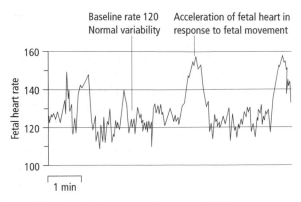

Baseline rate 120
Normal variability

Acceleration of fetal heart in
response to fetal movement

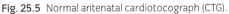

Fig. 25.5 Normal antenatal cardiotocograph (CTG).

Surveillance and intervention

To identify the SFD fetus, ultrasound measurements are used. Occasionally congenital malformations will be apparent and fetal blood sampling or amniocentesis may be used to exclude a chromosomal abnormality.

To identify the IUGR fetus, serial ultrasound and umbilical artery or fetal Doppler are used. These are necessary to exclude compromise in SFD fetuses.

To monitor the IUGR fetus, at least weekly umbilical artery Doppler (to detect deteriorating diastolic flow) is used, with daily CTG if the Doppler waveforms are severely abnormal.

The small but consistently growing fetus does not need intervention. The compromised fetus is normally delivered once maturity is attained (37 weeks), or if preterm is monitored closely with umbilical artery Doppler ± daily CTG, and delivered early if these are abnormal (www.ncl.ac.uk/nfmmg/guidelines/sga%20guide.html). Bedrest does not increase fetal growth, but admission or even delivery may be needed for other indications, particularly severe pre-eclampsia.

Small for dates (SFD) and intrauterine growth restriction (IUGR)

'*Small for dates*' means the fetus's weight or estimated weight is below the tenth/fifth/third centile

Intrauterine growth restriction implies compromise: growth has slowed or is less than is expected taking account of constitutional factors

---

The prolonged pregnancy

A pregnancy is prolonged if 42 weeks or more gestation are completed. However, the risk of perinatal mortality and morbidity starts increasing between 41 and 42 weeks. Prolonged pregnancy is more common if previous pregnancies have been prolonged, but the aetiology is poorly understood. If the dates are routinely checked using early ultrasound, only 6% of pregnancies are prolonged. Establishing the accuracy of dates therefore is essential.

The problem is that induced labour, particularly in nulliparous patients, may be unsuccessful and lead to Caesarean section. However, prolonged pregnancy increases the chances of fetal distress when labour does start: this also leads to an increased chance of a Caesarean section. The aim is to balance the risks of obstetric intervention against those of prolonged pregnancy.

By 41–42 weeks, this balance is in favour of induction of labour. This prevents one fetal death for every 500 women induced, and is associated with a *lower* Caesarean rate than expectant management (*NEJM* 1992; **326**: 1587). Induction before 41 weeks does not have this effect, and indeed is associated with increased intervention. It is therefore usual to induce labour at or after 41 weeks, but in appropriately counselled women who prefer not to be induced, or in nulliparous women with a very unfavourable cervix [→ p.212], surveillance with daily CTG is an acceptable alternative. 'Sweeping' the cervix helps spontaneous labour start earlier (*Cochrane* 2001: CD000451).

Management of the prolonged pregnancy

Check the gestation carefully; counsel patient appropriately
If correct, induction before 41 weeks is inappropriate unless complications are present

At 41 weeks:	Examine the patient vaginally and induce *unless* cervix very unfavourable (not ripe), OR Patient prefers to wait
If no induction:	Sweep cervix and arrange daily cardiotocography (CTG)
If CTG abnormal:	Deliver whatever the condition of the cervix, consider Caesarean

Antepartum death: stillbirth

Definition

Stillbirth is defined as delivery of a dead fetus after 24 weeks gestation. Prevention is a principal aim of fetal surveillance.

Aetiology

It is more frequent in the high-risk groups [→ p.171] unless surveillance is intensive. Most are described as unexplained [→ p.169]) (www.cemach.org.uk), but many, including these, are associated with IUGR (*BJOG* 1998; **105**: 524).

Clinical features

Most women complain of absent or reduced fetal movements; some present acutely with antepartum haemorrhage. The diagnosis is made with ultrasound.

Management

Delivery: Eighty per cent deliver spontaneously within 2 weeks, but labour is usually induced according to the mother's wishes. Prostaglandins rather than amniotomy are used for fear of introducing infection.

To find the cause: A postmortem (PM) fetal chromosome culture, histological examination and culture of the placenta, and a viral screen, glucose, lupus anticoagulant and anticardiolipin antibody testing [→ p.150] from the mother are advised. A Kleihauer test will detect occasional massive spontaneous fetomaternal transfusions. Adverse publicity has made PM examination difficult and consent is complicated, but valuable and sometimes previously unsuspected information can be gained. Limited examination or imaging techniques may be helpful where a full PM examination is declined. Any subsequent pregnancy is regarded as high risk.

Counselling and support. These are essential. As much preliminary explanation as possible is given by the obstetrician, who will counsel the couple when all test results are available. Referral to support groups is useful. The couple are encouraged to hold, photograph and to name the baby. A certificate of stillbirth is given; registration by the mother must take place within 42 days in the United Kingdom.

Further reading

Barker DJ, Gluckman PD, Godfrey KM *et al*. Fetal nutrition and cardiovascular disease in adult life. *Lancet* 1993; **341**: 938–41.

Bricker L, Neilson JP. Routine Doppler ultrasound in pregnancy. *Cochrane Database System Review (Online: Update Software)* 2000: CD001450.

Crowley P. Interventions for preventing or improving the outcome of delivery at or beyond term. *Cochrane Database System Review (Online: Update Software)* 2000; **2**: CD000170.

Harman CR, Baschat AA. Comprehensive assessment of fetal well being: which Doppler tests should be performed? *Current Opinion Obstetrics & Gynecology* 2003; **15**: 147–57.

Pattison N, McCowan L. Cardiotocography for antepartum fetal asessment. *Cochrane Database System Review (Online: Update Software)* 2000: CD001068.

Stanley F, Blair E, Alberman E. *Cerebral Palsies: Epidemiology and Causal Pathways*. Cambridge: Cambridge University Press, 2000.

Fetal Surveillance at a Glance

Screening for the high-risk pregnancy	Maternal, past obstetric and pregnancy history for risk factors
	Uterine artery Doppler at 23 weeks to identify some high-risk pregnancies
	Maternal alpha fetoprotein (AFP) or human chorionic gonadotrophin (HCG) levels at 16 weeks: treat as high risk if high in absence of an anomaly
	Antenatal care including, symphysis–fundal height measurements: refer for ultrasound if less than expected, and repeat at 2-week intervals if fetus small for dates
	'One-off' ultrasound, umbilical artery Doppler or cardiotocography (CTG) of little use
Methods of surveillance in the high-risk pregnancy	Fortnightly (max.) ultrasound to establish consistent growth
	Umbilical artery Doppler to identify the compromized fetus, if small for dates
	Cardiotocography on a daily basis in preterm compromised fetus, or to establish that fetus healthy at time of test
	Methods specific to disorder, e.g. blood pressure in pre-eclampsia

26 Abnormal Lie and Breech Presentation

Abnormal (transverse and oblique) lie

Definitions and epidemiology

The lie of the fetus describes the relationship of the fetus to the long axis of the uterus: if it is lying longitudinally within the uterus, the lie is longitudinal (Fig. 26.1a) and the *presentation* will be cephalic (head) or breech: either will be palpable at the pelvic inlet. If neither is present, the fetus must be lying across the uterus, with the head in one iliac fossa (oblique lie) or in the flank (transverse lie; Fig. 26.1b). Abnormal lie occurs at 1 in 200 births, but is more common earlier in the pregnancy.

Aetiology

Preterm labour is more commonly complicated by an abnormal lie than labour at full term. *Circumstances that allow more room to turn*, for example polyhydramnios [→ p.131] or multiparity (more lax uterus), are the most common causes, frequently resulting in an 'unstable' or continually changing lie. *Conditions that prevent turning*, e.g. fetal and uterine abnormalities and twin pregnancies, may also cause persistent transverse lie, as may *conditions that prevent engagement*, e.g. placenta praevia and pelvic tumours or uterine deformities (Fig. 26.2).

Complications

If the head or breech cannot enter the pelvis, labour cannot deliver the fetus. An arm or the umbilical cord (Fig. 26.3) may prolapse when the membranes rupture, and if neglected the obstruction eventually causes uterine rupture. Both fetus and mother are therefore at risk.

Management

Abnormal lie is common before 37 weeks and no action is required. After 37 weeks, the woman should be admitted to hospital in case the membranes rupture and an ultrasound scan performed to exclude particular identifiable causes, notably polyhydramnios and placenta praevia. External cephalic version (ECV [→ p.178]) is unjustified because the fetus usually turns back. Only if spontaneous version occurs and persists for more than 48 h should the woman be discharged. In the absence of pelvic obstruction, an abnormal lie will usually stabilize before 41 weeks. At this stage, the persistently abnormal lie is delivered by Caesarean, but in expert hands ECV and then amniotomy is occasionally successful.

Breech presentation

Definitions and epidemiology

The presentation refers to the part of the fetus that occupies the lower segment of the uterus or the pelvis. Presentation of the buttocks is breech presentation (Fig. 26.4). It occurs in 3% of term pregnancies, but, like the abnormal lie, is common earlier in the pregnancy and is therefore

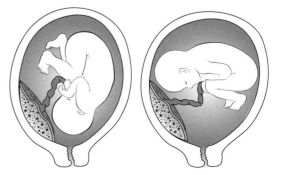

Fig. 26.1 (a) Longitudinal lie. (b) Transverse lie.

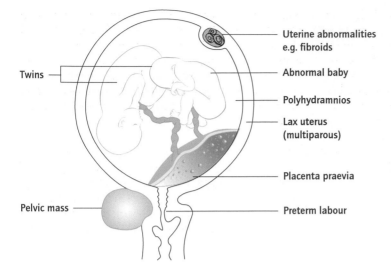

Uterine abnormalities
e.g. fibroids

Abnormal baby

Twins

Polyhydramnios

Lax uterus
(multiparous)

Placenta praevia

Pelvic mass

Preterm labour

Fig. 26.2 Causes of transverse lie and breech presentation.

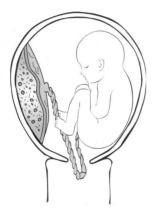

Fig. 26.3 Cord prolapse.

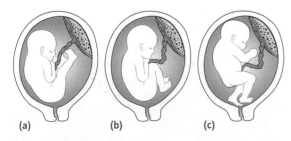

(a)   (b)   (c)

Fig. 26.4 Types of breech presentation. (a) Extended.
b) Flexed. (c) Footling.

more common (25%) if labour occurs prematurely. The extended breech (70%) has both legs extended at the knee. The flexed breech (15%) has both legs flexed at the knee. In the footling breech (15%, more common if preterm) one or both feet present below the buttocks.

Aetiology

No cause is found with most. A previous breech presentation has occurred in 8%. *Prematurity* is commonly associated with breech presentation. Conditions that prevent movement, such as *fetal* and *uterine abnormalities* or *twin pregnancies*, or that prevent engagement of the head, such as *placenta praevia*, *pelvic tumours* and *pelvic deformities* are more common (see Fig. 26.2).

Diagnosis

Breech presentation is commonly (30%) missed, but diagnosis is only important after 37 weeks or if the patient is in labour. Upper abdominal discomfort is common. The hard head is normally palpable and ballottable at the fundus. Ultrasound confirms the diagnosis, helps detection of a fetal abnormality, pelvic tumour or a placenta praevia and ensures the prerequisites for ECV are met.

Complications

Perinatal and long-term morbidity and mortality are increased. Fetal abnormalities are more common, but even 'normal' breech babies have higher rates of long-term neurological handicap (*BMJ* 1996; **312**: 1451), which is independent of the mode of delivery. In addition, labour has potential hazards. The relatively poor 'fit' of the breech or feet leads to an increased rate of cord prolapse [→ p.221]. The after-coming head may get trapped: in cephalic presentations a head that is too big or extended [→ p.189] will cause a cessation of progress in labour that is easily managed by Caesarean section, but with a breech only after the body has been delivered will the problem be evident. At this stage, a baby with a trapped head will rapidly die.

Management
External cephalic version (ECV)
After 37 weeks, an attempt is made to turn the baby to a cephalic presentation (Fig. 26.5). This is done without anaesthetic, but if the uterus is tight or with nulliparous women it is done with a uterine relaxant (tocolytic) (*Cochrane* 2002: CD000184). With both hands on the abdomen, the breech is disengaged from the pelvis and rotation in the form of a forward somersault is attempted. This is performed under ultrasound guidance and in hospital to allow immediate delivery if complications occur. Anti-D is given to rhesus-negative women [→ p.155]. The success rate is about 50%.

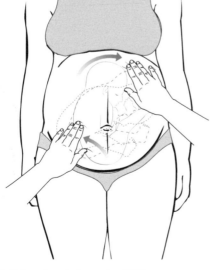

Fig. 26.5 External cephalic version (ECV).

Safety of ECV. The risk is minimal, provided care is taken (*J Matern Fetal Med* 1999; **8**: 203), although placental abruption and uterine rupture have been reported. The advantage is a reduction in breech presentation at term and therefore Caesarean or vaginal breech delivery (*Cochrane* 2000: CD000184). External cephalic version before 37 weeks does not have this effect and is not advised.

Contraindications to ECV. External cephalic version is not performed if the fetus is compromised [→ p.169], if vaginal delivery would be contraindicated anyway (e.g. placenta praevia), if there are twins, if the membranes are ruptured, or if there has been recent antepartum haemorrhage. One previous Caesarean section is not a contraindication.

Caesarean section
If ECV has failed or is contraindicated, the safest method of delivery for the singleton term breech is by Caesarean section (*Cochrane* 2001: CD000166). Parents should be counselled as to this, although the final decision rests with them. The increase in number of Caesarean sections required does not appear to increase maternal complications. This is because more than a third of attempts at vaginal breech delivery end in emergency Caesarean section, which carries even greater maternal risks than an elective procedure.

Nevertheless, some women are likely to still request vaginal breech birth, breech presentation is often diagnosed only in late labour and second twins often present as breech. Under such circumstances, vaginal breech delivery may still be appropriate, yet skills are being lost due to lack of experience of the procedure. Knowledge of the technique of vaginal breech delivery remains essential for any obstetrician and is therefore described.

Vaginal breech birth
Patient selection: Vaginal breech birth is probably yet more risky with a fetus >4.0 kg, with evidence of fetal compromise, an extended head or footling legs.
Intrapartum care: In about 30%, there is slow cervical dilatation in the first stage or poor descent in the second and Caesarean section is performed. Pushing is not encouraged until the buttocks are visible. Cardiotocography is advised. Epidural analgesia is common but not mandatory.
Breech delivery (Fig. 26.6) A difficult delivery is often the result of injudicious traction causing extension of the

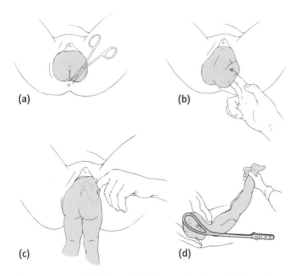

Fig. 26.6 Breech delivery. (a) As buttocks distend the perineum, perform the episiotomy. (b) A finger behind the knee delivers the legs. (c) A finger hooks each arm down. (d) Forceps deliver the head once the arms are delivered.

head. Once the buttocks distend the perineum, an episiotomy [→ p.207] is made. The fetus is delivered as far as the umbilicus, without traction. The legs can be flexed out of the vagina, whilst the back is kept anterior. Once the scapula is visible, the anterior and then the posterior arm is 'hooked' down by a finger over the shoulder sweeping it across the chest. Once the back of the neck is visible, an assistant holds the legs up whilst forceps are applied, and with the next contraction the head is lifted slowly out of the vagina.

An alternative method is the Mauriceau–Smellie–Veit manoeuvre: the operator supports the entire weight of the fetus on one palm and forearm, with his or her finger in its mouth to guide the head over the perineum and maintain flexion. With the same intent, his or her other hand presses against the occiput and an assistant applies suprapubic pressure.

Further reading

Hannah ME, Hannah WJ, Hewson SA *et al.* for the Term Breech Trial Collaborative Group. Planned Caesarean section versus planned vaginal birth for breech presentation at term: a randomised multicentre trial. *Lancet* 2000; **356**: 1375–83.

Impey L, Pandit M. Breech presentation in the new millenium. *Current Obstetrics & Gynaecology* 2001; **11**(5): 272–8.

Tunde-Byass MO, Hannah ME. Breech vaginal delivery at or near term. *Seminars in Perinatology* 2003; **27**(1): 34–45.

Transverse/Oblique Lie at a Glance	
Definition	Lie of fetus not parallel to long axis of uterus
Epidemiology	1 in 200 births
Aetiology	Preterm labour, polyhydramnios, multiparity, placenta praevia, pelvic mass, fetal or uterine abnormality, twins
Management	Admit if >37 weeks. Ultrasound to find cause If not stabilized by 41 weeks, or if pelvis obstructed, elective Caesarean

Breech Presentation at a Glance

Types	Extended (70%), flexed (15%), footling (15%)
Epidemiology	3% at term, more if preterm labour or previous breech presentation
Aetiology	Idiopathic, uterine/fetal anomalies, placenta praevia, pelvic mass, twins More common preterm

Complications	Increased perinatal mortality and morbidity due to:
	    Unknown but unrelated to vaginal delivery
	    Congenital anomalies
	    Intrapartum problems

Management	External cephalic version (ECV) after 37 weeks, 50% success. Not if antepartum haemorrhage, ruptured membranes, fetal compromise, twins Elective Caesarean section safest

Multiple Pregnancy

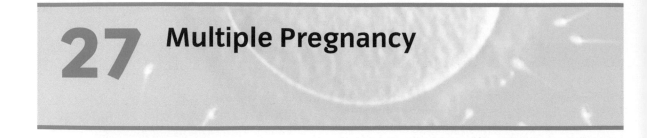

Epidemiology

Twins occur in 1 in 80 pregnancies, triplets in 1 in 1000. There is considerable geographic variation. The incidence is increasing because of subfertility treatment [→ p.73] and the increasing number of older mothers.

Types of multiple pregnancy

Dizygotic (DZ) twins (two-thirds of all multiple pregnancies) or triplets result from fertilization of different oocytes by different sperm (Fig. 27.1). Such fetuses may be of different sex and are no more genetically similar than siblings from different pregnancies.

Monozygotic (MZ) twins result from mitotic division of a single zygote into 'identical' twins. Whether they share the same amnion or placenta depends on the time at which division into separate zygotes occurred (see Fig. 27.1). Division before day 3 (approx. 30%) leads to twins

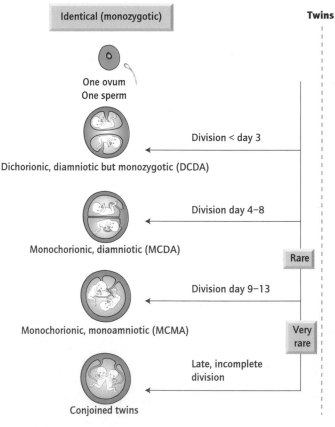

Fig. 27.1 Mechanisms of twinning.

with separate placentas and amnions (dichorionic diamniotic, DCDA). Division between days 4 and 8 (approx. 70%) leads to twins with a shared placenta but separate amnions (monochorionic diamniotic, MCDA). Later division is very rare and causes twins with a shared placenta and a single amniotic sac (monochorionic monoamniotic, MCMA). Incomplete division leads to conjoined twins. Monochorionic (MC) twins have a higher fetal loss rate, particularly before 24 weeks.

Aetiology

Assisted conception, genetic factors and increasing maternal age and parity are the most important factors, largely affecting DZ twinning. About 20% of all *in vitro* fertilization (IVF) [→ p.76] conceptions and 10% of clomiphene-assisted conceptions are multiple. Embryo transfer of more than two fertilized ova at IVF is now performed in the United Kingdom only under exceptional circumstances.

Diagnosis

Vomiting may be more marked in early pregnancy. The uterus is larger than expected from the dates and palpable before 12 weeks. Later in pregnancy, three or more fetal poles may be felt. Many are diagnosed only at ultrasound (Fig. 27.2): as this is now performed in most pregnancies, the diagnosis is seldom missed.

Complications

The perinatal mortality and long-term handicap rate of multiple pregnancies is greatly increased. Triplets fare even worse. Much of the risk is due to monochorionicity (see below).

Antepartum complications

Virtually all obstetric risks are exaggerated in multiple pregnancies (Fig. 27.3). *Preterm labour* is the main cause of perinatal mortality: 40% of twin and 80% of triplet pregnancies deliver before 37 weeks; 10% of twins deliver before 32 weeks. *Miscarriage* is more common. Some first-trimester bleeding occurs in 25% of all multiple pregnancies. *Congenital abnormalities* are two to four times more common. *Intrauterine growth restriction* (IUGR) is common. Twins usually grow at the same rate as singletons until about 28 weeks, but thereafter slower growth is normal (Fig. 27.4). However, growth may become discordant, usually as a result of placental insufficiency (e.g. associated with pre-eclampsia), but also as a result of the *twin–twin transfusion syndrome*. This is unique to MC twins and is diagnosed in 15%. The perinatal mortality is very high. It results from unequal blood distribution through vascular anastomoses of a MC placenta. The 'donor' twin usually develops anaemia, growth restriction and oligohydramnios. The 'recipient' twin may develop polycythaemia, cardiac failure and polyhydramnios. Both are at risk of *in utero* death and severely preterm delivery.

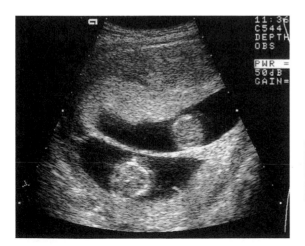

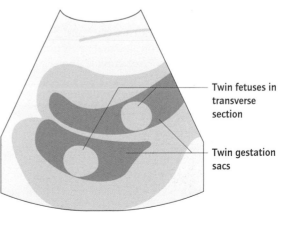

Twin fetuses in transverse section

Twin gestation sacs

Fig. 27.2 Ultrasound showing dichorionic twins in early pregnancy.

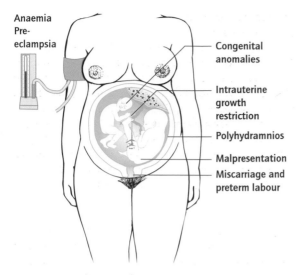

Fig. 27.3 Complications of twin pregnancies.

Polyhydramnios (6%) [→ p.131] and *antepartum haemorrhage* are both more common than with singletons.

Medical complications in pregnancy, particularly *gestational diabetes* and *pre-eclampsia*, are more frequent. *Anaemia* is more frequent, partly because of a greater increase in blood volume causing a dilutional effect and partly because more iron and folic acid are needed. Routine supplements of both are advised.

Intrapartum complications

Malpresentation of the first twin occurs in 20% (Fig. 27.5): this is an indication for Caesarean section. *Fetal distress* [→ p.199] in labour is more common. The *second twin* is particularly vulnerable after the first has been delivered because of an increased risk of cord prolapse, tetanic uterine contraction or placental abruption, and may present as a breech. *Postpartum haemorrhage* is more common (10%).

Complications of twin pregnancies
Perinatal mortality increased fourfold
Preterm labour and miscarriage
Congenital abnormalities
Placental insufficiency/intrauterine growth restriction (IUGR)
Twin–twin transfusion syndrome (monochorionic, MC, twins only)
Antepartum and postpartum haemorrhage
Pre-eclampsia, diabetes, anaemia
Malpresentation

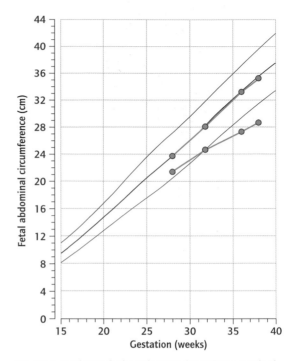

Fig. 27.4 Fetal growth chart showing discordant growth of twins.

Antepartum management

The pregnancy should be considered 'high risk': care should be consultant-led, although not every visit need be in the hospital. Iron and folic acid supplements are prescribed. Screening for chromosomal abnormalities is offered using nuchal translucency scanning [→ p.127]. Monochorionicity is most accurately diagnosed in the first trimester: the dividing membrane is thin and forms a 'T' as it meets the single placenta in perpendicular fashion. If the uterus is palpable abdominally before 12 weeks, early ultrasound scan is advised. Twins of opposite gender are always dizygous.

Selective reduction to a twin pregnancy at 12 weeks should be offered to those with triplets or higher order pregnancies. Whilst this increases early spontaneous miscarriage rates, it reduces the chances of preterm birth and therefore cerebral palsy and late fetal death (*BJOG* 1997; **104**: 1201).

Anomalies are sought at the 20-week scan. As IUGR is both more common and more difficult to detect in multiple pregnancies compared with singleton pregnancies, serial ultrasound examinations for growth are usually

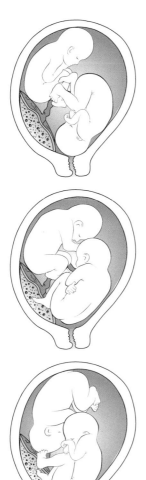

Fig. 27.5 Presentation of twins.

routinely performed at 28, 32 and 36 weeks. More frequent examination is usual for MC twins, higher order multiples, or if a problem is suspected. Twin–twin transfusion syndrome is managed in a fetal medicine centre by therapeutic amniocentesis of the recipient twin and piercing of the dividing membrane (septostomy), or with endoscopic laser vaporization of the placenta (*BJOG* 1998; **105**: 446) with severe disease.

Multiple pregnancies increase maternal tiredness and anxiety, and may result in financial problems. Postnatal home help should be discussed.

Intrapartum management
Mode of delivery

There is little evidence to support the increasing use of Caesarean section with twins. When the first fetus is cephalic, whatever the lie or presentation of the second (Fig. 27.5), vaginal delivery remains appropriate in the absence of other complications. Caesarean section is, however, the favoured route if the first fetus is a breech or a transverse lie, with triplets, if there have been antepartum complications, and, in some hospitals, with all MC twins. One previous Caesarean delivery should not contraindicate a subsequent vaginal delivery.

Method of delivery

It is common practice to induce labour in twins at about 38 weeks. Labour is not longer, but it can be augmented with oxytocin. Cardiotocography [→ p.199] is advised as the risk of intrapartum hypoxia is increased, particularly for the second twin. Epidural analgesia is not mandatory but is helpful as difficulty is occasionally encountered with delivery of the second twin. The first twin is delivered in the normal manner.

Delivery of the second twin

The lie is checked and external cephalic version (ECV) is performed if the lie is not longitudinal. Cardiotocography must continue. Oxytocin is started as contractions may decrease. Once the head or breech enters the pelvis, the membranes are ruptured and pushing again begins. Delivery is usually easy and achieved within 20 min of the first fetus. Excessive delay is associated with increased morbidity for the second twin, but excessive haste is equally dangerous. If the head does not descend, a malpresentation (particularly a brow) is likely and Caesarean section is very occasionally required. If fetal distress or cord prolapse occur, vaginal delivery can be expedited with a ventouse [→ p.216] or breech extraction. The latter must be performed under general or epidural anaesthesia, only by experienced personnel, and never with singleton breeches. It involves inserting a hand into the uterus, grasping the feet and guiding them down. After delivery, a prophylactic oxytocin infusion is used to prevent postpartum haemorrhage.

Further reading

Hogle KL, Hutton EK, McBrien KA, Barrett JF, Hannah ME. Cesarean delivery for twins: a systematic review and meta-analysis. *American Journal of Obstetrics and Gynecology* 2003; **188**: 220–7.

Russell RB, Petrini JR, Damus K, Mattison DR, Schwarz RH. The changing epidemiology of multiple births in the United States. *Obstetrics and Gynecology* 2003; **101**: 129–35.

Wee LY, Fisk NM. The twin–twin transfusion syndrome. *Seminars in Neonatology* 2002; **7**: 187–202.

Multiple Pregnancy at a Glance

Incidence	Twins 1.3%, triplets 0.1%; geographical variation	
Types	Dizygotic (DZ):	Different oocytes fertilized by different sperm
	Monozygotic (MZ):	Division of zygote after fertilization
	Dichorionic:	Two placentas
	Monochorionic (MC):	Shared placenta
Aetiology	Ovulation induction, genetic factors, increasing age and parity	
Diagnosis	Usually at ultrasound scan. Vomiting, 'large for dates', 3+ fetal poles	
Complications	Perinatal mortality increased, particularly if MC Most obstetric complications more common, particularly preterm labour and miscarriage, congenital abnormalities, placental insufficiency/intrauterine growth restriction (IUGR), antepartum and postpartum haemorrhage, pre-eclampsia, diabetes, anaemia and malpresentations. Twin–twin transfusion with MC twins	
Management	Antenatal: early diagnosis, identification of chorionicity. Consultant care. Iron and folic acid supplements Anomaly scan. Increased surveillance for pre-eclampsia, diabetes. Serial ultrasound at 28, 32 and 36 weeks. Caesarean section if first twin not cephalic and usual indications Labour: as for singletons. Cardiotocography. After first twin, lie of second twin checked: external cephalic version (ECV) if necessary. Oxytocin started. Amniotomy when presenting part engaged, then maternal pushing. Ventouse or breech extraction if fetal distress	

28 Labour 1: Mechanism—Anatomy and Physiology

Labour is the process whereby the fetus and placenta are expelled from the uterus, and it normally occurs between 37 and 42 weeks gestation. The diagnosis is made *when painful uterine contractions accompany dilatation and effacement of the cervix*. It is divided into stages. In the *first stage*, the cervix opens to 'full dilatation' to allow the head to pass through. The *second stage* is from full dilatation to delivery of the fetus. The *third stage* lasts from delivery of the fetus to delivery of the placenta.

Labour	
Diagnosis:	Painful contractions lead to dilatation of the cervix
First stage:	Initiation to full cervical dilatation
Second stage:	Full cervical dilatation to delivery of fetus
Third stage:	Delivery of fetus to delivery of placenta

Mechanical factors of labour

Three mechanical factors determine progress during labour:
1 The degree of force expelling the fetus (the powers).
2 The dimensions of the pelvis and the resistance of soft tissues (the passage).
3 The diameters of the fetal head (the passenger).

The powers (Fig. 28.1)

Once labour is established, the uterus contracts for 45–60 s about every 2–3 min. This pulls the cervix up (effacement) and causes dilatation, aided by the pressure of the head as the uterus pushes the head down into the pelvis. Poor uterine activity is a common feature of the nulliparous woman and in induced labour, [→ p.212] but is rare in multiparous women.

The passage
The bony pelvis
This has three principal planes. At its *inlet*, the transverse diameter is about 13 cm, wider than the 11-cm anteroposterior (AP) diameter (Fig. 28.2). The *mid-cavity* is almost round as the transverse and AP diameters are similar. At the *outlet*, the AP diameter (12.5 cm) is greater than the transverse diameter (11 cm). In the lateral wall of the round mid-pelvis, bony prominences called *ischial spines* are palpable vaginally. These are used as landmarks by which to assess the descent of the head on vaginal examination: the level of descent is called 'station' and is crudely measured in centimetres in relation to these 'spines'. Station 0 means the head is at the level of these spines; station +2 means it is 2 cm below and station −2 means it is 2 cm above (Fig. 28.3). A variety of pelvic shapes have been described, but diagnosis and therefore description of these is seldom useful in clinical practice.

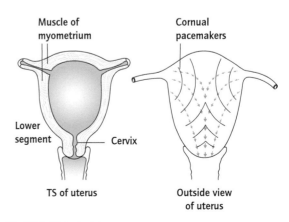

Fig. 28.1 The powers.

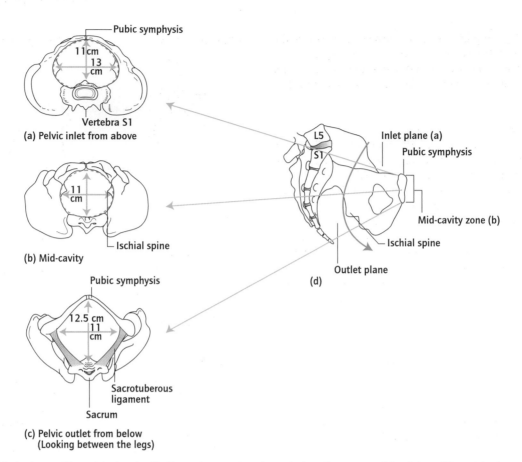

Pubic symphysis

11 cm
13 cm

Vertebra S1

(a) Pelvic inlet from above

11 cm

Ischial spine

(b) Mid-cavity

Pubic symphysis

12.5 cm
11 cm

Sacrotuberous ligament

Sacrum

(c) Pelvic outlet from below
(Looking between the legs)

L5
S1

Inlet plane (a)
Pubic symphysis

Mid-cavity zone (b)

Ischial spine

Outlet plane

(d)

Fig. 28.2 Anatomy of the pelvis showing the three planes, a, b and c, and where they are on a lateral view of the pelvis, d.

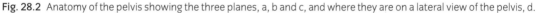

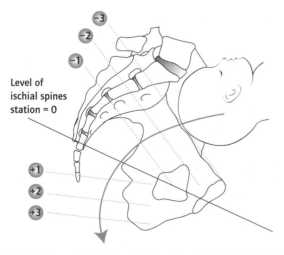

−3
−2
−1

Level of
ischial spines
station = 0

+1
+2
+3

Fig. 28.3 Descent of the head in labour in relation to the ischial spines.

The soft tissues

Cervical dilatation is a prerequisite for delivery and is dependent on contractions, the pressure of the fetal head on the cervix and the ability of the cervix to soften and allow distension. The soft tissues of the vagina and perineum need to be overcome in the second stage: the perineum often tears or is cut (episiotomy) to allow the head to deliver.

The passenger

The head is oblong in transverse section. Its bones are not yet fused and, on vaginal examination, spaces between them are palpable as sutures and fontanelles. The anterior fontanelle (bregma) lies above the forehead. The posterior fontanelle (occiput) lies on the back of the top of the head. Between these two is the area called the vertex. In front of the bregma is the brow (Fig. 28.4). Because the head is not round, several factors determine how easily it fits through the pelvic diameters.

Attitude

The attitude is the degree of flexion of the head on the neck (Fig. 28.5). The ideal attitude is maximal flexion, keeping the head bowed. This is called *vertex presentation*, and the presenting diameter is 9.5 cm, running from the anterior fontanelle to below the occiput at the back of the head. A small degree of extension results in a larger diameter. Extension of 90° causes a *brow presentation*, and a much larger diameter of 13 cm. A further 30° of extension (with the face looking parallel and away from the body) is a *face presentation*. Extension of the head can mean that the fetal diameters are too large to deliver vaginally.

Position

The position is the degree of rotation of the head on the neck (Fig. 28.6). If the sagittal suture is transverse, the oblong head will fit the pelvic inlet best. But at the outlet the sagittal suture must be vertical for the head to fit. The head must therefore normally rotate 90° during labour. It is usually delivered with the *occiput anterior*

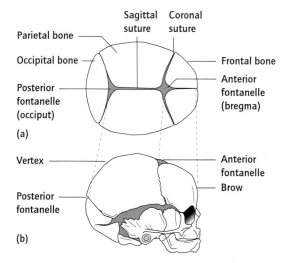

Fig. 28.4 (a) Fetal head from above, showing sutures and fontanelles. (b) Fetal head from the side.

Attitude of the head

What is palpable

Well flexed (vertex)

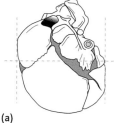

(a)

(b)

Deflexed

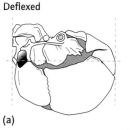

(a)

(b)

Extended (brow)

(a)

(b)

Hyperextended (face)

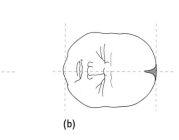

(a)

(b)

Fig. 28.5 Attitude of the fetal head showing how extension of the head changes the presenting diameter and what is palpable on vaginal examination.

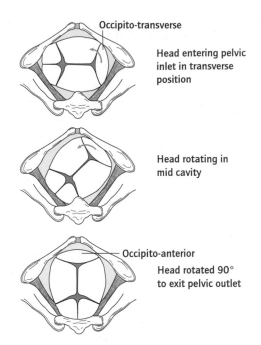

Occipito-transverse

Head entering pelvic inlet in transverse position

Head rotating in mid cavity

Occipito-anterior

Head rotated 90° to exit pelvic outlet

Fig. 28.6 View from below showing rotation of the head (position) according to the three planes of the pelvis.

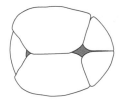

Fig. 28.7 Diagram of moulding showing compression and overlap of sutures.

or *caput*. It is relatively unusual for a normally formed head to be simply too big to pass through the bony pelvis (cephalopelvic disproportion), although a larger head may cause a longer and more difficult labour.

Terms describing the fetal head

Presentation is the part of the fetus that occupies the lower segment or pelvis: i.e. head (cephalic) or buttocks (breech)

Presenting part is the lowest part of the fetus palpable on vaginal examination: the lowest part of the head or breech. For a cephalic presentation, this can be the vertex, the brow or the face, depending on the attitude. For simplicity, these are often described as separate 'presentations'

Position of the head describes its rotation: occipito-transverse (OT), occipito-posterior (OP) or occipito-anterior (OA)

Attitude of the head describes the degree of flexion: vertex, brow or face

---

Movements of the head

Engagement in occipito-transverse (OT)
Descent and flexion
Rotation 90° to occipito-anterior (OA)
Descent
Extension to deliver
Restitution and delivery of shoulders

(occipito-anterior, OA). In 5% of deliveries it is occipito-posterior (OP) and more difficulty may be encountered. Persistence of the occipito-transverse (OT) position implies non-rotation and delivery without assistance is impossible.

Size of the head

The head can be compressed in the pelvis because the sutures allow the bones to come together and even overlap slightly. This slightly reduces the diameters of the head and is called *moulding* (Fig. 28.7). Pressure of the scalp on the cervix or pelvic inlet can cause localized swelling

Cervical dilatation: the 'stages' of labour

Initiation and diagnosis of labour

Involuntary contractions of uterine smooth muscle occur throughout the third trimester and are often felt as Braxton Hicks contractions. How this leads to labour is not fully understood, but the fetus has a role, and prostaglandin production has a crucial role both in reducing cervical resistance and increasing release of the hormone oxytocin from the posterior pituitary gland. This aids stimulation of contractions, which arise in one of the pacemakers situated at each cornu of the uterus.

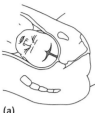

(a)

Engagement: The oblong-shaped head normally enters the pelvis in the occipito-transverse (OT) position, because the transverse diameter of the inlet is greater than the antero-posterior diameter.

(b)

Descent and flexion: The head descends into the round mid-cavity and flexes as the cervix dilates. Descent is measured by comparison with the level of the ischial spines [→187] and is called station.

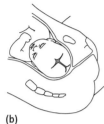

(c)

Rotation: In the mid-cavity, the head rotates 90°(internal rotation) so that the face is facing the sacrum and the occiput is anterior, below the symphisis pubis (occipito-anterior, OA). This enables it to pass through the pelvic outlet which has a wider antero-posterior than transverse diameter. In 5% of cases, the head rotates to occipito-posterior (OP).

(d)

Rotation completed, further descent: The perineum distends.

(e)

Extension and delivery.

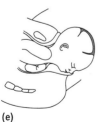

(f)

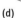

Restitution: The head then rotates 90° (external rotation) to the same position in which it entered the inlet, facing either right or left, to enable delivery of the shoulders.

Fig. 28.8(a–f) Movement of the head in labour.

Painful regular contractions lead to effacement and dilatation of the cervix. Effacement is when the normally tubular cervix is drawn up into the lower segment until it is flat (Fig. 28.9). This is commonly accompanied by a 'show' or pink/white mucus plug from the cervix and/or rupture of the membranes, causing release of liquor.

The first stage

This lasts from the diagnosis of labour until the cervix is dilated by 10 cm (fully dilated). The descent, flexion and internal rotation described occur to varying degree. If the membranes have not already ruptured, they normally do so.

The latent phase is where the cervix usually dilates slowly for the first 3 cm and may take several hours.

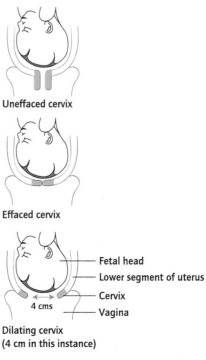

Uneffaced cervix

Effaced cervix

Fetal head

Lower segment of uterus

Cervix

4 cms

Vagina

Dilating cervix
(4 cm in this instance)

Fig. 28.9 Effacement and dilatation of the cervix.

The active phase follows: average cervical dilatation is at the rate of 1 cm/h in nulliparous women and about 2 cm/h in multiparous women. The first stage should not normally last longer than 12 h.

The second stage

This lasts from full dilatation of the cervix to delivery. Descent, flexion and rotation are completed and followed by extension as the head delivers.

The passive stage lasts from full dilatation until the head reaches the pelvic floor and the woman experiences the desire to push. Rotation and flexion are commonly completed. This stage may last a few minutes, but can be much longer.

The active stage is when the mother is pushing. The pressure of the head on the pelvic floor produces an irresistible desire to bear down, although epidural analgesia may prevent this. The woman gets in the most comfortable position for her, but not supine, and pushes with contractions. The fetus is delivered, on average, after 40 min (nulliparous) or 20 min (multiparous). This

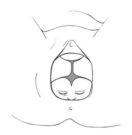

Fig. 28.10 Head delivery over the perineum by extension.

stage can be much quicker, but if it takes >1 h spontaneous delivery becomes unlikely.

Delivery

As the head reaches the perineum, it extends to come up out of the pelvis (Fig. 28.10). The perineum begins to stretch and often tears, but is cut (episiotomy) if progress is slow or fetal distress [→ p.199] is present. The head then restitutes, rotating 90° to adopt the transverse position in which it entered the pelvis. With the next contraction, the shoulders deliver: the anterior shoulder comes under the symphysis pubis first, usually aided by lateral body flexion in a posterior direction; the posterior shoulder is aided by lateral body flexion in an anterior direction. The rest of the body follows.

The third stage

This is the time from delivery of the fetus to delivery of the placenta. It normally lasts about 15 min and normal blood loss is up to 500 mL. Uterine muscle fibres contract to compress the blood vessels formerly supplying the placenta, which shears away from the uterine wall.

Further reading

Bernal AL. Overview of current research in parturition. *Experimental Physiology* 2001; **86**: 213–22.
Jaffe RB. Role of the human fetal adrenal gland in the initiation of parturition. *Frontiers of Hormone Research* 2001; **27**: 75–85.

Mechanism of Normal Labour at a Glance

When	37–42 weeks
Diagnosis	Contractions with effacement and dilatation of the cervix
First stage	Average duration 8 h, nulliparous; 4 h, multiparous Uterus contracts every 2–3 min Latent (<3 cm) and active (4–10 cm) phases Cervix dilates until the widest diameter of head passes through Head descends remaining flexed to maintain the smallest diameter (Variable descent occurs before labour: 'engagement') 90° rotation from occipito-transverse (OT) to occipito-anterior (OA) (or occipito-posterior, OP) begins Amniotic membranes usually rupture or are ruptured artificially
Second stage	Contractions continue Head descends and flexes further, rotation usually completed Pushing starts when head reaches pelvic floor (active second stage)
Delivery	Head now extends as it is delivered over perineum Head restitutes, rotating back to the transverse before the shoulders deliver
Third stage	Placenta is delivered. Average duration 15 min

29 Labour 2: Management

Monitoring progress: the partogram

Progress in labour is dependent on the powers, the passage and the passenger. A partogram (Fig. 29.1) is used to record progress in dilatation of the cervix (± descent of the head). This is assessed on vaginal examination and plotted against time. After the latent phase (i.e. at about 3 cm dilated) the usual minimum rate of dilatation is 1 cm/h: 'alert' and 'action' lines on the partogram indicate slow progress. This visual record therefore aids identification of abnormal progress and also forms a record of maternal vital signs, fetal heart rate (FHR) and liquor colour.

General measures to maintain progress

Continuous support during labour is associated with a reduction in operative delivery and the length of labour (*Cochrane* 2002: CD000199). This should be from the midwife as well as partner, or from non-medical supporters or 'doulas'. The impact of support is seldom remembered but reflects the importance of psychological well being on obstetric outcomes. Mobility should also be encouraged.

Nulliparous labour

The first stage. Slow progress in the nulliparous woman is usually due to inefficient uterine action, even if contractions are frequent or feel strong. Mobility, which should be encouraged, may help prevent this. Strengthening the powers artificially is called augmentation, and this can even sometimes correct passenger problems of attitude or position. This is performed with amniotomy; if this fails, artificial oxytocin is administered as a dilute solution and the dose is gradually increased (*Cochrane* 2000: CD000015).

This approach is safe because of the relative immunity of the nulliparous uterus to rupture. If full dilatation is not imminent within 12 h, the diagnosis is reconsidered

and Caesarean section is performed: problems with the passage or passenger are more likely and the immunity of the uterus to rupture is diminished.

The passive second stage. If descent is poor, oxytocin should be given and pushing delayed by up to 2 h. If an epidural has been used, the urge to push that is characteristic of the active second stage is diminished.

The active second stage. Pushing need not be directed unless an epidural is present. If the stage lasts longer than 1 h, spontaneous delivery becomes less likely because of maternal exhaustion; fetal hypoxia is also more common. If the head is distending the perineum, an episiotomy can be performed; if not, traction is often applied to the fetal head with a ventouse or forceps [→ p.216].

Multiparous labour

The first stage. Slow progress in the multiparous woman is rare. The multiparous uterus is seldom inefficient and the pelvic capacity has been 'proven' in the previous labour unless delivery has previously been by Caesarean section [→ p.213]. The cause is therefore likely to be the fetal head: its attitude or position, or because it is much bigger than before. In addition, the multiparous uterus is more prone to rupture than the nulliparous uterus. Augmentation of labour with oxytocin must be preceded by exclusion of a malpresentation.

The second stage. Instrumental delivery, though rarely needed, requires similar caution.

Progress in labour: problems and their treatment

The powers

'*Inefficient uterine action*' is the most common cause of slow progress in labour. Classifications are meaningless.

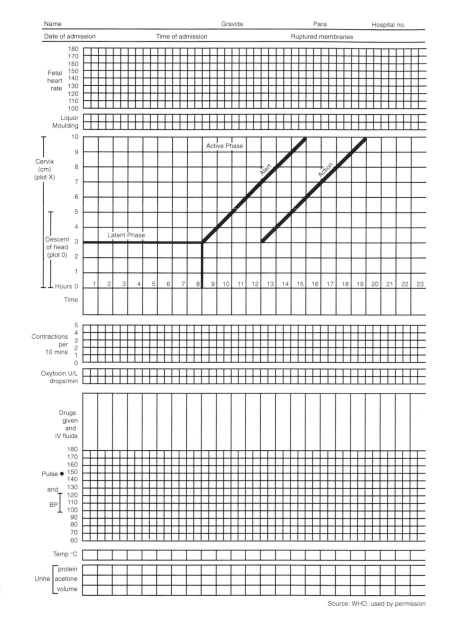

Fig. 29.1 World Health Organization partogram.

It is common in nulliparous women and in induced labour, but is rare in multiparous women. It is treated by augmentation, initially with amniotomy (Fig. 29.2) and then oxytocin (Fig. 29.3).

> ### Augmentation and induction
>
> Augmentation is the artificial strengthening of contractions in established labour
> Induction is the artificial initiation of labour

Hyperactive uterine action occurs with excessively strong or frequent or prolonged contractions. The FHR may be abnormal as placental blood flow is diminished and

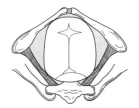

Fig. 29.4 The occipito-posterior (OP) position associated with extension of the head.

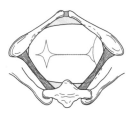

Fig. 29.5 The occipito-transverse (OT) position: delivery is impossible without rotation.

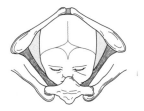

Fig. 29.6 Brow presentation.

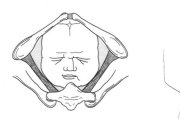

Fig. 29.7 Face presentation (chin is posterior).

normally only be diagnosed after labour has failed to progress and not with any accuracy before labour. Measuring the pelvis clinically or with X-rays or computed tomography (CT) scanning seldom helps. Cephalo-pelvic disproportion is slightly more likely with large babies, with very short women, or where the head in a nulliparous woman remains high at term. Elective Caesarean section is generally inappropriate in such women, but the term 'trial of labour' is sometimes thoughtlessly used.

Pelvic variants and deformities

Normal variants in pelvic shape have been extensively classified but this is seldom useful in practice. The 'gynaecoid' or ideal pelvis is found in 50–80% of Caucasian women. The 'anthropoid' pelvis (20%) has a narrower inlet, with a transverse diameter often less than the antero-posterior (AP) diameter. The android pelvis (5%) has a heart-shaped inlet and a funnelling shape to the mid-pelvis. In the platypelloid pelvis (10%) the oval shape of the inlet persists within the mid-pelvis.

Abnormal pelvic architecture is usually confined to developing countries where health and nutrition are poor. Rickets and osteomalacia, poorly healed pelvic fractures, spinal abnormalities (such as major degrees of kyphosis or scoliosis), poliomyelitis and congenital malformations are very rare in the West.

Other pelvic abnormalities

Rarely, a pelvic mass such as an ovarian tumour or uterine fibroid blocks the descent of the head. This will be palpable vaginally and Caesarean section is indicated.

The cervix

The role of the cervix is to prevent the fetus from literally dropping out before term: the rare cervical incompetence [→ p.158] causes painless preterm delivery. During normal labour, it is not simply the strength of contractions that removes this natural obstruction but a complex mechanism involving hydration of the cervical collagen. The cervix itself, in addition to the contractions, may determine the course of labour, but the clinical relevance of this remains poorly understood.

Care of the fetus

Permanent fetal damage attributable to labour is uncommon: only about 10% of cases of cerebral palsy are attributed solely to intrapartum problems. Nevertheless fetal death or damage, usually neurological, has devastating effects. There are several causes of damage:
1 Fetal hypoxia, commonly described as 'distress', is the best known.
2 Infection in labour, e.g. Group B streptococcus [→ p.134].
3 Meconium aspiration leads to chemical pneumonitis.
4 Trauma is rarely spontaneous and more commonly due to obstetric intervention, e.g. forceps.
5 Fetal blood loss [→ p.166].

Fetal distress

Definition

The term 'fetal distress' is a clinical diagnosis made by indirect methods. It should be defined as *hypoxia that might result in fetal damage or death if not reversed or the fetus delivered urgently*, but the term is widely abused. In reality hypoxia is simply the best known cause of intrapartum fetal damage and its effects are unpredictable and vary considerably. The convention is that a pH of <7.20 in the fetal scalp blood (see below) indicates significant hypoxia.

Aetiology

Why hypoxia occurs is poorly understood. Contractions temporarily reduce placental perfusion and may compress the umbilical cord, so longer labours and those with excessive time (>1 h) spent pushing are more likely to produce hypoxia. Acute hypoxa in labour can be due to placental abruption, hypertonic uterine states and the use of oxytocin, prolapse of the umbilical cord and maternal hypotension.

Epidemiology

Prediction of the 'at-risk' fetus is imprecise. Intrapartum risk factors include long labour, meconium, the use of epidurals and oxytocin; antepartum factors include the high-risk pregnancy. Fetuses with these risk factors are usually monitored in labour with cardiotocography (CTG).

Diagnosing fetal distress

As hypoxia is a relatively rare cause of handicap, the effects of attempts to prevent it will be limited.

The diagnosis of fetal distress is usually made from the finding of significant fetal acidosis (scalp pH < 7.20) or ominous FHR abnormalities. The following are methods employed in the detection of fetal distress.

Colour of the liquor: meconium

Meconium is the bowel contents of the fetus that stains the amniotic fluid. It is rare in preterm fetuses but common (30%) after 42 weeks. Meconium very diluted in amniotic fluid is seldom significant, but with undiluted meconium ('pea-soup') perinatal mortality is increased fourfold. Nevertheless, the presence or absence of meconium is not a reliable indicator of fetal well being (*Obstet Gynecol* 2003; **102**: 89). It is an indication for caution because (i) the fetus may aspirate it, causing meconium aspiration syndrome and (ii) because hypoxia is more likely.

Fetal heart rate (FHR) auscultation

The heart is auscultated every 15 min with a Pinard's stethoscope (Fig. 29.8) or a hand-held Doppler for 60 s after a contraction. The distressed or potentially distressed fetus normally exhibits abnormal heart rate patterns, which can be heard. This method of intrapartum fetal surveillance is appropriate for low-risk pregnancies, and if abnormalities are detected, CTG is indicated.

Cardiotocography (CTG)

Cardiotocography records the FHR on paper, either from a transducer placed on the abdomen or from a clip or probe in the vagina attached to the fetal scalp. Another transducer synchronously records the uterine contractions. Interpretation is complex and difficult, requiring experience. A combination of abnormal patterns increases the likelihood of fetal distress. There are several important features:

Baseline rate: This should be 110–160 beats per minute. *Tachycardias* are associated with fever, fetal infection,

and partial motor blockade from the upper abdomen downwards is the norm. It is therefore suitable both for the entire labour as well as obstetric procedures.

Advantages

This is the only method in labour that can make women pain-free and is very popular. It can also be advised on purely medical grounds, if labour is long, to help reduce blood pressure in hypertensive women, to abolish a premature urge to push, and as analgesia for instrumental delivery or Caesarean section.

Contraindications to epidural analgesia

Sepsis
Coagulopathy or anticoagulant therapy (unless low-dose heparin)
Active neurological disease
Spinal abnormalities
Hypovolaemia

Disadvantages

Increased midwifery supervision is needed to check the blood pressure and pulse regularly. The woman is bedbound, although low-dose regimes in combination with spinal blockade allow some mobility. Reduced bladder sensation causes urinary retention. Maternal fever is more common. The Caesarean section rate is not increased, although instrumental delivery rates appear to be (*Cochrane* 2000: CD000331), particularly if the passive second stage is not modified [→ p.206]. Transient hypotension (*BJOG* 2002; **109**: 274) is minimized if intravenous fluid is given first. Transient fetal bradycardias are also common, but seldom precipitate fetal distress. There is little evidence for an association between epidural analgesia and back pain after delivery.

Major complications of technique

'Spinal tap' (0.5%) is inadvertent puncture of the dura mater causing leakage of CSF and often a severe headache. This can be treated by the administration of a 'blood patch' to seal the leak. Very rarely, inadvertent intravenous injection produces convulsions and cardiac arrest. Or inadvertent injection of local anaesthetic into the CSF combined with progression up the spinal cord causes 'total spinal analgesia' and respiratory paralysis.

Epidural analgesia is very safe in expert hands but needs increased midwifery care and modification of the second stage of labour.

Problems with epidurals

Spinal tap
Total spinal analgesia
Hypotension
Local anaesthetic toxicity
Higher instrumental delivery rate
Poor mobility
Urinary retention
Maternal fever

Mental health in labour

Environment: This need not be too clinical. Resuscitation equipment can be hidden. Music and privacy may help. More women now choose to deliver at home [→ p.208]. *The birth attendant*: The continuous presence of a midwife is reassuring. This reduces the length of labour, the use of analgesia, and the augmentation and Caesarean section rates (*Cochrane* 2002: CD000199). Continuous support, explanation and encouragement are needed.

The partner or accompanying person is an important potential source of support for the woman. He/she may need support too.

Control: Women have differing expectations of labour. Some want labour to be safe, quick and reasonably painless. Others have definite views, either because they view labour as a positive experience rather than a means to an end or because they have preconceptions based on other people's experiences. They should be encouraged to write their views on a 'birth plan', which can be discussed so that expectations are realistic and the woman does not regard deviation from the plan as failure. Most requests in uncomplicated labour can then be safely accommodated as most labours need little or no intervention. If an unwanted intervention becomes necessary, adequate explanation is important.

Physical health in labour

Observations: The temperature, pulse and blood pressure should be monitored. If abnormal, or the circumstances predispose to abnormalities (e.g. epidural), measurement should be more frequent. Hypotension associated with epidural analgesia will respond to intravenous fluids ± ephedrine; hypertension should be treated as antenatally.

Pyrexia in labour: This is best defined as >37.5°C. This is associated with an increased risk of neonatal illness and is not always a result of chorioamnionitis. It is more common with epidural analgesia and prolonged labour. Cultures of the vagina, urine and blood are taken. Intravenous antibiotics and antipyretics are normally administered.

Hydration: Dehydration in labour is common and women should be encouraged to drink water. Intravenous fluid is also necessary if an epidural is used or if labour is prolonged.

Stomach and food: Eating is often discouraged because stomach contents can be aspirated (Mendelson's syndrome) if a general anaesthetic is required. Ranitidine is often given to reduce the stomach acidity. However, general anaesthesia should rarely be used in obstetric practice, and routine starvation of women in labour is inhumane.

Mobility and delivery positions: Freedom of movement is encouraged. Most women deliver semi-recumbent: squatting, kneeling or the left-lateral position all increase the dimensions of the pelvic outlet. Pregnant women should never lie flat on their back: the gravid uterus compresses the main blood vessels, reducing cardiac output and causing hypotension, and often fetal distress. This is called aortocaval compression (Fig. 29.13) and in the supine position it is prevented by maintaining at least 15° left lateral tilt.

The urinary tract: Neglected retention of urine can irreversibly damage the detrusor muscle [→ p.55]. An epidural usually removes bladder sensation. The woman must be encouraged to micturate frequently in labour; if she has an epidural, catheterization may be needed. Routine catheterization of all, however, is unnecessary.

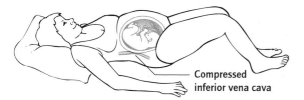

Fig. 29.13 Aortocaval compression. If the patient is allowed to lie flat on her back, the inferior vena cava is compressed.

Conduct of labour

Initiation of labour

The woman is advised to admit herself or to call the midwife if painful contractions are regular and at 5–10 min intervals, or if the membranes have ruptured. A brief history of the pregnancy and past obstetric history is taken, and temperature, blood pressure, pulse and urinalysis are recorded. The presentation is checked and a vaginal examination is performed to check for cervical effacement and dilatation to confirm the diagnosis of labour. The degree of descent is also assessed. The colour of any leaking liquor is noted. Every 15 min, the fetal heart is listened to for 1 min following a contraction; if the pregnancy is high risk or meconium is seen, a CTG [→ p.199] is started. Routine shaving or the administration of an enema are obsolete.

The diagnosis of labour

Painful contractions with effacement and dilatation of cervix
Painful contractions with show and/or ruptured membranes suggestive

---

First stage of labour (Fig. 29.14)
The mother

The mother is made comfortable and encouraged to remain mobile. The supine position is avoided. Continuous support, attention and explanation are needed. Analgesia is given as requested: commonly this is epidural. The vital signs and fluid balance are monitored; catheterization is often needed if an epidural is used, but it should not be routine.

The fetus

The colour of the liquor is observed. The fetal heart is auscultated for 60 s after a contraction every 15 min; or it is monitored with CTG if the pregnancy is 'high risk', a heart rate abnormality is detected, or if labour is longer than about 5 h. If the heart rate pattern is abnormal, the fetus may be hypoxic. Oxygen, intravenous fluid and the left lateral position (to avoid aortocaval compression) are used. Any oxytocin is usually stopped. If the abnormal heart rate pattern persists, a fetal scalp blood sample is taken. If there is fetal distress (i.e. scalp blood pH <

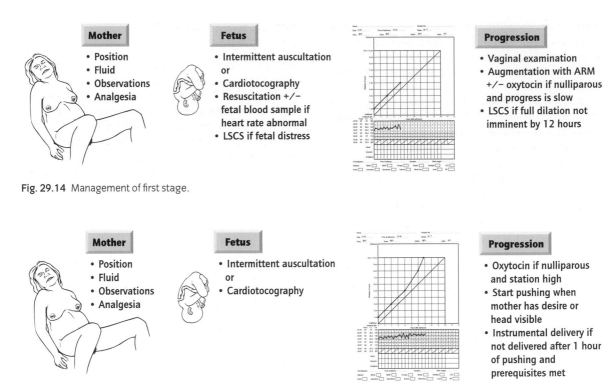

Fig. 29.14 Management of first stage.

Fig. 29.15 Management of second stage.

7.20), expedition of delivery in the first stage can only be accomplished by Caesarean section.

Progress

Progress is assessed by 2–4-hourly vaginal examination. Dilatation is estimated digitally in centimetres; descent of the head is measured by its relationship to the ischial spines: these measurements are recorded on the partogram. Slow dilatation after the latent phase (<1 cm/h) is normally an indication for artificial rupture of the membranes (ARM or amniotomy). If progress continues to be slow, oxytocin is used in a nulliparous woman, but in a multiparous woman a malpresentation or malposition must be carefully excluded first. If the cervix is not fully dilated by 12 h, Caesarean delivery is usually appropriate unless delivery can be anticipated in the next hour or two.

Second stage of labour (Fig. 29.15)

If an epidural is *in situ*, it is normal to wait at least an hour before pushing, and oxytocin is administered if the woman is nulliparous and descent is poor. If there is no epidural, 'non-directed' pushing is encouraged only when the mother has the desire or the head is visible. If numb from an epidural, the mother is encouraged to push about three times for about 15 s during each contraction. If the baby is not delivered after 1 h of pushing, instrumental vaginal delivery is normally indicated. Fetal distress is normally diagnosed in the same manner as for the first stage, but expedition of delivery is usually possible with the ventouse or forceps. Careful assessment is required to ensure that all the prerequisites [→ p.217] for this are met.

Normal delivery

As the head approaches the perineum, the attendant's hands are scrubbed and gloved and the perineum is cleaned. The mother should be however she feels most comfortable, but *not* flat on her back. The routine use of an episiotomy has no benefit (*Cochrane* 2000: CD000081) and episiotomy should be reserved for where there is fetal distress, progress is slow or a large tear is likely. If episiotomy is to be performed, the perineum is infiltrated with 1% lidocaine (lignocaine) and a 3-cm cut is made with scissors from the centre of the fourchette to the (mother's) right side of the perineum (Fig. 29.16).

A swab is pushed against ('guarding') the perineum as the head distends it, and the patient is asked to stop pushing and to pant slowly. This enables a controlled and slow delivery of the head and reduces perineal damage. Once all the head is delivered, the airways are sucked out if meconium is present. The head then restitutes. With the next contraction, maternal pushing and gentle downward traction on the head lead to delivery of the anterior shoulder; traction is then directed upwards to deliver the posterior shoulder, once again guarding the perineum. Unless it requires resuscitation, the baby is delivered onto the mother's bare abdomen and kept warm; the umbilical cord need not be clamped and cut immediately (Fig. 29.17).

Third stage of labour (Fig. 29.18)

Oxytocin is administered intramuscularly to help the uterus contract once the shoulders are delivered (*BJOG* 1996; **103**: 1068) (not until after the last fetus if it is a multiple pregnancy). Once placental separation is evident from lengthening of the cord and the passage of blood, continuous gentle traction on the cord allows delivery of the placenta (controlled cord traction). At the same time, the left hand pushes down suprapubically to prevent uterine inversion [→ p.223]. If the placenta cannot be delivered after an hour, it should be 'manually removed' with a hand in the uterus under general or spinal anaesthesia. The placenta is checked for missing cotyledons and the vagina and perineum for tears.

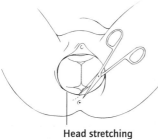

Head stretching the perineum

Fig. 29.16 Episiotomy.

Perineal trauma and suturing (Fig. 29.19)

The perineum is intact in about a third of nulliparous women and in half of multiparous women. A *first-degree tear* involves minor damage to the fourchette and is not normally repaired. *Second-degree tears* and *episiotomies* involve perineal muscle. They are sutured with subcuticular dexon or vicryl (*Cochrane* 2000: CD000006) using lidocaine if the perineum is not already anaesthetized. *Third-degree tears* involve the external anal sphincter as well and occur in 2.5% of deliveries. Forceps and large

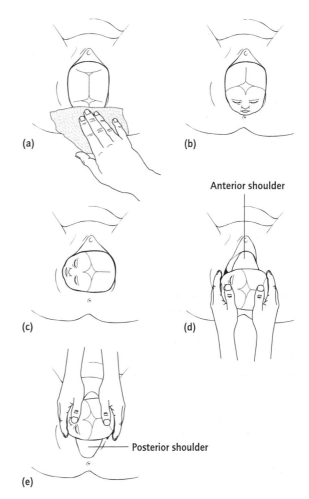

(a) (b)

Anterior shoulder

(c) (d)

Posterior shoulder

(e)

Fig. 29.17 Normal delivery. (a) 'Guarding' the perineum as the head distends it. (b) The head delivers. (c) The head restitutes. (d) The anterior shoulder is delivered by gentle downward traction until the next contraction. (e) The posterior shoulder is delivered by gentle upward traction.

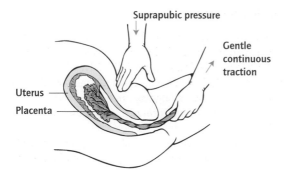

Fig. 29.18 Management of third stage. Delivery of the placenta.

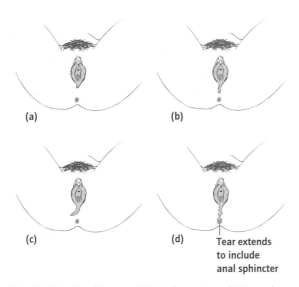

Fig. 29.19 Perineal trauma. (a) First-degree tear. (b) Second-degree tear. (c) Mediolateral episiotomy. (d) Third-degree tear.

babies are the main risk factors. The sphincter is repaired under epidural or spinal anaesthetic. *Fourth-degree* tears also involve the anal mucosa. A rectal and vaginal examination excludes sutures that are too deep and retained swabs respectively. The mother is then cleaned, made comfortable and encouraged to breastfeed if she wishes. Maternal observation should continue for several hours.

Natural approaches to labour

Childbirth is a major life event. Whilst safety is the most important factor, it is usually taken for granted. The ex-

perience can be 'negative' for other reasons, particularly if the woman is immobile and attached to monitors or 'drips'. This can even have medical consequences such as postnatal depression. Whilst the safety of childbirth has increased, this cannot all be attributed to the increased 'medicalization' that has occurred in the last few years, much of which has been without scientific basis. There is increasing pressure among women to be allowed more choice and participation in decisions about their labours: now that labour is safer, we should try to make it more rewarding.

Home birth

Progress and fetal condition are monitored in the normal way and non-epidural analgesia may be administered. If intervention is required, the woman is transferred to hospital. It is suitable for low-risk, preferably multiparous women, and in those with a planned, rather than inadvertent home birth, safety does not appear to be compromised. Suitable plans for transport into hospital are important, should this become necessary.

Water birth (Fig. 29.20)

The labour and delivery are conducted in a large bath of water maintained at 37°C. Water is relaxing and analgesic. The baby is delivered under water and does not breathe until brought rapidly to the surface. It is used for motivated low-risk women, provided that trained personnel are available. Intermittent auscultation and vaginal examinations are easily performed under water. There is inadequate evidence regarding the safety of this method.

Fast labour: 'active management'

This was developed to reduce the length of labour. The principles apply to nulliparous women and are: (i) early diagnosis of labour, (ii) 2-hourly vaginal examinations, (iii) early correction of slow progress with amniotomy and oxytocin (augmentation), and (iv) Caesarean section by 12 h if delivery is not imminent. In addition, there is one-to-one midwifery care, a comprehensive antenatal education programme and continuous audit. Early augmentation minimizes the effect of inefficient uterine action. This shortens labour and the 'latent phase' [→ p.191] so long as it is only used once the cervix is fully effaced. Prolonged labour is rare and Caesarean and vaginal operative delivery rates are low.

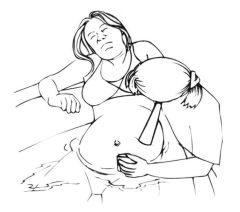

Fig. 29.20 Water birth.

The policy has been criticised. The length of labour is undoubtedly reduced, however, trials have failed to show a consistent reduction in Caesarean sections (*NEJM* 1995; **333**: 745). Perhaps the most important aspects are consistent methods of care, continuous audit and the fact that only senior midwifery and medical staff make management decisions.

Avoiding labour: Caesarean section for maternal request

For a discussion, see page 219.

Criteria for home birth
Woman's request
'Low risk' on basis of antenatal or past obstetric and medical complications
37–41 weeks
Cephalic presentation
Clear liquor
Normal fetal heart rate (FHR)
All maternal observations normal

Further reading

Bewley S, Cockburn J. The unethics of 'request' Caesarean section. *BJOG: an International Journal of Obstetrics and Gynaecology* 2002; **109**: 593–6.

Eltzschig HK, Lieberman ES, Camann WR. Regional anesthesia and analgesia for labor and delivery. *The New England Journal of Medicine* 2003; **348**: 319–32.

Friedman EA. Primigravid labor: a graphicostatistical analysis. *Obstetrics and Gynecology* 1955; **6**: 567–89.

Hodnett ED. Caregiver support for women during childbirth. *Cochrane Database System Review (Online: Update Software)* 2002; **1**: CD000199.

Hodnett ED. Home-like versus conventional institutional settings for birth. *Cochrane Database System Review (Online: Update Software)* 2001; **4**: CD000012.

Hodnett ED. Pain and women's satisfaction with the experience of childbirth: a systematic review. *American Journal of Obstetrics and Gynecology* 2002; **186**(Suppl. 5): S160–72.

National Institute of Clinical Excellence (NICE). The use of electronic fetal monitoring. *Inherited Guideline C.* 2001. www.nice.org.uk

Nelson KB. Infection, inflammation and the risk of cerebral palsy. *Current Opinion in Neurology* 2000; **13**: 133–9.

Royal College of Obstetricians and Gynaecologists. *The Royal College of Obstetricians and Gynaecologists Statement 2001: Birth in Water.* London: The Royal College of Obstetricians and Gynaecologists Press, 2001. www.rcog.org.uk

Thacker SB, Stroup D, Chang M. Continuous electronic heart rate monitoring for fetal assessment during labor. *Cochrane Database System Review (Online: Update Software)* 2001; **2**: CD000063.

World Health Organization. Partograph in management of labour. World Health Organization Maternal Health and Safe Motherhood Programme. *Lancet* 1994; **343**: 1399–404.

Slow Progress in Labour at a Glance

Definitions	'Slow labour' is progress slower than 1 cm/h after latent phase 'Prolonged labour' is >12 h duration after latent phase	
Epidemiology	Common in nulliparous women; rare in multiparous	
Aetiology	Powers:	Inefficient uterine action
	Passenger:	Fetal size, disorder of rotation, e.g. occipito-transverse (OT), occipito-posterior (OP) Disorder of flexion, e.g. brow
	Passage:	Cephalo-pelvic disproportion, rarely cervical resistance
Management	Nulliparous:	Amniotomy; oxytocin
	Multiparous:	Amniotomy; oxytocin if malpresentation/malposition excluded
	If this fails:	Caesarean section if first stage Instrumental delivery if second stage (if prerequisites met)

Occipito-posterior (OP) Position at a Glance

Definition	Abnormality of rotation, with face upwards. Some extension common
Epidemiology	5% of deliveries, more common in early labour
Aetiology	Idiopathic, inefficient uterine action, pelvic variants
Features	Slow labour. Back pain, early desire to push. Occiput posterior on vaginal examination
Management	Nil required if progress normal If slow progress, amniotomy and oxytocin If these fail in first stage, Caesarean section If second stage, >1 h of pushing, instrumental delivery if criteria met

Fetal Monitoring in Labour at a Glance

Modes of fetal injury	Hypoxia, meconium aspiration, trauma, infection/?inflammation, blood loss
Fetal distress	Hypoxia that may result in fetal damage or death if not reversed or the fetus delivered urgently
High-risk situations	Fetal conditions, e.g. intrauterine growth restriction (IUGR), prolonged pregnancy Medical complications, e.g. diabetes and pre-eclampsia Intrapartum factors: long labours, presence of meconium

Monitoring methods	Intermittent auscultation (IA), inspection for meconium:
	
	If IA abnormal or high-risk situation: cardiotocography (CTG)
	
	    Normal features: rate 110–160, accelerations, variability >5 beats per minute
	
	    Abnormal features: tachy- or bradycardias, decelerations, reduced variability
	
	If CTG abnormal: resuscitate, fetal blood sample

Intervention	If fetal blood sample abnormal, delivery by quickest route:
	    Caesarean section if first stage
	    Instrumental vaginal delivery if second stage and criteria met

Pain Relief in Labour at a Glance

Types	Non-medical:	Support, transcutaneous electrical nerve stimulation (TENS), water
	Medical:	Entonox, opiates, epidural
Epidural	Injection of local anaesthetic into epidural space:	
	Advantages:	Best pain relief. Prevents premature pushing
	Disadvantages:	Increased supervision, maternal fever, reduced mobility, increased instrumental delivery rate, hypotension, urinary retention
	Complications:	Spinal tap, 'total spinal analgesia', local anaesthetic toxicity
	Contraindications:	Sepsis, coagulopathy, active neurological disease, hypovolaemia, spinal abnormalities, cardiac outflow obstruction

Labour 3: Special Circumstances

Induction of labour

Labour that is started artificially is induced. It is different from augmentation [→ p.195], when the contractions of established labor are strengthened. Theoretically, induction is performed in situations where allowing the pregnancy to continue would expose the fetus and/or mother to risk greater than that of induction. In practice, there are many instances when labour is induced and quantification of risk is virtually impossible.

Methods of induction

Whether induction is successful depends on the state, or 'favourability', of the cervix. This is related to 'consistency', the degree of effacement or early dilatation, how low in the pelvis the head is (station) and the cervical position (anterior or posterior within the vagina). These are often scored out of 10, as the 'Bishop's score': the lower the score, the more unfavorable the cervix (Fig. 30.1). Transvaginal assessment of cervical length may also be used (*Ultrasound Obstet Gynecol* 2001; **18**: 623).

Induction with prostaglandins

Prostaglandin E_2 (PGE$_2$) gel (normally 2 mg) is inserted into the posterior vaginal fornix. Misoprostol [→ p.97] is cheaper and slightly more effective but, as hyperstimulation is more common (*Cochrane* 2003: CD000941), concerns regarding safety remain. Medical induction is the best method in most nulliparous women, and in multiparous women when the cervix is very unfavorable. It either starts labour, or the 'favourability' of the cervix is improved and amniotomy is used.

Induction with amniotomy ± oxytocin

The forewaters are ruptured with an instrument called an amnihook. An oxytocin infusion is then usually started within 2 h if labour has not ensued (*Cochrane* 2001: CD003250). Oxytocin is used alone if spontaneous rupture of the membranes has already occurred [→ p.214].

Methods of induction	
Medical:	Prostaglandins/misoprostol
	Oxytocin (after membrane rupture)
Surgical:	Amniotomy

Natural induction

Cervical sweeping involves passing a finger through the cervix and 'stripping' between the membranes and the lower segment of the uterus (Fig. 30.2). At 40 weeks, this reduces the chance of induction and postdates pregnancy (*Cochrane* 2001: CD000451). However, it can be uncomfortable.

Indications for induction

In practice the decision to induce, and the choice of method and timing, are dependent on each individual case.

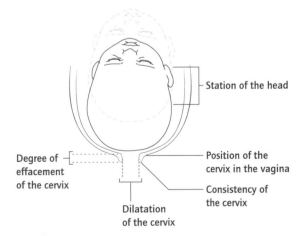

Fig. 30.1 The Bishop's score.

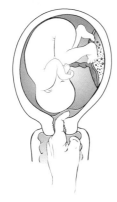

Fig. 30.2 Sweeping the membranes. A finger is inserted through the cervix and rotated: the membranes are peeled off the lower segment.

Fetal indications include high-risk situations such as prolonged pregnancy [→ p.174], suspected IUGR or compromise [→ p.169], antepartum hemorrhage, poor obstetric history and prelabour term rupture of the membranes [→ p.214].

Materno–fetal indications, where both mother and fetus should benefit, include pre-eclampsia and maternal disease such as diabetes. *Maternal indications* are social reasons and *in utero* death.

Common indications for induction
Prolonged pregnancy
Suspected growth restriction
Prelabour term rupture of the membranes
Pre-eclampsia
Medical disease: hypertension and diabetes

Complications

Labour may fail to start or be slow due to inefficient uterine activity. The risk of instrumental delivery or Caesarean section is probably higher, even allowing for the higher-risk pregnancies. Paradoxically, over-activity of the uterus can occur. This hyperstimulation is rare but can result in fetal distress and even uterine rupture. The umbilical cord can prolapse [→ p.221] at amniotomy. Postpartum hemorrhage (PPH) is more likely, as is intrapartum and postpartum infection. Iatrogenic prematurity can follow, by accident (incorrect gestation) or design.

Contraindications

Absolute contraindications include acute fetal compromise, abnormal lie, placenta praevia, or pelvic obstruction such as a pelvic mass, or pelvic deformity causing cephalo-pelvic disproportion. It is usually considered inappropriate after more than one Caesarean section.

Relative contraindications include one previous Caesarean section and prematurity.

Labour after a previous Caesarean section

Many Caesarean sections are elective procedures done solely because a Caesarean was performed previously. After two Caesareans, or if there is a vertical uterine scar, vaginal delivery is not usually attempted in the United Kingdom as scar rupture [→ p.221] is more common.

Factors influencing vaginal delivery after one Caesarean section

About 60–80% of all women who had a Caesarean in their last pregnancy will achieve a vaginal delivery if allowed to labour (*BMJ* 1987: 1645). The indication for the original Caesarean has only a small influence: if performed for slow progress, success rates are the lowest; if for breech, they are the highest. No factor is entirely predictive of success, but repeat Caesarean in labour is more likely if the woman has not also previously had a vaginal delivery, or the second fetus is larger or if the head is not engaged.

Safety of vaginal delivery after Caesarean section

In women who have had a previous Caesarean, maternal morbidity and mortality are lower with a vaginal delivery than with a repeat elective Caesarean. Many women are more emotionally satisfied, although some fear another labour. Costs are much lower. The principal risk is that another Caesarean will be required after several hours of labour, and this has a higher maternal morbidity and is unpleasant. Rupture of the uterine scar (Fig. 30.3) occasionally occurs (0.5%), although this contributes little to overall perinatal mortality. The risk of

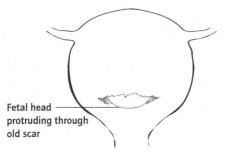

Fetal head protruding through old scar

Fig. 30.3 Rupture of scar from previous Caesarean section.

rupture is related to the thickness of the lower uterine segment (*Lancet* 1996; **347**: 281).

Deciding on mode of delivery with a previous Caesarean section

Women should be fully appraised of the risks of labour in this situation. In the absence of robust evidence, it is usual for them to decide on the mode of delivery.

Management of labour after a Caesarean section

Hospital delivery and cardiotocography (CTG) are advised because of the risk of scar rupture. Epidural analgesia is safe, but induction and augmentation require caution and labour should not be prolonged. Scar rupture usually presents as fetal distress, sometimes accompanied by pain, cessation of contractions, vaginal bleeding, and even maternal collapse. Immediate laparotomy and Caesarean is indicated if rupture is suspected.

Prelabour term rupture of the membranes

In 10% of women after 37 weeks, the membranes rupture before the onset of labour. The reason is unknown in the majority of patients. This is to be distinguished from prelabour *preterm* rupture of the membranes [→ p.160], when the fetus is not mature.

Diagnosis of prelabour term rupture of the membranes

Typically, there is a gush of clear fluid, which is followed

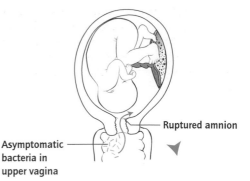

Ruptured amnion

Asymptomatic bacteria in upper vagina

Fig. 30.4 Ascending infection can complicate prelabour rupture of the membranes.

by an uncontrollable intermittent trickle. This is occasionally initially confused with urinary incontinence. The diagnosis, however, is seldom in doubt, although the finding of reduced liquor volume on ultrasound may help. A few have only a "hindwater" rupture: that is, liquor is definitely leaking, but membranes remain present in front of the fetal head.

Risks of prelabour term rupture of the membranes

Only 20% of women do not labour spontaneously within 24 h of membrane rupture. At this stage prematurity is not a problem. Cord prolapse is rare and usually a complication of transverse lie or breech presentation. There is a small but definite risk of neonatal infection: this is increased by vaginal examination (Fig. 30.4), the presence of Group B streptococcus and increased duration of membrane rupture (*AmJOG* 1998; **179**: 635).

Management

Confirmation is made by collection of liquor. The lie and presentation are checked. Digital vaginal examination is usually avoided, but may be performed in a sterile manner if there is a risk of cord prolapse (abnormal lie or fetal distress); a vaginal swab is used to screen for infection. Cardiotocography is performed. Induction of labour at this stage, with oxytocin rather than PGE_2 (*Cochrane* 2000: CD000159), is probably safer for the neonate (*NEJM* 1996; **334**: 1005) but is seldom practised. More often the onset of spontaneous labour is awaited, at least up to 24 h. The maternal pulse, temperature and fetal heart rate are measured every 4 h. After

18 h, it is usual to prescribe antibiotics as a prophylaxis against Group B streptococcus [→ p.134] unless the presence of this bacterium in the vagina and rectum has recently been excluded using swabs. The presence of meconium or evidence of infection warrants immediate induction.

Further reading

Flamm BL. Vaginal birth after Caesarean (VBAC). *Best Practice & Research. Clinical Obstetrics & Gynecology* 2001; **15**: 81–92.

Hannah ME, Ohlsson A, Farine D *et al.* Induction of labor compared with expectant management for prelabor rupture of the membranes at term. TERMPROM Study Group. *The New England Journal of Medicine* 1996; **334**: 1005–10.

Rayburn WF, Zhang J. Rising rates of labor induction: present concerns and future strategies. *Obstetrics and Gynecology* 2002; **100**: 164–7.

Delivery after Caesarean Section at a Glance

Incidence	Many still undergo elective Caesarean; usual practice if >1
Success	60–80% vaginal delivery rate if labour attempted
Contraindications	Vertical uterine scar; usual indications for Caesarean
Safety	Emergency Caesarean section risk 20–40% Fetal mortality not increased; maternal morbidity lower Scar rupture rate 0.5%
Management	Cardiotocography (CTG), careful monitoring of progress

Induction of Labour at a Glance

Definition	Labour is started artificially	
Methods	Vaginal prostaglandin E_2 (PGE_2)/misoprostol; amniotomy and oxytocin	
Main indications	Fetal:	Prolonged pregnancy, prelabor term spontaneous rupture of membranes (SROM), intrauterine growth restriction (IUGR)
	Materno–fetal:	Pre-eclampsia, diabetes
	Maternal:	Social
Contraindications	Absolute acute fetal distress, where elective Caesarean indicated Relative: previous lower segment Caesarean section (LSCS); unfavourable cervix	
Complications	LSCS, other interventions in labour, longer labour, hyperstimulation, postpartum hemorrhage (PPH)	

Prelabour Term Rupture of the Membranes at a Glance

Definition	Membranes rupture after 37 weeks before the onset of labour
Incidence	10%: 80% start labour in <24 h
Features	Gush of fluid. Check temperature, lie/presentation. Avoid vaginal examination
Investigations	Cardiotocography (CTG), high vaginal swab (HVS)
Management	Antibiotics if >18 h duration. Consider immediate induction or wait 24 h

31 Instrumental and Operative Delivery

Forceps or ventouse delivery

These allow the use of traction if delivery needs to be expedited in the second stage of labour. The shape of the pelvis will only allow delivery if the occiput is anterior [→ p.189], or occasionally posterior. Rotation is therefore sometimes also needed. No instrument can drag a fetus that is too large through the pelvis, and technique and judgement are required. The aim is to shorten a long second stage or make labour safer for the fetus or mother.

Ventouse

Also known as the vacuum extractor, this consists of a rubber or metal cap, connected to a handle; the cap is fixed near the fetal occiput by suction (Fig. 31.1). Traction during maternal pushing will deliver the occipito-anterior (OA) positioned head, but also usually allows the shape of the pelvis to simultaneously rotate a malpositioned head to the OA position. The ventouse is the instrument of choice for most instrumental deliveries, the metal ventouse being most suitable for more difficult deliveries.

Obstetric forceps

These come in pairs that fit together for use. Each has a 'blade', shank, lock and handle. When assembled, the blades fit around the fetal head and the handles fit together (Fig. 31.2). The lock prevents them from slipping apart. *Non-rotational forceps* grip the head in whatever position it is and allow traction. They are therefore only suitable when the occiput is anterior. These forceps have a 'cephalic' curve for the head and a 'pelvic curve' which follows the sacral curve. *Rotational forceps* have no pelvic curve and enable a malpositioned head to be rotated by the operator to the OA position, before traction is applied.

Safety of ventouse and forceps

Failure: Both methods of delivery can fail: this is more common with the ventouse, particularly if the cup is placed inaccurately.

Maternal complications and the need for analgesia are greater with forceps (*Cochrane* 2000: CD000224), but use of either instrument can cause vaginal laceration, blood loss or third-degree tears [→ p.207] (*BJOG*

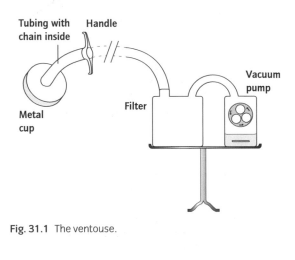

Fig. 31.1 The ventouse.

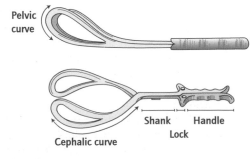

Fig. 31.2 Forceps.

1996; **103**: 845). Cervical and uterine tears are very rare.

Fetal complications are slightly worse with the ventouse. An unsightly 'chignon', a swelling of the area of scalp that was drawn into the cup by suction is usual. It diminishes over a period of hours, but a mark may be visible for days. Scalp lacerations, cephalhaematomata and neonatal jaundice are more common with the ventouse. Facial bruising, facial nerve damage and even skull and neck fractures occasionally occur with injudicious use of forceps, and prolonged traction by either instrument is dangerous.

Indications for instrumental vaginal delivery

Prolonged second stage is the most common indication. Instrumental vaginal delivery is usual if 1 h of pushing (active second stage) has failed to deliver the baby. If the mother is exhausted it may be performed earlier. The length of passive second stage is less important.

Fetal distress: This is more common in the second stage: delivery can be expedited.

Prophylactic use of instrumental vaginal delivery is indicated to prevent pushing in some women with medical problems such as severe cardiac disease or hypertension. *In a breech* delivery [→ p.179], forceps are often applied to the after-coming head to control the delivery.

Types of instrumental vaginal delivery

The type of delivery (and to a certain extent the instrument itself) is determined by the *position* and *descent* of the head. If moderate traction does not produce immediate and progressive descent, Caesarean section is indicated. 'High' forceps deliveries (the head is still palpable abdominally) are dangerous and obsolete.

Low-cavity delivery

The head is well below the level of the ischial spines, bony prominences palpable vaginally on the lateral wall of the mid-pelvis [→ p.187] and is usually OA (Fig. 31.3a). A pudendal block [→ p.203] with perineal infiltration is usually sufficient analgesia.

Mid-cavity delivery

The head is still not palpable abdominally, but is at or just below the level of the ischial spines (Fig. 31.3a). Epidural or spinal anaesthesia are usual. The position may be OA, occipito-transverse (OT) or occipito-

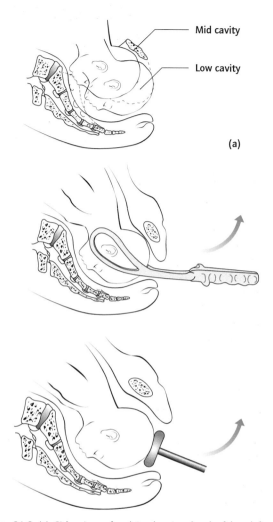

Fig. 31.3 (a) Side view of pelvis showing level of head for mid-cavity and low-cavity forceps delivery. (b) Forceps and ventouse in position on the fetal head showing direction of traction.

posterior (OP): the latter two are malpositions and can be corrected by manual rotation or using the ventouse. The OP position is occasionally corrected by rotation 180° with rotational (Kielland's) forceps and delivered. Few operators now use these forceps, preferring the safer, but sometimes less successful, ventouse (Fig. 31.3b). If there is any doubt that delivery will be successful, it is attempted in the operating theatre, with full preparations for a Caesarean section. This is called a 'trial' of forceps or ventouse.

Common indications for ventouse or forceps delivery
Prolonged active second stage Maternal exhaustion Fetal distress in second stage

Prerequisites for instrumental vaginal delivery

Both forceps and the ventouse are potentially dangerous instruments and their use is subject to stringent conditions. *The head must not be palpable abdominally* (therefore deeply engaged); on vaginal examination the head must be *at or below the level of the ischial spines. The cervix must be fully dilated*: the second stage must have been reached (occasional exceptions are made by experts delivering with the ventouse for fetal distress). *The position of the head must be known*: incorrect placement of forceps or ventouse may cause fetal and maternal trauma as well as result in failure. There must be *adequate analgesia*. The *bladder should be empty*: catheterization is normally required. The operator must be skilled and delivering for a *valid reason*.

Prerequisites for ventouse or forceps delivery
Head not palpable abdominally Head at/below ischial spines on vaginal examination Cervix fully dilated Position of head known Adequate analgesia Valid indication for delivery Bladder empty

Instrumental delivery rates

A 'normal' vaginal delivery usually produces less blood loss, requires less analgesia and is safer and more pleasant for mother and baby unless a valid indication for intervention is present. In the United Kingdom, approximately 20% of nulliparous and 2% of multiparous women are delivered by forceps or ventouse. The need for instrumental delivery can be reduced in several ways: encouragement from midwives; altering maternal position; antenatal education; using oxytocin for slow progress in the second stage; and allowing a longer passive second stage when an epidural is present.

Caesarean section

Delivery by Caesarean section occurs for 15–25% of babies in the developed world. The usual operation is the lower segment operation (lower segment Caesarean section; LSCS), in which the abdominal wall is opened with a suprapubic transverse incision and the lower segment of the uterus is also incised transversely to deliver the baby (Fig. 31.4). Very occasionally, the uterus is incised vertically and this is called a classical Caesarean section. After delivery of the placenta, the uterus and abdomen are sutured. A trial (CAESAR) examining different surgical techniques is in progress.

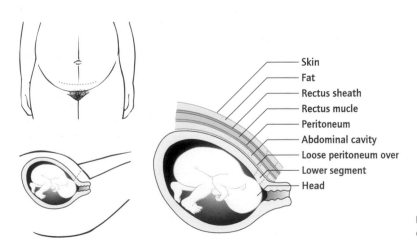

Skin
Fat
Rectus sheath
Rectus mucle
Peritoneum
Abdominal cavity
Loose peritoneum over
Lower segment
Head

Fig. 31.4 Layers of the abdominal wall for delivery of fetus by Caesarean section.

Safety of Caesarean section

Serious complications are rare. However, the mother is at increased risk compared to vaginal delivery. Blood transfusion may be needed; infection of the uterus or wound occurs in up to 20% of women. Prophylactic antibiotics reduce the incidence of infection (*Cochrane* 2002: CD000933). Elective Caesarean is associated with fewer complications than an emergency procedure. Overall, approximately 1 in 5000 women will die after a Caesarean.

Indications

Emergency Caesarean section
This is performed in labour.

Prolonged first stage of labour is diagnosed when full dilatation is not imminent by 12 h, or earlier if labour was initially rapid. Occasionally, full dilatation is achieved but not all the criteria for instrumental delivery are met. Most commonly, it is due to abnormalities of the 'powers': inefficient uterine action. The 'passenger' (malposition or malpresentation) or 'passage' (pelvic abnormalities and cephalo-pelvic disproportion) can also contribute [→ p.197].

Fetal distress is diagnosed from abnormalities of the fetal heart rate, normally in conjunction with fetal blood sampling [→ p.199]. A Caesarean section is performed if it is the quickest route of delivery for the baby.

Elective Caesarean section
This is performed to avoid labour. It is normally performed at 39 weeks gestation to reduce the risk of neonatal lung immaturity (*BJOG* 1995; **102**: 101).

Absolute indications are placenta praevia, severe antenatal fetal compromise, uncorrectable abnormal lie, previous vertical Caesarean section and gross pelvic deformity.

Relative indications include: breech presentation, twin pregnancy, diabetes mellitus and other medical diseases, previous Caesarean section, older nulliparous patients and maternal request.

When delivery is needed before 34 weeks, it is usual to perform a Caesarean section rather than induce labour. The most common indications are severe pre-eclampsia and severe intrauterine growth restriction.

Elective Caesarean for maternal request
This is becoming increasingly common. The ethics surrounding this are complex (*BJOG* 2002; **109**: 593). As emergency Caesarean sections in labour have become commonplace it is not surprising that some women would rather have the Caesarean without several hours of labour first. Most requests can be addressed by reassurance: if this fails, most obstetricians now agree to the procedure.

Common reasons for Caesarean section	
Emergency:	Failure to progress in labour
	Fetal distress
Elective:	Previous Caesarean section(s)
	Breech presentation

Caesarean section rates

The high rate is only partly related to the decrease in perinatal mortality [→ p.23], and is causing increasing concern among doctors and consumer groups. It is essential to distinguish between elective and emergency Caesarean section when discussing rates. Attempts to reduce the rate should concentrate on training for both doctors and midwives, more senior interest in the Delivery Ward and increased support for women in labour.

Further reading

Miksovsky P, Watson WJ. Obstetric vacuum extraction: state of the art in the new millennium. *Obstetrical Gynecological Survey* 2001; **56**: 736–51.

O'Grady JP, Pope CS, Hoffman DE. Forceps delivery. *Best Practice & Research. Clinical Obstetrics & Gynecology* 2002 **16**: 1–16.

Royal College of Obstetricians and Gynaecologists. *The National Sentinel Caesarean Section Audit.* London: The Royal College of Obstetricians and Gynaecologists Press, 2001.

Forceps and Ventouse at a Glance

Descriptions	Ventouse attaches by suction, allowing traction with rotation Non-rotational forceps grip and allow traction Rotational forceps grip, allow rotation and then traction
Rates	20%, nulliparous; 2%, multiparous
Indications	Prolonged second stage, fetal distress in second stage, when maternal pushing contraindicated
Prerequisites	Cervix fully dilated, position of head known, head deeply engaged and mid-cavity or below, adequate analgesia, empty bladder, valid indication
Complications	Maternal trauma: Lacerations, haemorrhage
	Fetal trauma: Lacerations, bruising, facial nerve injury, hypoxia if prolonged delivery

Caesarean Section at a Glance

Descriptions	Lower segment (>99%); classical (vertical) rare
Rates	15–25%
Common indications	Elective: Breech presentation, previous lower segment Caesarean section (LSCS), placenta praevia
	Emergency: Failure to advance, fetal distress
Complications	Haemorrhage, uterine/wound sepsis, thromboembolism, anaesthetic

32 Obstetric Emergencies

Shoulder dystocia

This is difficulty in delivering the shoulders after the head has delivered. The obstruction is at the pelvic inlet. If untreated, the baby will quickly die from asphyxia. It occurs in approximately 1 in 200 deliveries. Risk factors include a previous history, maternal diabetes and a large fetus, particularly where the abdominal circumference is much greater than the head circumference ('asymmetric macrosomia'). Others risk factors include instrumental vaginal delivery and prolonged pregnancy or labour. It is difficult to predict shoulder dystocia with adequate specificity to justify prophylactic Caesarean section, but where there is a previous history or a large baby in a diabetic, elective Caesarean is usual.

Senior aid is summoned. An episiotomy is performed. Suprapubic pressure is applied, combined with moderate downward traction on the head. If this fails, the legs are hyperextended onto the abdomen (McRoberts' manoeuvre). If this fails, the operator's hand is inserted into the vagina (hence the need for an episiotomy) and the operator's hand grasps the posterior arm and rotates the shoulder through 180°, so delivering the shoulder anteriorly below the subpubic arch. Excessive traction on the neck can damage the brachial plexus, resulting in Erb's (waiter's tip) palsy, but this usually resolves (Fig. 32.1).

Cord prolapse

This is when, after the membranes have ruptured, the umbilical cord descends below the presenting part (Fig. 32.2). Untreated, the cord will be compressed or go into spasm and the baby will rapidly become hypoxic.

It occurs in 1 in 500 deliveries. Risk factors include preterm labour, breech presentation, abnormal lie and twin pregnancy. More than half occur at artificial amniotomy. The diagnosis is usually made when the fetal heart rate becomes abnormal or the cord is palpated vaginally or appears at the introitus.

Initially the presenting part must be prevented from compressing the cord: it is pushed up by the examining

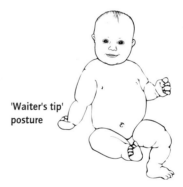

Fig. 32.1 Erb's palsy of right arm in characteristic 'waiter's tip' position.

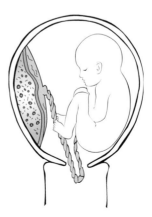

Fig. 32.2 Cord prolapse (here associated with flexed breech presentation).

finger, or the patient is asked to go on 'all fours'. If the cord is out of the introitus, it should be kept warm and moist but not forced back inside. The fetus should then be delivered by the fastest safe route. Caesarean section is normally used, but instrumental vaginal delivery is appropriate if the cervix is fully dilated and the head is low. With prompt treatment, fetal mortality is rare.

Amniotic fluid embolus

This is when liquor enters the maternal circulation, causing sudden dyspnoea, hypoxia and hypotension, often accompanied by seizures. Acute right-sided heart failure is evident. It occurs in 1 in 80 000 pregnancies, but is a significant cause of maternal mortality because 80% die. If the woman survives for 30 min, she will rapidly develop disseminated intravascular coagulation (DIC), and often pulmonary oedema and adult respiratory distress syndrome (ARDS). Commonly associated with uterine hyperstimulation in parous women, it can occur at any time during a pregnancy and prevention is almost impossible.

Resuscitation is with oxygen and fluid under central venous monitoring, and cardiopulmonary resuscitation (CPR) if appropriate. Blood for clotting, full blood count and cross-match is taken. Blood and fresh frozen plasma (FFP) will be required. The patient is transferred to an intensive care unit.

Uterine rupture

The uterus can tear *de novo* (Fig. 32.3) or an old scar (e.g. from a Caesarean section) can open. Rupture occurs in 1 in 1500 pregnancies, and in 1 in 200 women who have had a lower segment Caesarean section (LSCS). Principal risk factors include labour after a previous Caesarean section or other uterine surgery, particularly a classical (vertical [→ p.218]) Caesarean or myomectomy [→ p.22]. Neglected obstructed labour is rare in the West but is a common obstetric emergency in developing countries. Rupture of a LSCS scar has a lower perinatal and maternal mortality than primary ruptures or those from a classical Caesarean: the lower segment is not very vas-

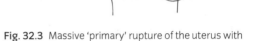

Fig. 32.3 Massive 'primary' rupture of the uterus with extrusion of the fetus.

cular and heavy blood loss and extrusion of the fetus into the abdomen are less likely.

Preventive measures include caution when using oxytocin in women with a previous Caesarean section, and elective Caesarean section in women with a uterine scar not in the lower segment. The diagnosis is suspected from fetal heart rate abnormalities or a constant lower abdominal pain; vaginal bleeding, cessation of contractions and maternal collapse may also occur.

Blood for clotting, haemoglobin and cross-match is taken. Intravenous fluid and then blood are given. Laparotomy must be performed urgently: the baby is delivered and the uterus either repaired or removed.

Maternal convulsions

Epileptiform seizures are most commonly the result of maternal epilepsy or eclampsia [→ p.139], but can also be due to hypoxia from any cause. The airway is cleared with suction and oxygen administered. Cardiopulmonary resuscitation may be required. The patient is not restrained but is prevented from hurting herself. In the absence of cardiopulmonary collapse, diazepam will normally stop the fit in the first instance. However, it is wise to assume the worst, i.e. that the fit is due to eclampsia, until this is excluded by the absence of suggestive examination and laboratory findings. Magnesium sulphate is not useful for non-eclamptic seizures and is therefore inappropriate where the diagnosis is uncertain, but it is superior to diazepam in the eclamptic woman (*Lancet* 1995; **345**: 1455).

Uterine inversion

This is when the fundus inverts into the uterine cavity (Fig. 32.4). It usually follows traction on the placenta and occurs in 1 in 20000 deliveries. Haemorrhage, pain and profound shock are normal. A brief attempt is made immediately to push the fundus up via the vagina. If impossible, a general anaesthetic is given and replacement performed with hydrostatic pressure of several litres of warm saline, which is run past a clenched fist at the introitus into the vagina.

Local anaesthetic toxicity

Excessive doses or inadvertent intravenous doses of local anaesthetic can cause transient cardiac, respiratory and neurological consequences, occasionally resulting in cardiac arrest. Prevention is most important; treatment involves resuscitation and even intubation until the effects have worn off.

Other emergencies

These are discussed elsewhere:
- Massive antepartum haemorrhage [→ p.162]
- Massive postpartum haemorrhage [→ pp.226, 264]
- Pulmonary embolus [→ p.151]
- Total spinal analgesia [→ p.203].

Further reading

Chamberlain G, Steer P. ABC of labour care: obstetric emergencies. *BMJ* 1999; **318**: 1342–5.

Christoffersson M, Kannisto P, Rydhstroem H, Stale H, Walles B. Shoulder dystocia and brachial plexus injury: a case-control study. *Acta Obstetricia et Gynecologica Scandinavica* 2003; **82**:147–51.

Eden RD, Parder RT, Gall SA. Rupture of the pregnant uterus: a 53-year review. *Obstetrics and Gynecology* 1986; **68**: 671–4.

Murphy D, MacKenzie I. The mortality and morbidity associated with umbilical cord prolapse. *British Journal of Obstetrics and Gynaecology* 1995; **102**: 826–30.

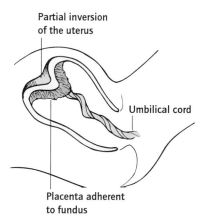

Partial inversion of the uterus

Umbilical cord

Placenta adherent to fundus

Fig. 32.4 Inverted uterus.

Aetiology (Fig. 33.2)

Uterine causes account for 80%. The uterus fails to contract properly, either because it is 'atonic' or because there is a retained placenta [→ p.207], or part of the placenta. Atony is more common with prolonged labour, with grand multiparity and with overdistension of the uterus (polyhydramnios and multiple pregnancy) and fibroids. Blood loss exceeds 500 mL at many Caesarean sections.

Vaginal causes account for about 20%. Bleeding from a perineal tear or episiotomy is obvious, but a high vaginal tear must be considered, particularly after an instrumental vaginal delivery.

Cervical tears are rare, but associated with precipitate labour and instrumental delivery.

Coagulopathy is rare. Congenital disorders, anticoagulant therapy or disseminated intravascular coagulation (DIC) all cause PPH.

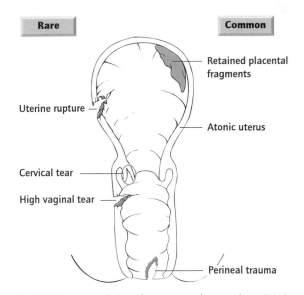

Fig. 33.2 Causes and sites of postpartum haemorrhage (PPH).

Risk factors for postpartum haemorrhage (PPH)
Previous history
Previous Caesarean delivery
Coagulation defect or anticoagulant therapy
Instrumental or Caesarean delivery
Retained placenta
Antepartum haemorrhage
Polyhydramnios and multiple pregnancy
Grand multiparity
Uterine malformation or fibroids
Prolonged and induced labour

Prevention

Routine use of oxytocin in the third stage of labour reduces the incidence of PPH by 60%. Oxytocin is as effective as ergometrine (*Cochrane* 2001: CD001808) which often causes vomiting and is contraindicated in hypertensive women.

Clinical features

Blood loss should be minimal after delivery of the placenta. An enlarged uterus (above the level of the umbilicus) suggests a uterine cause. The vaginal walls and cervix are inspected for tears. Occasionally blood loss may be abdominal: there is collapse without overt bleeding.

Management

To resuscitate, the patient is nursed flat, intravenous access is obtained, blood is cross-matched and blood volume is restored with colloid.

A retained placenta should be removed manually if there is bleeding, or if it is not expelled by normal methods within 60 min of delivery.

To identify and treat the cause of bleeding, vaginal examination is performed to exclude the rare uterine inversion and the uterus is bimanually compressed. Vaginal lacerations are often palpable. Uterine causes are common and oxytocin and/or ergometrine is given intravenously to contract the uterus if trauma is not obvious. If this fails, an examination under anaesthetic (EUA) is performed: the cavity of the uterus is explored manually for retained placental fragments and the cervix and vagina inspected for tears, which should be sutured. If uterine atony persists, prostaglandin $F_{2\alpha}$ ($PGF_{2\alpha}$) is injected into the myometrium; surgery (hysterectomy or internal iliac artery ligation), brace suture (*BJOG* 1997; **104**: 372) or uterine artery embolization are used if this fails.

Other problems of the puerperium

Secondary PPH

Secondary PPH is 'excessive' blood loss occurring between 24 h and 6 weeks after delivery. It is due to endometritis [→ p.64], with or without retained placental tissue, or, rarely, incidental gynaecological pathology or gestational trophoblastic disease [→ p.100]. The uterus is enlarged and tender with an open internal cervical os. Vaginal swabs and an ultrasound are performed. A full blood count is taken, and cross-match in severe cases. Milder cases usually respond to antibiotics, but if these fail, or bleeding is heavy, an evacuation of retained products of conception (ERPC [→ p.104]) is required. Histological examination of the evacuated tissues will exclude gestational trophoblastic disease.

Postpartum pyrexia

This is a maternal fever of ≥38°C in the first 14 days. *Infection* is the most common cause. Genital tract sepsis (endometritis) is a major cause of maternal mortality, in addition to the long-term consequences of pelvic infection [→ p.65]. It is most common after Caesarean section: prophylactic antibiotics considerably reduce this. Group A streptococcus, staphylococcus and *Escherichia coli* are the most important pathogens in severe cases. The lochia may be offensive and the uterus is enlarged and tender. Urinary infection (10%), chest infection, mastitis, perineal infection and wound infection after Caesarean section are also common (Fig. 33.3). Careful examination of the abdomen, breasts, any intravenous access sites, chest and legs is required. Blood, urine, high vaginal and fetal cultures are taken. Broad-spectrum antibiotics are given. *Deep vein thrombosis* (DVT) often causes a low-grade pyrexia.

Thromboembolic disease

Deep vein thrombosis or pulmonary embolism is a leading cause of maternal mortality, although less than 0.5% of women are affected. Half the deaths are postnatal, usually after discharge from hospital. Early mobility and hydration is important for all women. Risk factors, prevention and treatment are discussed elsewhere [→ p.151].

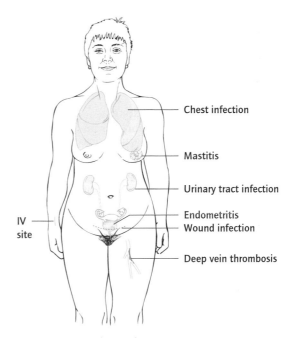

Fig. 33.3 Causes and sites of postpartum pyrexia.

Psychiatric problems of the puerperium

'Third day blues', consisting of temporary emotional lability, affects 50% of women. Support and reassurance are required.

Postnatal depression affects 10% of women but most do not present and receive no help. Questionnaires are helpful in identifying this extremely important problem, but screening is difficult (*Acta Psychiatr Scand* 2003; **107**: 10). Depression is more common in women who are socially or emotionally isolated, with a previous history, or after pregnancy complications. Postpartum thyroiditis [→ p.149] should be considered. The severity is variable, but symptoms include tiredness, guilt and feelings of worthlessness. Treatment involves social support and psychotherapy. Antidepressants (*Cochrane* 2001: CD002018) are used in conjunction with these. Suicide is now a major cause of death postpartum.

Puerperal psychosis affects 0.2% of women and is characterized by abrupt onset of psychotic symptoms, usually around the fourth day. It is more common in primigravid women with a family history. Treatment involves psychiatric admission and major tranquillizers, after ex-

Other Common Serious Problems of the Puerperium at a Glance

Secondary postpartum haemorrhage (PPH)	Due to endometritis ± retained placental tissue Give antibiotics, do evacuation of retained products of conception (ERPC) if no improvement
Pyrexia	Endometritis, wound, perineal, urine, breast, chest infection, thromboembolism Do cultures and give antibiotics
Urinary incontinence	20%. Exclude fistula and retention. Usually improves with time. Do urine culture and arrange physiotherapy
Urinary retention	Due to epidural or delivery, particularly forceps Catheterize for at least 24 h
Faecal incontinence	4%. Exclude rectovaginal fistula. Can be due to anal sphincter or pudendal nerve damage; associated with third-degree tears and forceps. Treat with physiotherapy ± sphincter repair
Postnatal depression	10%. Identification difficult. Support, psychotherapy, drugs
Thrombosis	0.5%. Major cause of mortality. Prophylaxis if high risk. Intravenous heparin then low-molecular-weight heparin (LMWH)

Birth Statistics and Audit

Audit

This is the process whereby clinical care is systematically and critically analysed: comparing what *should be done* with what *is being done* allows changes to be made to what *will be done*. Practice can then be re-analysed, in a completion of the 'audit cycle'. The *Report on Confidential Enquiries into Maternal Deaths in the UK* and the *Report on Confidential Enquiry into Stillbirths and Deaths in Infancy (CESDI)* are examples of audit in obstetrics. These have recently been amalgamated into the Confidential Enquiry into Maternal and Child Health (www.chemach.org.uk). These reports analyse, criticize and make recommendations; reports of later years examine their impact. On a local level, maternal and perinatal mortality are rare, and examination of 'near-miss maternal mortality', perinatal morbidity and intervention in pregnancy and labour are often more useful.

Perinatal mortality

Definitions and terms in the United Kingdom

Stillbirth occurs when a fetus is delivered after 24 completed weeks gestation showing no signs of life. *Neonatal death* is defined as death occurring within 28 days of delivery; *early neonatal death* occurs within 7 days of delivery.
Miscarriage occurs when a fetus is born with no signs of life before 24 weeks of gestation (however, if a fetus is delivered before 24 weeks, shows signs of life but subsequently dies, it is classified as a neonatal death).
The perinatal mortality rate is the sum of stillbirths and early neonatal deaths per 1000 total births.

The 'corrected' perinatal mortality rate excludes those stillbirths and early neonatal deaths that are due to congenital malformations. Different countries have different definitions concerning gestation and/or birthweight, so comparisons can be misleading. In 1992, in line with improvements in neonatal care, the earliest gestation defined as a stillbirth changed from 28 to the current 24 weeks in the United Kingdom. This is reflected in Fig. 34.1.

Perinatal mortality rate

In developed countries the perinatal mortality rate has been declining since the 1930s: in the United Kingdom it has declined from >50.0 to 7.9 per 1000 births in 1999 (not Scotland, where data is collected separately) (Fig. 34.1). The lowest rates are found in Scandinavian countries and the highest in Bangladesh and Central Africa.

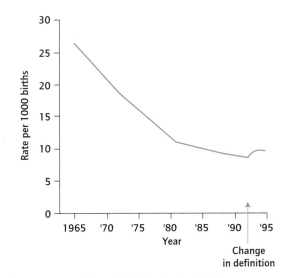

Fig. 34.1 Perinatal mortality in England and Wales.

35 Legal Issues in Obstetrics and Gynaecology

The United Kingdom's national annual insurance reserve estimate to cover the cost of clinical negligence litigation rose from £1 million in 1974/75 to £446 million in 2001/02. Patients are more informed, they expect more, and they do not expect that pregnancy, as a normal life event, could go wrong. Funding options have also changed, with increased availability of legal expenses insurance and claimants' solicitors offering conditional fee agreements. In addition, the amount of compensation awarded has increased to keep track with inflation: in a successful clinical negligence claim the combined general and future damages awarded to look after the future care needs of a child with cerebral palsy can be £3 million or over. There is no evidence, however, that more substandard practice is occurring.

Clinical negligence

To establish that a doctor has been negligent, it must be established both that (i) the doctor was in breach of his or her duty of care, either by act or omission, and that (ii) this was on the balance of probabilities the most likely cause of harm. The standard of care required is governed by the *Bolam* principle: 'A doctor is not guilty of negligence if he or she has acted in accordance with the practice accepted as proper by a responsible body of medical men skilled in that particular art' (Bolam vs. Friern Hospital 1957).

Establishing causation is particularly difficult in obstetrics. When an infant is born in poor condition and subsequently develops cerebral palsy, it is labour, as the most recent and apparently dangerous event, which is frequently blamed. Furthermore, patients frequently perceive labour-related events to be preventable. Hypoxia in labour, however, probably accounts for only 10% of cases of cerebral palsy [→p.169]. Guidelines to help establish whether hypoxia in labour is to blame have been drawn up (*BMJ* 1999; **319**:1054), although they bear little relationship to whether cases are settled (*BJOG* 2003; **110**: 6).

Legal claims are funded by the Clinical Negligence Scheme for Trusts (CNST) insurance scheme, with Trusts paying quarterly insurance premiums to the National Health Service (NHS) Litigation Authority, which is responsible for payments to claimants. The insurance premium is fixed after an annual audit of compliance against nationwide CNST standards and previous claims history. There is a separate CNST standard for obstetrics in recognition of the fact that it is a high-risk area of clinical practice.

Concerned at the spiralling costs of clinical negligence litigation, the Chief Medical Officer has proposed two NHS redress schemes, still at consultation stage, that may be available to patients in addition to civil litigation and the NHS complaints procedure. The second NHS redress scheme for neurologically damaged children suggests that there would be no need to establish fault or negligence to give compensation to severely neurologically impaired babies. A national panel of experts would assess severity of impairment and causation.

Clinical governance

The Chief Executive of a Trust now carries responsibility for the quality of medical care. Every Trust must have mechanisms to ensure the quality of care, identify faults and improve the service, and report annually on this. 'Clinical governance' has been developed, ostensibly to ensure the safety of patients and staff, and is described as 'a framework through which NHS organisations are accountable for continuously improving the quality of their services and safeguarding high standards of care by creating an environment in which excellence in clinical care will flourish'. Roughly translated, it means 'do a good job and prove it'.

Clinical governance incorporates the implementation of evidence-based and 'effective' practice. Evidence-based guidelines for the management of common clinical situations have been drawn up, including guidance from the National Institute for Clinical Excellence

(NICE; www.nice.org.uk), although they cannot entirely dictate the management of every clinical situation. It is easier to defend clinical practice if guidelines have been followed; equally, where a clear deviation has occurred, negligence is more likely to be alleged unless a clear reason for the deviation in practice is documented. Clinical governance also encompasses audit of clinical practice.

Risk management

Risk management aims to reduce risk of patient harm. Each NHS Trust has an incident reporting system to report adverse incidents: the organization has to routinely review, learn and, if necessary, change clinical practice or systems to try to prevent these from occurring again. Clinical Negligence Scheme for Trusts assessors audit NHS Trusts annually for evidence of working practices, protocols and guidelines that show good risk management systems.

NHS complaints procedure

The NHS complaints procedure specifies time limits for the acknowledgement, investigation and resolution of a complaint. If unsatisfied with a Trust's response, a complainant may request an independent assessment of their complaint with ultimate recourse to the Complaints Ombudsman. Many people seeking compensation cite a fear of other people experiencing the same situation or that communication after an adverse event was poor. Successful local resolution of a complaint can reduce the likelihood of litigation.

Consent

When negligent outcome is alleged it is common for patients to allege that they were not aware of the risks associated with the medical treatment. The Department of Health (DoH) consent forms now require discussion and documentation of the benefits, risks and side effects of treatment. When such risks are rare in the general patient population they must still be mentioned if they are serious for a specific patient.

Confidentiality

The doctor has a moral, professional, contractual and legal duty to maintain patient confidentiality. No details can be disclosed to a third party, including a relative, without the patient's consent. The Data Protection Act 1998 extends this duty to ensuring adequate protection and storage of information, such as patient records and communications. Confidentiality can be breached only in exceptional circumstances where the health and safety of others would otherwise be at serious risk.

Avoiding litigation
Communication
Consent
Clear documentation
Candour

Avoiding litigation

Besides ensuring you do your best medically, including referring to other more experienced colleagues if you are unsure, remembering the 4 'C's will help prevent allegations of negligence. *Consent* must be thorough and this, and any discussion with or examination of a patient, must be *clearly documented*. Each entry in the notes must be legible, dated and signed, preferably with the doctor's name printed. *Communication* before and during treatment is essential, but even after an adverse event has occurred, an adequate explanation, with *candour*, may be all that patients require.

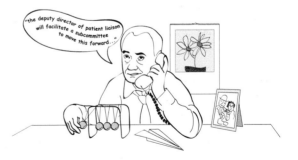

Further reading

Clements RV. *Risk Management* and *Litigation in Obstetrics and Gynaecology*. London: RSM Press, 2001.

www.cgsupport.nhs.uk for information on clinical governance.

Gynaecology Management Section

Management of bleeding or pain in early pregnancy

Fundamentals   Exclude ectopic pregnancy; ensure viability of intrauterine pregnancy

Causes	**Chapter reference**
Miscarriage	Chapter 14
Ectopic pregnancy	
Rarer: Molar pregnancy	**Where to see**
Gynaecological	Gynaecology 'on call'
	Gynaecology ward
	Theatre

Resuscitation   If collapse or heavy vaginal loss, intravenous (i.v.) access, give colloid and cross-match blood

History   Review of gynaecological history. Nature of pain and bleeding? Past pelvic operations? Ectopics? Pelvic inflammatory disease (PID)? Sexually transmitted infection (STIs)?

Examination

General:	Anaemia, blood pressure (BP), pulse
Abdomen:	Tenderness, rebound tenderness
Pelvis:	Size of uterus, cervical excitation, adnexal mass/tenderness, cervical os open/closed (insert i.v. line first if ?ectopic)

Investigations   Pregnancy test; ultrasound scan of pelvis (transvaginal if <7 weeks), full blood count (FBC), 'group and save' (G&S)

Management

If threatened:	Usually allow home if bleeding light
If missed:	Do evacuation of retained products of conception (ERPC)
If inevitable/incomplete:	Patient bleeding heavily: give ergometrine intramuscularly (i.m.), do ERPC Patient not bleeding heavily: consider waiting
If complete:	(Empty uterus, history/examination) Allow home
If molar pregnancy:	Do ERPC, check histology and human chorionic gonadotrophin beta-subunit (β-HCG) and refer to centre
If certain ectopic:	Do laparoscopy, consider methotrexate if criteria met

If unsure but possible ectopic (uterus empty on USS):
Admit, i.v. access, do β-HCG: If >1000 IU, do laparoscopy; if <1000 IU, repeat 48 h later
                                            If rise <66%, do laparoscopy. Repeat USS after 1 week if negative

After miscarriage or ectopic pregnancy:
Give anti-D if patient rhesus negative. Offer counselling or referral to support group

Management of urinary incontinence

Fundamentals   Incontinence is neither normal nor incurable, but treatment depends on the degree of disability caused

Causes	**Chapter reference**
Genuine stress incontinence (GSI)	Chapter 8
Overactive bladder	
Rarer: Chronic retention	**Where to see**
Fistula	Gynaecology clinic
	Urodynamics lab
	Physiotherapy departments
	Theatre

History   Review of gynaecological history. Incontinence with 'stress' or urgency?
What about daytime frequency? Nocturia? Enuresis? Haematuria? Dysuria? What is the fluid intake? How much is the patient's life affected?

Examination

General:	Weight, chest problems (chronic cough)
Abdomen:	Exclude masses, urinary retention
Pelvis:	Exclude pelvic mass. Look for leak when coughing, prolapse, particularly of bladder neck (use Sims' speculum)

Investigations   Do mid-stream urine (MSU) sample and urine dipstick
Ultrasound or post-micturition catheterization
Urinary diary: nocturia with small volumes suggests overactive bladder
Consider methylene blue/intravenous pyelogram (IVP) if possible fistula (continuous incontinence)
If no overflow/fistula/infection, do cystometry

Management

If cystometry normal, GSI likely: refer for physiotherapy ± surgery
If detrusor contractions: overactive bladder likely: give terodiline

Management of vaginal discharge

Fundamentals	Discharge is usually physiological or infective. Attention to detail prevents the diagnosis of 'intractable' discharge from being made

Causes	**Chapter references**
Candidiasis	Chapters 4 & 10
Bacterial vaginosis (BV)	
Atrophic vaginitis	**Where to see**
Cervical eversion/ectropion	Gynaecology clinic
Trichomoniasis (TV)	Genito-urinary medicine clinic
Rarer: Malignancy	Microbiology lab
Foreign body	

History	Review of gynaecological history. Ask about: Colour? Odour? Timing? Irritation? Ask regarding: Pelvic pain? Sexual intercourse? Superficial dyspareunia? Bloody discharge suggests malignancy of cervix or endometrium

Examination	Pelvis:	Palpate for pelvic masses/tenderness
	Speculum:	Cervix: look for eversion/ectropion
	Vaginal walls:	Redness/irritation, atrophy, discharge

Investigations	Cervical smear, high vaginal swab (HVS) and cervical swab (including *Chlamydia*) Take a slide and examine do whiff test, pH with litmus paper

Table of discharge and diagnosis

Cause	Itching	Discharge	pH	Redness	Odour	Treatment
Ectropion/eversion	No	Clear	Normal	No	Normal	Cryotherapy
Bacterial vaginosis	No	Grey/white	Raised	No	Fishy	Antibiotics
Candidiasis	Yes	'Cottage cheese'	Normal	Yes	Normal	Imidazole
Trichomonas	Yes	Grey/green	Raised	Yes	Yes	Antibiotics
Malignancy	No	Red/brown	Variable	No	Yes	Biopsy
Atrophic	No	Clear	Raised	Yes	No	Oestrogen

Management

If whiff test and swabs negative, infective cause unlikely:
Treat atrophic vaginitis with oestrogen cream (or hormone replacement therapy, HRT, if postmenopausal)
Treat cervical ectropion/eversion with cryotherapy or diathermy
Reassure if physiological

If infection present:
If candidiasis:	Use clotrimazole pessary, and if recurrent, oral fluconazole
If bacterial vaginosis (BV):	Use clindamycin cream or metronidazole
If sexually transmitted infection (STI):	Treat appropriately and arrange contact tracing

Management of the subfertile couple

Fundamentals	Consider basic criteria for fertility. Refer rapidly for assisted conception if failed treatment, especially if older woman

Common causes
Polycystic ovary syndrome (PCOS)
Hypothalamic hypogonadism
Hyperprolactinaemia
Male factor
Pelvic inflammatory disease (PID)
Endometriosis

Chapter references
Chapters 9, 10 & 11

Where to see
Gynaecology clinic
Fertility clinic or *in vitro* fertilization (IVF) unit
Andrology clinic
Theatre

Initial assessment

History		Counselling is essential. See the couple together. Prescribe folic acid
		Review of gynaecological and medical history. Menstruation? Exercise? Smoking? Eating habits? Coitus? (History from male if semen analysis abnormal)
Examination	General:	Health, blood pressure (BP), weight, hirsutism
	Pelvic:	Look for masses or reduced mobility
Investigations	Blood:	Check for ovulation: mid-luteal progesterone
		Cause for anovulation: follicle-stimulating hormone (FSH), luteinizing hormone (LH) (days 1–3), thyroid function, prolactin
		Check rubella immunity before pregnancy
	Semen analysis	
	Ultrasound:	Mid-cycle for follicle development and PCOS

Review

Results should be ready, and treatment can begin. Two or more causes may be found

If anovulation:	Reconsider weight gain or loss from history/examination
If prolactin (PRL) raised:	Repeat and if persistent/high, do computed tomography (CT) of pituitary. Start bromocriptine
If thyroid function tests (TFTs) abnormal:	Treat appropriately
If PCOS:	Give clomiphene and check mid-luteal progesterone in two subsequent cycles
If FSH, LH low:	(Oestradiol low also) Start gonadotrophins
If FSH and LH high:	Recheck several times. If consistent, probable premature menopause: offer egg donation
If semen analysis abnormal, repeat:	
If mild abnormalities:	Alteration in personal habits, testicular cooling
If marked abnormality:	Examine male, do FSH, LH and refer to andrologist
If oligospermic:	Where no treatable cause found, consider IVF (intracytoplasmic sperm injection, ICSI) after testicular sperm aspiration (TESA)
If all above normal:	Laparoscopy: dye test (or hysterosalpingogram)

Management of the subfertile couple *continued*

If fallopian tube damage:

If both tubes blocked:	IVF
If peritubal adhesions:	Surgery (divide) at time of laparoscopy
If endometriosis:	Surgery (diathermy/laser) at time of laparoscopy

Subsequent management

General	Confirm ovulation with ultrasound scan (USS) and mid-luteal progesterone
If PCOS	Metformin, or ovarian diathermy at laparoscopy, if still anovulatory If still unsuccessful: consider IVF

Once situation optimized, e.g. previously anovulatory patient ovulating on treatment, wait 6 months. If pregnancy still not achieved or cause unexplained, consider intrauterine insemination (IUI)/IVF

Management of acute pelvic pain

Fundamentals	Alleviate pain; identify and treat cause, particularly ectopic pregnancy, pelvic inflammatory disease (PID), pelvic masses

Common causes
Ectopic pregnancy
Septic/incomplete miscarriage
Ovarian cyst accident
Pelvic inflammatory disease, endometriosis
Renal tract infection/calculus
Appendicitis
Ovarian malignancy if older
None found

Chapter references
Chapters 5, 8–10 & 14

Where to see
Gynaecology 'on call'
Gynaecology clinic
Theatre

History	Review of gynaecological history. Timing? Nature/site of pain? Menstruation? Dyspareunia? Sexual/contraceptive history? Gastrointestinal symptoms/anorexia?

Examination		
	General:	Appearance, temperature, blood pressure (BP), pulse, anaemia, shock
	Abdomen:	Site and degree of tenderness, bowel sounds
	Pelvis:	Masses, cervical excitation, adnexal tenderness, discharge

Investigations	Pregnancy test, swabs for culture if negative, ultrasound, full blood count (FBC), mid-stream urine (MSU) sample

Differentiation between common causes of acute pelvic pain

	Ovarian cyst accident	Ectopic	Pelvic inflammatory disease (PID)	Appendicitis
Initial pain	Unilateral	Unilateral	Bilateral	Right-sided
Bleeding	Occasional	Usual	Often	Unusual
Discharge	Occasional	Bloody	Usual	No
Fever	Low grade	No	Often	Low grade
Peritonism	Often	Often	Often	Usual
Pregnancy test	Usually negative	Positive	Negative	Negative
Ultrasound	Usually shows cyst	Empty uterus	Normal	Normal

Management

Give analgesia, admit, nil by mouth

If probable ectopic:	Laparoscopy
If ovarian cyst:	Laparoscopy
If PID:	Antibiotics
If unsure:	Where pregnancy test negative, admit, observe, give antibiotics empirically, and do laparoscopy if no improvement

Management of chronic pelvic pain

Fundamentals   Exclude pathological causes with history and laparoscopy, offer support if apparently not pathological. Rare in postmenopausal women: consider malignancy

Causes
Endometriosis
Chronic pelvic inflammatory disease (PID)
Irritable bowel syndrome (IBS)
Urinary tract: Infection/calculi
Pelvic pain syndrome
Rarer: Residual ovary
　　　　Adhesions
　　　　Pain clinics
　　　　Counselling sessions

Chapter references
Chapters 9 & 10

Where to see
Gynaecology clinic

History   Review of gynaecological history. Is pain cyclical? Dyspareunia? Bowel habit and effect of opening
bowels on pain (IBS)? Discuss effect on patient's life, and stress/life events
Ask about previous pelvic infection or surgery

Examination   General: Health, weight, appearance, mental state

Abdomen: Tenderness, masses

Pelvis: Tenderness, masses

Investigations   Ultrasound scan (USS), laparoscopy, mid-stream urine (MSU) sample
Do high vaginal swab (HVS) and cervical swab

Differentiation between causes of chronic pelvic pain

	Organic cause more likely	Organic cause less likely
Age	Older	Younger
Pain	Cyclical Consistent relieving factors	Non-cyclical
Previous history	Not investigated	Multiple admissions/operations
Drugs	Hormones helped	Hormones no help Patient asks for opiates

Management

If features of IBS:	Antispasmodics and refer to dietician ± gastroenterologist
If other symptoms or signs (e.g. abnormal bleeding):	Investigate and treat appropriately
Perform laparoscopy:	In all patients without obvious bowel/psychiatric disease
If organic cause:	Treat appropriately [→·p.59]
If adhesions at laparoscopy:	Cut but ascribe pain to them with caution
If laparoscopy negative:	If intractable pain try gonadotrophin-releasing hormone (GnRH) agonists
If successful:	Reconsider cause: consider total abdominal hysterectomy and bilateral salpingo-oöphorectomy (TAH + BSO) if family complete
If unsuccessful:	Pain management programmes, psychotherapy or counselling

Management of chronic dyspareunia

Fundamentals	Differentiate between deep and superficial dyspareunia, exclude organic, and consider pyschological factors

Causes

Deep causes:
Endometriosis
Chronic pelvic inflammatory disease (PID) pelvic mass
Irritable bowel

Superficial causes:
Vagina/vulval infection
Surgery; childbirth
Psychological
Also: Vulval dysplasias; atrophic vaginitis

Chapter references
Chapters 6 & 9

Where to see
Gynaecology clinic

History	Review of gynaecological/obstetric history. Dyspareunia deep or superficial? Timing? Sexual history? Other symptoms? What is patient's reaction to problem?	
Examination	General:	Mental state
	Abdominal:	Masses, tenderness
	Pelvic:	If superficial, inspect vulva and vagina: pinpoint tender area If deep, uterine mobility, adnexal and uterosacral tenderness/thickening
Investigations	Superficial:	High vaginal swab (HVS) and cervical swab
	Deep:	Laparoscopy

Management

Superficial dyspareunia:

If painful ulceration:	Often herpes simplex	Contact tracing, aciclovir
If discoloration:	Vulval condition, e.g. vulvar intraepithelial neoplasia (VIN)	Biopsy, then treat
If vaginal discharge:	Trichomoniasis, candidiasis	Take swabs, treat
If thin red epithelium:	Atrophic vaginitis	Topical oestrogen/hormone replacement therapy (HRT)
If mass:	Vaginal cyst, Bartholin's abscess	Surgery
If normal:	Psychological/vaginismus	Gradual dilatation; psychotherapy
If recent surgery/birth:		Unless obvious abnormality, wait 6 months before surgery (e.g. Fenton's repair)

Deep dyspareunia:

Do laparoscopy:	If organic cause found:	Treat (fibroids/retroverted uterus are rare as causes)
	If pelvis normal:	Treat as chronic pelvic pain [→ p.59]; consider psychotherapy

Management of the abnormal smear

Fundamentals	Cervical screening programmes reduce the incidence of cervical carcinoma

Chapter reference
Chapter 4

Where to see
Gynaecology clinic
Colposcopy clinic
Pathology lab

History	Review of gynaecological history. Contraception and sexual intercourse? Menstruation? Cervical smear history? Vaginal discharge? Smoking?
Examination	To exclude coincidental disease or advanced carcinoma

Management

If smear is:

Mild dyskaryosis/borderline nuclear abnormalities (BNA):	Repeat in 6 months, colposcopy if persistent
Moderate dyskaryosis:	Do colposcopy
Severe dyskaryosis:	Urgent colposcopy
Columnar atypia/cervical glandular intraepithelial neoplasia (CGIN):	Colposcopy, hysteroscopy

If colposcopy suggests:

Cervical intraepithelial neoplasia (CIN) I/human papilloma virus (HPV):	Do biopsy, repeat smear in 6 months
CIN II–III:	Large loop excision of transformation zone (LLETZ)
Invasion:	Diagnostic cone biopsy

If histology shows:

CIN I–III:	Repeat smear in 6 months
Invasion <3 mm:	Stage 1a(i): do cone biopsy
Deeper/lymph invasion:	Treat as cervical carcinoma

Obstetric Management Section

Management of common problems in the antenatal clinic

Fundamentals   Listen to the patient. Beware of unexplained proteinuria or reduced fetal movements

Chapter references
Chapters 20, 21 & 24–26

Where to see
Antenatal clinic
Antenatal ward
Ultrasound department

Management

If reduced fetal movements:
Check fetal size, consider ultrasound scan (USS) for growth. Do cardiotocography (CTG). Warn about continuing surveillance of movements [→ p.170]

Possible ruptured membranes (spontaneous rupture of membranes, SROM):
Ask regarding contractions. If history suggestive of SROM, admit to hospital for confirmation [→ p.214]. Check presentation. Do sterile speculum examination of posterior vaginal fornix to look for fluid. Avoid digital examination unless contractions

Hypertension but blood pressure (BP) <170/110, no proteinuria:
Possible early/mild pre-eclampsia. Recheck BP and urinalysis twice a week and refer for USS. Do full blood count (FBC), urea and electrolytes (U&E), liver function tests (LFTs)

Hypertension, BP ≥170/110, 1+ proteinuria:
Admit to hospital and manage as pre-eclampsia [→ p.137]

Symphysis –fundal height >2 cm below number of weeks at 24 weeks or more:
Arrange USS for size, and umbilical artery Doppler if small size confirmed

Antepartum haemorrhage:
Admit to hospital. Do CTG

Abnormal lie:
If <37 weeks: review at 37 weeks
If ≥37 weeks: admit to hospital and do USS [→ p.177]

Breech after 37 weeks:
Refer for USS and consider external cephalic version

Pregnancy at or beyond 41 weeks:
Recheck gestation. Offer cervical sweep. Consider induction. If not, daily CTG

Suspected polyhydramnios:
Do USS: if confirmed, look for fetal anomaly on ultrasound and do timed glucose [→ p.145]

Management of the small-for-dates fetus

Fundamentals   Perinatal mortality is higher with lower birthweight, but most mortality is of apparently normally grown fetuses

Common causes
Constitutional factors
Idiopathic
Maternal disease, e.g. pre-eclampsia
Smoking

Chapter references
Chapters 20, 21 & 25

Where to see
Antenatal clinic
Ultrasound department

History   Review of obstetric and medical history. Previous birthweight? Smoking? Complications (e.g. pre-eclampsia)? Vaginal bleeding? Fetal movements?

Examination   General: Blood pressure and urinalysis

Abdominal: Symphysis–fundal height

Investigations   Ultrasound scan (USS); umbilical artery (UA) Doppler, cardiotocography (CTG)

To identify the small-for-dates fetus
'Low-risk' pregnancy:
Measure symphysis–fundal height. If <2 cm less than gestation, refer for USS

'High-risk' pregnancy:
As above and serial USS measurement of fetal growth at 28, 32 and 36 weeks

Management

If ultrasound shows:
Size >10th centile: Continue usual antenatal care
Size <10th centile: Do UA Doppler. Look for fetal/maternal disease, e.g. pre-eclampsia

If Doppler shows:
Normal resistance: Repeat USS and UA Doppler every 2 weeks

High resistance: If >37 weeks, do CTG and induce
                     If <37 weeks, repeat twice weekly

Severe abnormality: If >34 weeks, CTG and deliver
                        If <34 weeks, fetal Doppler, steroids, daily CTG

If CTG shows: Normal: do daily
                      Abnormal: deliver (lower segment Caesarean section, LSCS, if <34 weeks)

Management of hypertension in pregnancy

Fundamentals   Pre-eclampsia is common, is unpredictable, and can kill the mother and the fetus. Monitor both

Causes
Pregnancy-induced: Pre-eclampsia and transient
Underlying: Essential and secondary

Chapter references
Chapters 17, 20 & 25

Where to see
Antenatal ward
High-dependency ward
Antenatal clinic

History   Review of obstetric history. Risk factors for pre-eclampsia? Headache? Epigastric pain? Visual disturbances?

Examination   General: Recheck blood pressure (BP) and urinalysis. Look for epigastric tenderness, oedema, radio-femoral delay and renal bruits. Examine fundi

Abdominal: Symphisis–fundal height

Investigations   Do urea and electrolytes (U&E), full blood count (FBC), liver function tests (LFTs), uric acid, 24-h urine for protein (if > trace proteinuria) and vanillylmandelic acid (VMA). Ultrasound scan (USS) for growth, umbilical artery (UA) Doppler, cardiotocography (CTG)

Management

As outpatient:
If BP < 170/110 and <0.5 g/24 h proteinuria
Do twice weekly BP and urinalysis, fortnightly USS for fetal growth, UA Doppler

Admission:
If BP ≥ 170/110 or >0.5 g/24 h proteinuria, or if symptoms or fetal compromise

Treat BP if:
BP ≥ 170/110: Admit, give nifedipine. If controlled, start methyldopa. If not, repeat

Delivery:
If eclampsia: Give magnesium sulphate, stabilize [→ p.141]. CTG. Deliver

If other complications: Stabilize. CTG. Deliver

If no complications: If proteinuria and >34–36 weeks, admit, daily CTG, induction
                         If proteinuria and <34 weeks, steroids, monitor daily as inpatient including CTG, deliver (lower segment Caesarean section, LSCS) if deterioration
                         If no proteinuria and BP < 170/110, consider delivery at term

After delivery: Treat BP ≥ 170/110, fluid balance; FBC, U&E, LFTs. Keep in hospital for 5 days

Management of abnormal or unstable lie at term

Fundamentals	Only abnormal at term: exclude pathological cause, beware cord prolapse. Most turn to cephalic and deliver normally

Common causes Lax multiparous uterus Abnormal uterus Pelvic obstruction, e.g. placenta praevia Polyhydramnios	**Chapter reference** Chapter 26 **Where to see** Antenatal ward

History	Review of obstetric history. Diabetic? Multiparous?	
Examination	Abdominal:	Palpation of lie, liquor volume, fetal size
	Vaginal:	(If not placenta praevia) Exclude pelvic mass
Investigations	Ultrasound scan (USS):	Liquor volume, fetal/uterine abnormality, placental site

Management

If lie not longitudinal <37 weeks:	Re-check at 37 weeks
If lie not longitudinal >37 weeks:	Admit and stay, unless cephalic for >48 h
If lie never longitudinal:	Lower segment Caesarean section (LSCS) at 39 weeks
If lie abnormal/unstable >41 weeks:	LSCS

Management of breech presentation

Fundamentals   Breech presentation at term is associated with increased risk. External cephalic version reduces the incidence of breech delivery and Caesarean section

Causes
Idiopathic
Abnormal fetus
Pelvic obstruction
Twins
Uterine anomaly

Chapter reference
Chapter 26

Where to see
Antenatal clinic
Ultrasound department
Labour ward

History   Review of obstetric history. Check gestation

Examination   Abdominal: Confirm presentation

Vaginal: (If not placenta praevia)

Investigation   Ultrasound scan (USS) to confirm, look for abnormalities, placenta praevia, suitability for external cephalic version (ECV)

Management

If <37 weeks: Review at 37 weeks

If >37 weeks: Attempt ECV if no contraindication

If contraindication: Lower segment Caesarean section (LSCS) at 39 weeks, check presentation first

If successful: Manage as normal

If unsuccessful: LSCS at 39 weeks, check presentation first

Management of antepartum haemorrhage

Fundamentals Resuscitate mother first, beware concealed haemorrhage, deliver baby if fetal distress or heavy maternal blood loss

Common causes
Placenta praevia
Placental abruption
Undiagnosed

Chapter reference
Chapter 24

Where to see
Antenatal ward
Theatre
Labour ward

Resuscitation If patient shocked, or heavy vaginal bleeding, or pain
Insert intravenous (i.v.) access, give colloid, cross-match blood and check full blood count (FBC), urea and electrolytes (U&E), clotting (consider uncross-matched blood)
Nurse in left lateral position, oxygen, consider central venous pressure (CVP)

History Review of obstetric history, if placental site is known. Pain (constant/contractions)? Volume and colour of blood loss?

Examination General: Colour, pulse, blood pressure (BP)

Abdomen: Tenderness, uterine activity, size and presentation, head engagement

Pelvis: Vaginal examination (VE) (if placenta praevia excluded)

Investigations Cardiotocography (CTG) (immediate), ultrasound scan (USS) to determine placental site
Catheterize (hourly urine output), bloods as above

Management

The shocked patient must receive full resuscitation [→ p.263]

Placenta praevia:
Shock/heavy bleeding or >37 weeks: Lower segment Caesarean section (LSCS), give blood.
Watch for postpartum haemorrhage (PPH)

Blood loss stopped, <37 weeks: Give steroids if <34 weeks, anti-D if Rhesus negative
Keep in hospital; LSCS at 39 weeks

Placental abruption or undiagnozed bleed:
CTG abnormal: Emergency LSCS

Fetus dead: Anticipate coagulopathy and transfuse blood
Induce labour. Consider CVP line

CTG normal, >37 weeks: Induce unless small painless bleed

CTG normal, <37 weeks: Steroids if <34 weeks, anti-D if Rhesus negative
Serial USS

Recurrent small painless bleeds without placenta praevia:
Inspect cervix, do colposcopy. Serial USS

Management of prelabour rupture of the membranes

Fundamentals   Beware of infection; if present, deliver whatever gestation

Causes	**Chapter references**
Idiopathic	Chapters 23 & 30
Infection	
	Where to see
	Antenatal ward

History   Review of obstetric history. Gestation? Colour of fluid? Contractions?

Examination	General:	Temperature, pulse
	Abdomen:	Lie, presentation, engagement, tenderness
	Vaginal:	Only if abnormal lie or presentation. Can pass sterile speculum

Investigations   Cardiotocography (CTG), high vaginal swab (HVS), ultrasound scan (USS) for growth, liquor volume if preterm

Management

If infection: (Fever/ tachycardia/ abdominal tenderness/ offensive liquor)
Antibiotics and deliver whatever gestation

If <37 weeks: Do 4-hourly pulse, temperature, and fetal heart rate. Give steroids if <34 weeks. Give erythromycin. Induce labour at 37 weeks

If >37 weeks: If meconium, induce immediately
Induction usual but may prefer to wait. Give antibiotics if >18 h

Management of induction of labour

Fundamentals   Induction can fail. Easier to do in multiparous than nulliparous

Common indications	**Chapter reference**
Prolonged pregnancy	Chapter 30
Prelabour term spontaneous rupture of membranes (SROM)	
Medical conditions in pregnancy	**Where to see**
Intrauterine growth restriction (IUGR)	Labour ward

History   Review of obstetric history. Check gestation, indication

Examination   Abdominal: Check longitudinal lie and cephalic presentation

Vaginal: To assess cervical 'ripeness'

Investigation   Cardiotocography (CTG)

Management

Cervix unripe: Give prostaglandin E_2 (PGE_2) usually in evening
Artificial rupture of membranes (ARM) next morning, oxytocin if no labour in 2 h

Cervix ripe: Do ARM and await labour. Oxytocin if no labour in 2 h

CTG in labour. Anticipate slow progress initially and maintain encouragement

Management of slow progress in labour

Fundamentals	Oxytocin safe in nulliparous women, beware slow progress in multiparous

Causes

Powers:	Inefficient uterine action	**Chapter references**
Passenger:	Occipito-posterior (OP) position, brow or face	Chapters 28 & 29
Passage:	Cephalo-pelvic disproportion	
		Where to see
		Labour ward

History   Review of obstetric history. Parity, induction?

Look at partogram: length of labour, cervical dilatation

If slow progress in second stage, has passive stage been ignored?

Examination

General:	Temperature, pain relief, hydration
Abdomen:	Note fetal size, degree of engagement
Vaginal:	Cervical dilatation, station of head, position and attitude, moulding

Investigations   Cardiotocography (CTG)

Management

First stage:
Consider mobilization if delay not extreme and mother willing

If nulliparous:	Do artificial rupture of membranes (ARM); start oxytocin if no further dilatation 2 h later
If multiparous:	Do ARM; start oxytocin 2 h later if no malposition
Both:	Do lower segment Caesarean section (LSCS) if no increase in rate of dilatation within 4 h of oxytocin

Second stage:

If nulliparous:	Anticipate if head high: start oxytocin and delay pushing by 1 h
If multiparous:	No oxytocin: anticipate malposition or presentation
Both:	Push for 1 h; then instrumental delivery if prerequisites met; LSCS if not

Management of suspected fetal distress in labour

Fundamentals	Resuscitate first. Most suspected fetal distress cases are false alarms. Consider fetal blood sampling (FBS) unless bradycardia, when act quickly

Causes	**Chapter reference**
Unknown	Chapter 29
Chronic fetal compromise	
Prolonged labour; rapid labour	**Where to see**
Acute intrapartum events, e.g. cord prolapse	Labour ward

Resuscitation (of fetus)	Lie patient in left lateral, oxygen and stop any oxytocin infusion
	Intravenous (i.v.) fluid

History	Review of obstetric history and labour: Is it high risk, induced?
	Why is fetal distress suspected (i.e. abnormal cardiotocography, CTG, or pH of FBS). Flat on her back? Epidural or oxytocin?

Examination	General:	Take blood pressure, temperature
	Abdominal:	Uterine tenderness
	Vaginal:	Assess for cord prolapse and assess progress of labour

Management

If recent epidural insertion:	Increase i.v. fluid
If cord prolapse or bradycardia:	Urgent delivery (lower segment Caesarean section (LSCS) unless full dilatation)
If other CTG abnormality:	Do FBS and analyse pH
If pH <7.20:	Urgent delivery, LSCS unless full dilatation
If pH <7.25, ≥7.20:	Repeat FBS at 30 min
If CTG abnormality worsens/persists:	Repeat FBS at 30 min

Management of collapse on the labour ward

Fundamentals	Request senior help early and involve anaesthetic staff. Haemorrhage is the most common cause

Causes

Haemorrhage:	Intra-abdominal/revealed		**Chapter references**
Also:	Eclampsia or severe pre-eclampsia		Chapters 20, 21, 24, 32 & 33
	Total spinal, local anaesthetic toxicity		
	Pulmonary or amniotic fluid embolus		**Where to see**
	Maternal cardiac disease		Labour ward
			High-dependency unit

Resuscitation	Clear airway, oxygen. Cardiopulmonary resuscitation (CPR) if necessary. Intravenous (i.v.) access If seizures, give diazepam; magnesium sulphate if eclampsia

History	Review of obstetric and medical history. Eye-witness account, ante/postpartum? Vaginal bleeding? Pain? Seizures?

Examination	General:	Colour, pulse, temperature, blood pressure, sweating Lungs/heart
	Abdominal:	Uterine and abdominal tenderness; fetal lie

Investigations	Cross-match, clotting, full blood count (FBC), urea and electrolytes (U&E), liver function tests (LFTs). Cardiotocography (CTG) if fetus undelivered

Management

Antepartum:

If bleeding heavy:	Placenta praevia or abruption [→ p.162] likely
If not but pale/tachycardic:	Abruption/uterine rupture [→ pp.164, 222] are likely

Postpartum:

If bleeding heavy:	Atonic uterus/retained placenta, or laceration [→ p.226] likely
If not, but pale/tachycardic:	Uterine rupture or atonic uterus full of blood

If sudden cardiorespiratory embarrassment:
Consider pulmonary embolus [→ p.151], amniotic fluid embolus [→ p.222], total spinal [→ p.203] or cardiac decompensation in cardiac disease

If seizures:
Consider eclampsia [→ p.139], epilepsy or cardiorespiratory embarrassment

Management of massive postpartum haemorrhage (PPH)

Fundamentals Blood loss may be faster than you can replace, so find cause. Call for senior and anaesthetic help early

Causes
Uterine atony
Retained placental parts
Perineal/vaginal trauma
Also: Cervical laceration
          Uterine rupture
          Coagulopathy

Chapter references
Chapters 32 & 33

Where to see
Labour ward
Theatre
Postnatal ward

Resuscitation Is placenta delivered? If not, do so. Lie patient flat, give oxygen; intravenous (i.v.) access, colloid or O-negative blood if *in extremis*. Compress uterus bimanually

---

History Review of obstetric history. Pain? Mode of delivery?

Examination

General: Pallor, pulse, blood pressure

Abdominal: Size of uterus, abdominal tenderness

Vaginal: For bimanual compression. Exclude uterine inversion, palpate and inspect for vaginal tears

---

Investigations Blood for full blood count (FBC), urea and electrolytes (U&E), clotting, cross-match

---

Management

If perineal/vaginal trauma: Suture

If uterus poorly contracted: Give ergometrine and oxytocin infusion

If bleeding persistent: Examination under anaesthetic (EUA): uterine cavity, cervix and vagina
Remove placental tissue manually if present

If uterine atony confirmed: Intra-myometrial prostaglandin $F_{2\alpha}$ ($PGF_{2\alpha}$) if oxytocics fail

If uterine bleeding persists: Laparotomy, with hysterectomy or ligation of the internal iliac arteries (senior obstetrician only), consider brace suture or embolization

After: Check clotting, full blood count (FBC). Watch fluid balance and oxygen saturation. Oxytocin infusion

---

Principles of blood volume replacement
Normovolaemia is the priority
Stop the source of bleeding
Use central venous pressure (CVP) monitoring to prevent fluid overload
Use fresh frozen plasma (FFP) if >5 U of blood are needed

Management of postpartum pyrexia

Fundamentals	Full investigation and treatment prevents the high mortality and morbidity previously associated with this problem

Causes	**Chapter references**
Uterine infection	Chapters 21 & 33
Wound infection	
Urine infection	**Where to see**
Also: Thromboembolism, mastitis	Postnatal ward
Chest infection	
Perineal infection	

History	Review of obstetric and medical history. Mode of delivery? Prolonged spontaneous rupture of membranes (SROM)? Pyrexia in labour? Pain? Cough? Shortness of breath? Dysuria?

Examination	General:	Temperature, pulse, blood pressure
	Abdomen:	Uterine or loin tenderness
	Vaginal:	Uterine tenderness, cervical os open?
	Other:	Breasts, legs, chest, perineum/wound, intravenous (i.v.) sites

Investigations	Routine:	Full blood count (FBC); blood, urine and high vaginal swab (HVS) cultures
	If appropriate:	Sputum, wound swab cultures; venogram

Management

If endometritis:	Antibiotics, review after culture sensitivity. Do evacuation of retained products of conception (ERPC) if not improving <24 h
If wound infection:	Keep clean and give antibiotics
If chest infection:	Antibiotics and arrange physiotherapy
If mastitis:	Antibiotics and consider possibility of breast abscess
If suspected deep vein thrombosis (DVT):	Intravenous heparin. Organize venogram/investigations for pulmonary embolus [→ p. 151]

Index

Note: page numbers in *italics* refer to figures and boxes. **Bold** shows the main area where a topic is discussed.